AAOS

Special Events Medical Services

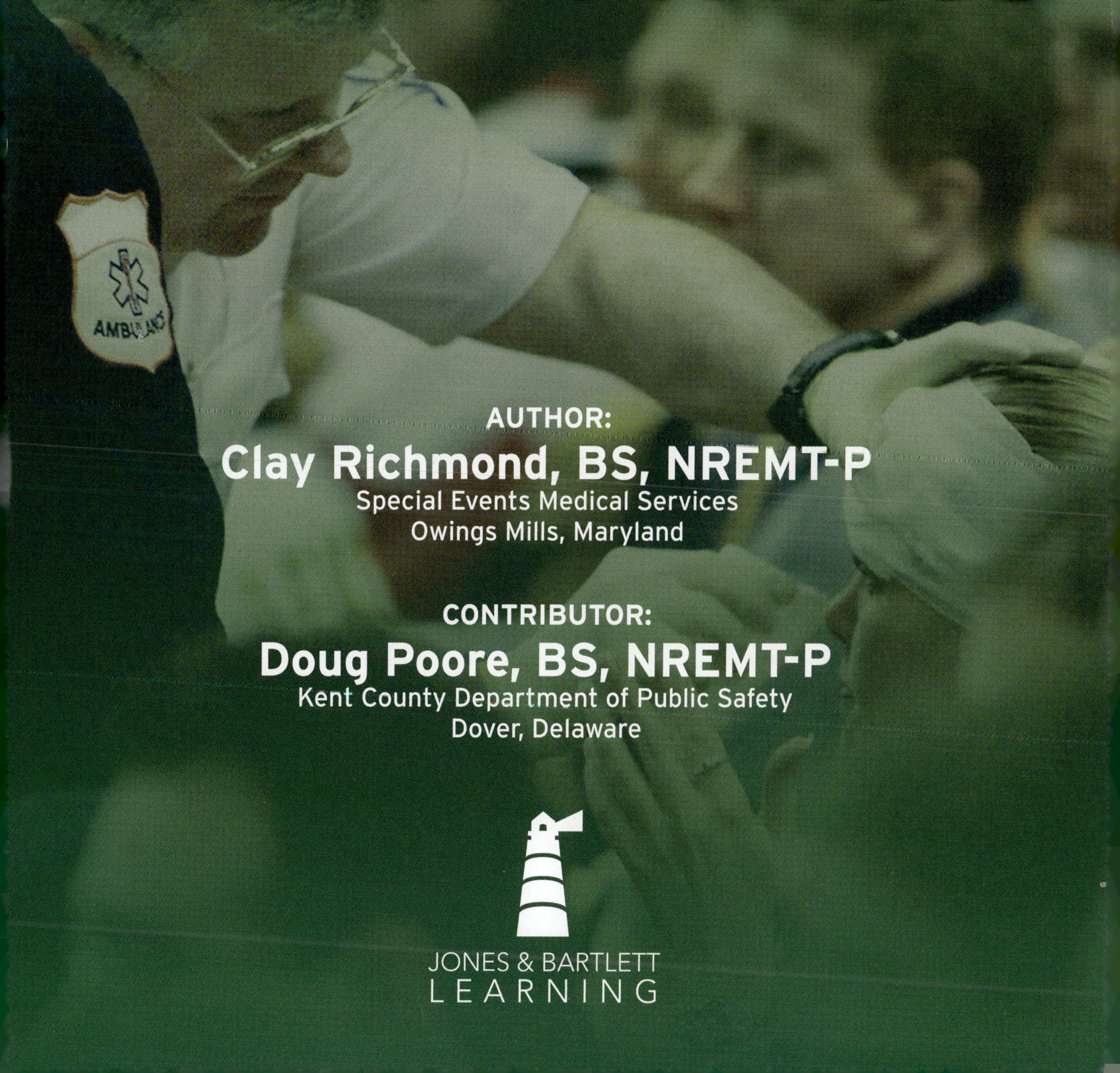

AUTHOR:
Clay Richmond, BS, NREMT-P
Special Events Medical Services
Owings Mills, Maryland

CONTRIBUTOR:
Doug Poore, BS, NREMT-P
Kent County Department of Public Safety
Dover, Delaware

JONES & BARTLETT
LEARNING

World Headquarters
Jones & Bartlett Learning
40 Tall Pine Drive
Sudbury, MA 01776
978-443-5000
info@jblearning.com
www.jblearning.com

Jones & Bartlett Learning Canada
6339 Ormindale Way
Mississauga, Ontario L5V 1J2
Canada

Jones & Bartlett Learning International
Barb House, Barb Mews
London W6 7PA
United Kingdom

Substantial discounts on bulk quantities of Jones & Bartlett Learning publications are available to corporations, professional associations, and other qualified organizations. For details and specific discount information, contact the special sales department at Jones & Bartlett Learning via the above contact information or send an email to specialsales@jblearning.com.

AAOS
American Academy of Orthopaedic Surgeons

Editorial Credits
Chief Education Officer: Mark W. Wieting
Director, Department of Publications: Marilyn L. Fox, PhD
Managing Editor: Barbara A. Scotese

Jones & Bartlett Learning books and products are available through most bookstores and online booksellers. To contact Jones & Bartlett Learning directly, call 800-832-0034, fax 978-443-8000, or visit our website, www.jblearning.com.

Production Credits
Chairman, Board of Directors: Clayton E. Jones
Chief Executive Officer: Ty Field
President: James Homer
Publisher: Kimberly Brophy
Acquisitions Editor—EMS: Christine Emerton
Managing Editor: Carol B. Guerrero
Production Manager: Jenny L. Corriveau
Director of Sales, Public Safety Group—Matthew Maniscalco
Director of Marketing: Alisha Weisman
V.P., Manufacturing and Inventory Control: Therese Connell
Composition: Shepherd, Inc.
Cover and Title Page Design: Kristin E. Parker
Photo and Permissions Associate: Emily Howard
Cover and Title Page Image: © Jim Bourg/Reuters
Printing and Binding: Courier
Cover Printing: Courier

The procedures and protocols in this book are based on the most current recommendations of responsible medical sources. The American Academy of Orthopaedic Surgeons and the publisher, however, make no guarantee as to, and assume no responsibility for, the correctness, sufficiency, or completeness of such information or recommendations. Other or additional safety measures may be required under particular circumstances.

This textbook is intended solely as a guide to the appropriate procedures to be employed when rendering emergency care to the sick and injured. It is not intended as a statement of the standards of care required in any particular situation, because circumstances and the patient's physical condition can vary widely from one emergency to another. Nor is it intended that this textbook shall in any way advise emergency personnel concerning legal authority to perform the activities or procedures discussed. Such local determinations should be made only with the aid of legal counsel.

The patients and providers described in the cases throughout this textbook are fictitious.

Additional illustration and photographic credits appear on page 239, which constitutes a continuation of the copyright page.

To order this product, use ISBN: 1-4496-0077-8

Library of Congress Cataloging-in-Publication Data
Richmond, Clay L.
Special events medical services / Clay L. Richmond.
p. ; cm.
ISBN-13: 978-0-7637-5842-4
ISBN-10: 0-7637-5842-6
1. Emergency medical services. 2. Special events. I. Title.
[DNLM: 1. Emergency Medical Services. 2. Disaster Planning. 3. Mass Casualty Incidents—prevention & control. WX 215 R533s 2011]
RA645.5.R53 2011
362.18—dc22
2009049564

6048
Printed in the United States of America
14 13 12 11 10 10 9 8 7 6 5 4 3 2 1

Contents

Resource Preview

Chapter Resources

Special Events Medical Services is designed to teach the basic principles of how to preplan for providing emergency medical services at a special event. Features that reinforce and expand on essential information include:

You Are the SEMS Provider case studies Two case studies are presented in each chapter, allowing the reader to become familiar with the logistics, challenges, and practical aspects of providing EMS at a special event. Each case includes critical-thinking questions to help the student synthesize the concepts he or she has learned. Chapters conclude with answers to the questions posed within the cases.

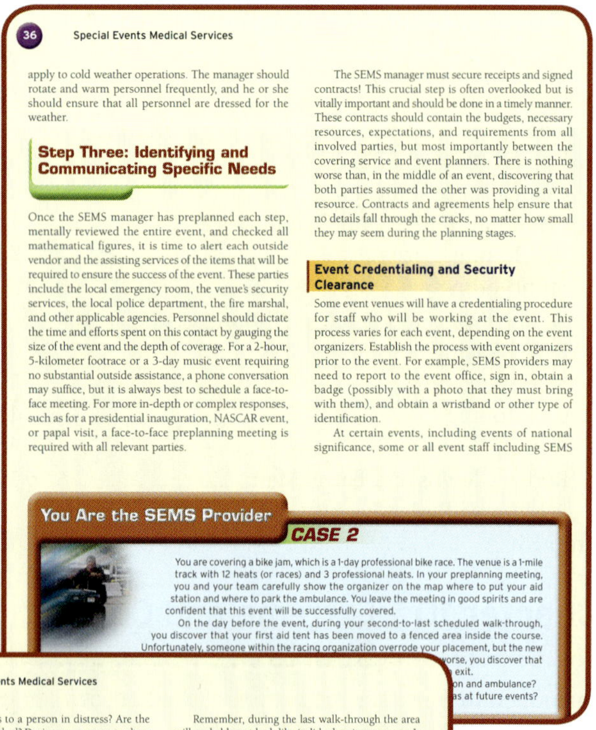

36 Special Events Medical Services

apply to cold weather operations. The manager should rotate and warm personnel frequently, and he or she should ensure that all personnel are dressed for the weather.

Step Three: Identifying and Communicating Specific Needs

Once the SEMS manager has preplanned each step, mentally reviewed the entire event, and checked all mathematical figures, it is time to alert each outside vendor and the assisting services of the items that will be required to ensure the success of the event. These parties include the local emergency room, the venue's security services, the local police department, the fire marshal, and other applicable agencies. Personnel should dictate the time and efforts spent on this contact by gauging the size of the event and the depth of coverage. For a 2-hour, 5-kilometer footrace or a 3-day music event requiring no substantial outside assistance, a phone conversation may suffice, but it is always best to schedule a face-to-face meeting. For more in-depth or complex responses, such as for a presidential inauguration, NASCAR event, or papal visit, a face-to-face preplanning meeting is required with all relevant parties.

The SEMS manager must secure receipts and signed contracts! This crucial step is often overlooked but is vitally important and should be done in a timely manner. These contracts should contain the budgets, necessary resources, expectations, and requirements from all involved parties, but most importantly between the covering service and event planners. There is nothing worse than, in the middle of an event, discovering that both parties assumed the other was providing a vital resource. Contracts and agreements help ensure that no details fall through the cracks, no matter how small they may seem during the planning stages.

Event Credentialing and Security Clearance

Some event venues will have a credentialing procedure for staff who will be working at the event. This process varies for each event, depending on the event organizers. Establish the process with event organizers prior to the event. For example, SEMS providers may need to report to the event office, sign in, obtain a badge (possibly with a photo that they must bring with them), and obtain a wristband or other type of identification.

At certain events, including events of national significance, some or all event staff including SEMS

You Are the SEMS Provider — CASE 2

You are covering a bike jam, which is a 1-day professional bike race. The venue is a 1-mile track with 12 heats (or races) and 3 professional heats. In your preplanning meeting, you and your team carefully show the organizer on the map where to put your aid station and where to park the ambulance. You leave the meeting in good spirits and are confident that this event will be successfully covered.

On the day before the event, during your second-to-last scheduled walk-through, you discover that your first aid tent has been moved to a fenced area inside the course. Unfortunately, someone within the racing organization overrode your placement, but the new ... orse, you discover that ... exit.

... on and ambulance?

... as at future events?

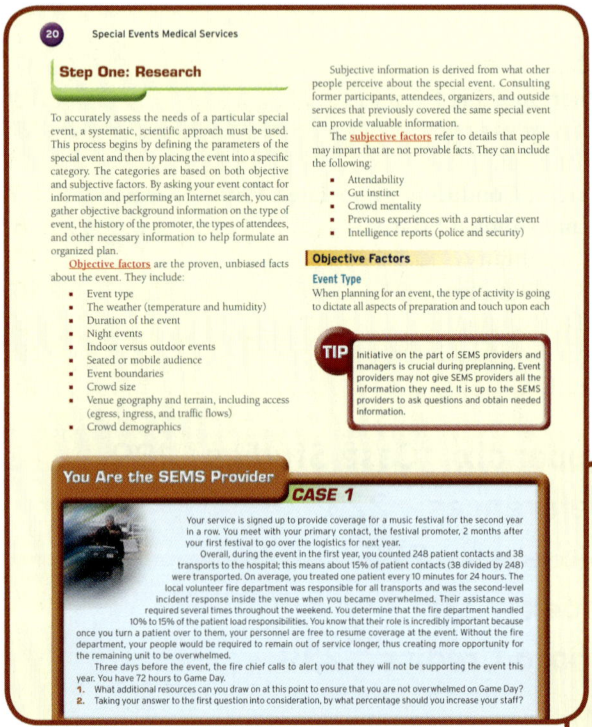

20 Special Events Medical Services

Step One: Research

To accurately assess the needs of a particular special event, a systematic, scientific approach must be used. This process begins by defining the parameters of the special event and then by placing the event into a specific category. The categories are based on both objective and subjective factors. By asking your event contact for information and performing an Internet search, you can gather objective background information on the type of event, the history of the promoter, the types of attendees, and other necessary information to help formulate an organized plan.

Objective factors are the proven, unbiased facts about the event. They include:

- Event type
- The weather (temperature and humidity)
- Duration of the event
- Night events
- Indoor versus outdoor events
- Seated or mobile audience
- Event boundaries
- Crowd size
- Venue geography and terrain, including access (egress, ingress, and traffic flows)
- Crowd demographics

Subjective information is derived from what other people perceive about the special event. Consulting former participants, attendees, organizers, and outside services that previously covered the same special event can provide valuable information.

The subjective factors refer to details that people may impart that are not provable facts. They can include the following:

- Attendability
- Gut instinct
- Crowd mentality
- Previous experiences with a particular event
- Intelligence reports (police and security)

Objective Factors

Event Type

When planning for an event, the type of activity is going to dictate all aspects of preparation and touch upon each

TIP Initiative on the part of SEMS providers and managers is crucial during preplanning. Event providers may not give SEMS providers all the information they need. It is up to the SEMS providers to ask questions and obtain needed information.

You Are the SEMS Provider — CASE 1

Your service is signed up to provide coverage for a music festival for the second year in a row. You meet with your primary contact, the festival promoter, 2 months after your first festival to go over the logistics for next year.

Overall, during the event in the first year, you counted 248 patient contacts and 38 transports to the hospital; this means about 15% of patient contacts (38 divided by 248) were transported. On average, you treated one patient every 10 minutes for 24 hours. The local volunteer fire department was responsible for all transports and was the second-level incident response inside the venue when you became overwhelmed. Their assistance was required several times throughout the weekend. You determine that the fire department handled 10% to 15% of the patient load responsibilities. You know that their role is incredibly important because once you turn a patient over to them, your personnel are free to resume coverage at the event. Without the fire department, your people would be required to remain out of service longer, thus creating more opportunity for the remaining unit to be overwhelmed.

Three days before the event, the fire chief calls to alert you that they will not be supporting the event this year. You have 72 hours to Game Day.

1. What additional resources can you draw on at this point to ensure that you are not overwhelmed on Game Day?
2. Taking your answer to the first question into consideration, by what percentage should you increase your staff?

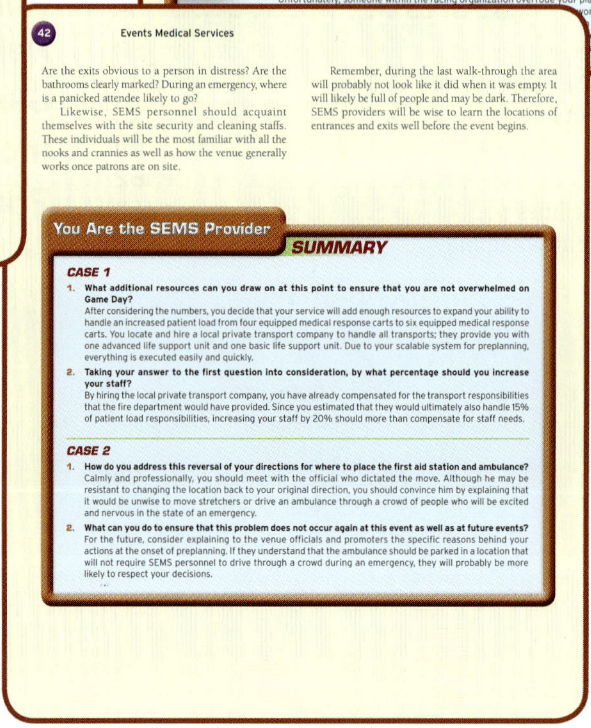

42 Events Medical Services

Are the exits obvious to a person in distress? Are the bathrooms clearly marked? During an emergency, where is a panicked attendee likely to go?

Likewise, SEMS personnel should acquaint themselves with the site security and cleaning staffs. These individuals will be the most familiar with all the nooks and crannies as well as how the venue generally works once patrons are on site.

Remember, during the last walk-through the area will probably not look like it did when it was empty. It will likely be full of people and may be dark. Therefore, SEMS providers will be wise to learn the locations of entrances and exits well before the event begins.

You Are the SEMS Provider — SUMMARY

CASE 1

1. **What additional resources can you draw on at this point to ensure that you are not overwhelmed on Game Day?**
   After considering the numbers, you decide that your service will add enough resources to expand your ability to handle an increased patient load from four equipped medical response carts to six equipped medical response carts. You locate and hire a local private transport company to handle all transports; they provide you with one advanced life support unit and one basic life support unit. Due to your scalable system for preplanning, everything is executed easily and quickly.
2. **Taking your answer to the first question into consideration, by what percentage should you increase your staff?**
   By hiring the local private transport company, you have already compensated for the transport responsibilities that the fire department would have provided. Since you estimated that they would ultimately also handle 15% of patient load responsibilities, increasing your staff by 20% should more than compensate for staff needs.

CASE 2

1. **How do you address this reversal of your directions for where to place the first aid station and ambulance?**
   Calmly and professionally, you should meet with the official who dictated the move. Although he may be resistant to changing the location back to your original direction, you should convince him by explaining that it would be unwise to move stretchers or drive an ambulance through a crowd of people who will be excited and nervous in the state of an emergency.
2. **What can you do to ensure that this problem does not occur again at this event as well as at future events?**
   For the future, consider explaining to the venue officials and promoters the specific reasons behind your actions at the onset of preplanning. If they understand that the ambulance should be parked in a location that will not require SEMS personnel to drive through a crowd during an emergency, they will probably be more likely to respect your decisions.

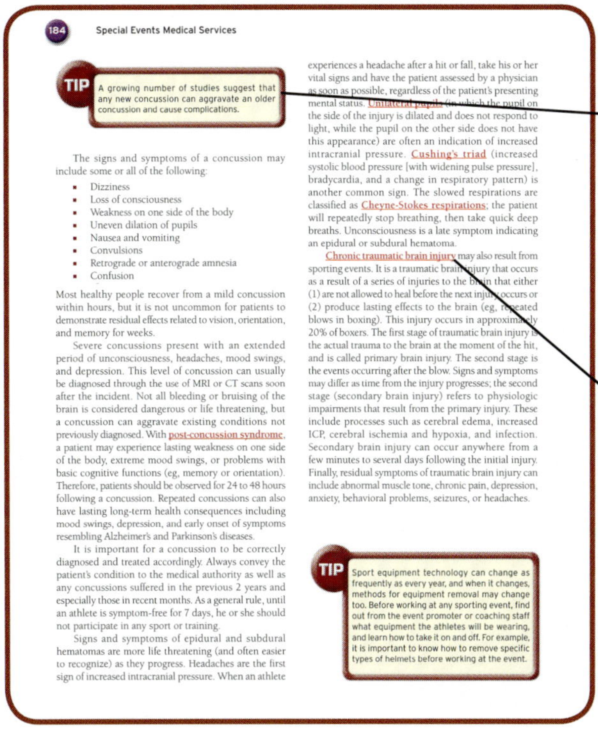

184 Special Events Medical Services

TIP A growing number of studies suggest that any new concussion can aggravate an older concussion and cause complications.

The signs and symptoms of a concussion may include some or all of the following:

- Dizziness
- Loss of consciousness
- Weakness on one side of the body
- Uneven dilation of pupils
- Nausea and vomiting
- Convulsions
- Retrograde or anterograde amnesia
- Confusion

Most healthy people recover from a mild concussion within hours, but it is not uncommon for patients to demonstrate residual effects related to vision, orientation, and memory for weeks.

Severe concussions present with an extended period of unconsciousness, headaches, mood swings, and depression. This level of concussion can usually be diagnosed through the use of MRI or CT scans soon after the incident. Not all bleeding or bruising of the brain is considered dangerous or life threatening, but a concussion can aggravate existing conditions not previously diagnosed. With post-concussion syndrome, a patient may experience lasting weakness on one side of the body, extreme mood swings, or problems with basic cognitive functions (eg, memory or orientation). Therefore, patients should be observed for 24 to 48 hours following a concussion. Repeated concussions can also have lasting long-term health consequences including mood swings, depression, and early onset of symptoms resembling Alzheimer's and Parkinson's diseases.

It is important for a concussion to be correctly diagnosed and treated accordingly. Always convey the patient's condition to the medical authority as well as any concussions suffered in the previous 2 years and especially those in recent months. As a general rule, until an athlete is symptom-free for 7 days, he or she should not participate in any sport or training.

Signs and symptoms of epidural and subdural hematomas are more life threatening (and often easier to recognize) as they progress. Headaches are the first sign of increased intracranial pressure. When an athlete experiences a headache after a hit or fall, take his or her vital signs and have the patient assessed by a physician as soon as possible, regardless of the patient's presenting mental status. Unilateral pupils (in which the pupil on the side of the injury is dilated and does not respond to light, while the pupil on the other side does not have this appearance) are often an indication of increased intracranial pressure. Cushing's triad (increased systolic blood pressure [with widening pulse pressure], bradycardia, and a change in respiratory pattern) is another common sign. The slowed respirations are classified as Cheyne-Stokes respirations; the patient will repeatedly stop breathing, then take quick deep breaths. Unconsciousness is a late symptom indicating an epidural or subdural hematoma.

Chronic traumatic brain injury may also result from sporting events. It is a traumatic brain injury that occurs as a result of a series of injuries to the brain that either (1) are not allowed to heal before the next injury occurs or (2) produce lasting effects to the brain (eg, repeated blows in boxing). This injury occurs in approximately 20% of boxers. The first stage of traumatic brain injury is the actual trauma to the brain at the moment of the hit, and is called primary brain injury. The second stage is the events occurring after the blow. Signs and symptoms may differ as time from the injury progresses; the second stage (secondary brain injury) refers to physiologic impairments that result from the primary injury. These include processes such as cerebral edema, increased ICP, cerebral ischemia and hypoxia, and infection. Secondary brain injury can occur anywhere from a few minutes to several days following the initial injury. Finally, residual symptoms of traumatic brain injury can include abnormal muscle tone, chronic pain, depression, anxiety, behavioral problems, seizures, or headaches.

TIP Sport equipment technology can change as frequently as every year, and when it changes, methods for equipment removal may change too. Before working at any sporting event, find out from the event promoter or coaching staff what equipment the athletes will be wearing, and learn how to take it on and off. For example, it is important to know how to remove specific types of helmets before working at the event.

Tip boxes Highlight key points and practical advice from SEMS providers.

Vocabulary Terms are easily identified within the chapter, and defined at the end of each chapter, as well as in a complete glossary at the end of the book.

Ready for Review Summarizes chapter content in a comprehensive bulleted list.

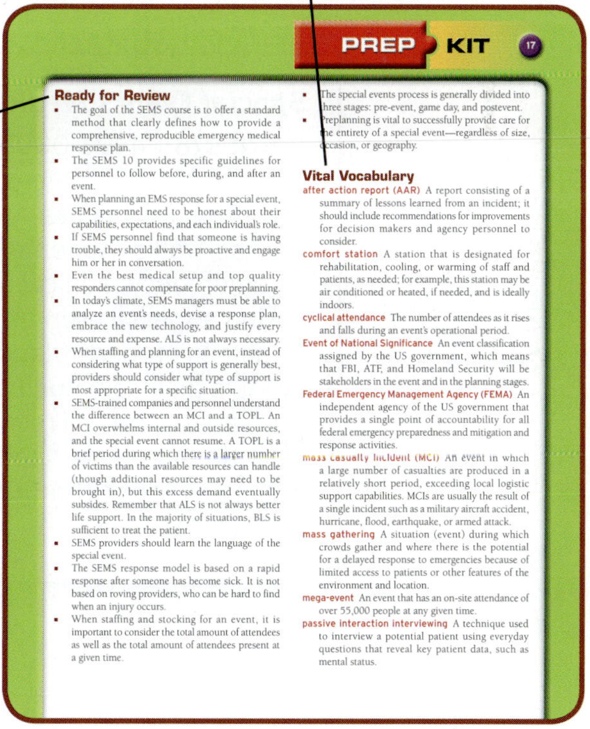

PREP KIT 17

Ready for Review

- The goal of the SEMS course is to offer a standard method that clearly defines how to provide a comprehensive, reproducible emergency medical response plan.
- The SEMS 10 provides specific guidelines for personnel to follow before, during, and after an event.
- When planning an EMS response for a special event, SEMS personnel need to be honest about their capabilities, expectations, and each individual's role.
- If SEMS personnel find that someone is having trouble, they should always be proactive and engage him or her in conversation.
- Even the best medical setup and top quality responders cannot compensate for poor preplanning.
- In today's climate, SEMS managers must be able to analyze an event's needs, devise a response plan, embrace the new technology, and justify every resource and expense. ALS is not always necessary.
- When staffing and planning for an event, instead of considering what type of support is generally best, providers should consider what type of support is most appropriate for a specific situation.
- SEMS-trained companies and personnel understand the difference between an MCI and a TOPL. An MCI overwhelms internal and outside resources, and the special event cannot resume. A TOPL is a brief period during which there is a larger number of victims than the available resources can handle (though additional resources may need to be brought in), but this excess demand eventually subsides. Remember that ALS is not always better life support. In the majority of situations, BLS is sufficient to treat the patient.
- SEMS providers should learn the language of the special event.
- The SEMS response model is based on a rapid response after someone has become sick. It is not based on roving providers, who can be hard to find when an injury occurs.
- When staffing and stocking for an event, it is important to consider the total amount of attendees as well as the total amount of attendees present at a given time.
- The special events process is generally divided into three stages: pre-event, game day, and postevent.
- Preplanning is vital to successfully provide care for the entirety of a special event—regardless of size, occasion, or geography.

Vital Vocabulary

after action report (AAR) A report consisting of a summary of lessons learned from an incident; it should include recommendations for improvements for decision makers and agency personnel to consider.

comfort station A station that is designated for rehabilitation, cooling, or warming of staff and patients, as needed; for example, this station may be air conditioned or heated, if needed, and is ideally indoors.

cyclical attendance The number of attendees as it rises and falls during an event's operational period.

Event of National Significance An event classification assigned by the US government, which means that FBI, ATF, and Homeland Security will be stakeholders in the event and in the planning stages.

Federal Emergency Management Agency (FEMA) An independent agency of the US government that provides a single point of accountability for all federal emergency preparedness and mitigation and response activities.

mass casualty incident (MCI) An event in which a large number of casualties are produced in a relatively short period, exceeding local logistic support capabilities. MCIs are usually the result of a single incident such as a military aircraft accident, hurricane, flood, earthquake, or armed attack.

mass gathering A situation (event) during which crowds gather and where there is the potential for a delayed response to emergencies because of limited access to patients or other features of the environment and location.

mega-event An event that has an on-site attendance of over 55,000 people at any given time.

passive interaction interviewing A technique used to interview a potential patient using everyday questions that reveal key patient data, such as mental status.

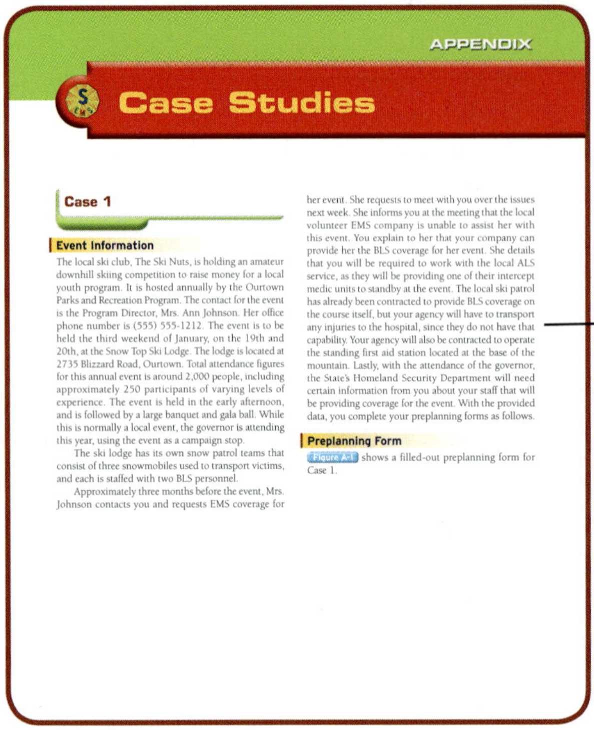
APPENDIX

Case Studies

Case 1

Event Information

The local ski club, The Ski Nuts, is holding an amateur downhill skiing competition to raise money for a local youth program. It is hosted annually by the Ourtown Parks and Recreation Program. The contact for the event is the Program Director, Mrs. Ann Johnson. Her office phone number is (555) 555-1212. The event is to be held the third weekend of January, on the 19th and 20th, at the Snow Top Ski Lodge. The lodge is located at 2735 Blizzard Road, Ourtown. Total attendance figures for this annual event is around 2,000 people, including approximately 250 participants of varying levels of experience. The event is held in the early afternoon, and is followed by a large banquet and gala ball. While this is normally a local event, the governor is attending this year, using the event as a campaign stop.

The ski lodge has its own snow patrol teams that consist of three snowmobiles used to transport victims, and each is staffed with two BLS personnel.

Approximately three months before the event, Mrs. Johnson contacts you and requests EMS coverage for her event. She requests to meet with you over the issues next week. She informs you at the meeting that the local volunteer EMS company is unable to assist her with this event. You explain to her that your company can provide her the BLS coverage for her event. She details that you will be required to work with the local ALS service, as they will be providing one of their intercept medic units to standby at the event. The local ski patrol has already been contracted to provide BLS coverage on the course itself, but your agency will have to transport any injuries to the hospital, since they do not have that capability. Your agency will also be contracted to operate the standing first aid station located at the base of the mountain. Lastly, with the attendance of the governor, the State's Homeland Security Department will need certain information from you about your staff that will be providing coverage for the event. With the provided data, you complete your preplanning forms as follows.

Preplanning Form

Figure A-1 shows a filled-out preplanning form for Case 1.

Case Study Appendix Five in-depth cases walk readers through how to fill out the master preplanning form, plan staffing levels and transport units, and apply critical-thinking skills to sample incidents that could occur.

Special Events Medical Services Online Course

ISBN: 978-1-4496-0005-1

The *Special Events Medical Services (SEMS) Online Course* walks students through the process of creating an emergency medical response plan and implementing it during a special event. From staffing to setup, students will be able to properly plan for and manage any type of special event in their community. Upon successful completion of the course, students will receive a Course Completion Certificate from the American Academy of Orthopaedic Surgeons. An access code for the *SEMS Online Course* is packaged in each textbook.

Acknowledgments

The American Academy of Orthopaedic Surgeons, Jones & Bartlett Learning, and the author would like to thank the contributors and reviewers of this book.

Contributors

Mark A. Buck, MS, ATC, EMT-IV
Saint Thomas Emergency Medical Services
Nashville, Tennessee

Heather Goddard, NREMT-P
Howard County, Maryland

J. Kevin Janney, BA, NREMT-P
Assistant Chief, EMS Director
Navy Region Mid-Atlantic Fire & Emergency Services
Norfolk, Virginia

Doug Poore, BS, NREMT-P
Kent County Department of Public Safety
Dover, Delaware

Reviewers

Jeffrey L. Benincosa, EMT
Somerset Training Center
Friedens, Pennsylvania

Leila Chandler
Paramedic Clinical Tutor
South Western Ambulance Service
Plymouth, Devon
England

Darryl Conway, MA, ATC, EMT-B
University of Maryland—College Park
College Park, Maryland

Scott Cook, BAS, CCEMT-P
Director of Education, Delta Ambulance
Waterville, Maine
Adjunct Instructor, Southern Maine Community College
South Portland, Maine

Lonnie Creager, EMT-P
Paramedic Instructor
Navarro College
Waxahachie, Texas

Joshua D. Crisp
Director
Regional Emergency Services Training Center
Gaston College
Dallas, North Carolina

T. Kevin Crump, NREMT-P, CCEMT-P
Partner
Vital Response Education & Consulting
Fort Worth, Texas

Lana G. Duff
Paramedic, Operations Manager
Rossville, Georgia

Audrey Finkel Esposito, MS, EMT-P
Silver Cross Hospital EMS Education Program
Lisle, Illinois

Julia Diane R. Fox, MSc, NREMT-P, PI
Program Director, EMS Education
Clarian Health Partners, Methodist Hospital
Emergency Response Training Institute
Indianapolis, Indiana

Ed Gannon, AS, EMT-P
Derry Fire Department/Pinkerton Academy
Auburn, New Hampshire

Marisa Hanson
Clinical Coordinator
MedStar EMS
Fort Worth, Texas

Donell Harvin, MPA, MPH, EMT-P
Adjunct Professor, Advisory Board Member
Reganhard Center for Emergency Response Studies
John Jay College of Criminal Justice
New York, New York

Victor Robert Hernandez, BA, EMT-P
Sierra College, Tahoe Truckee Campus
Truckee, California

Dave Howe, BS, CEM
Emergency Manager, Safety Instructor
Dublin, California

Paul Kattenhorn
Clinical Operations General Manager
East of England Ambulance Service (EEAS)
Stevenage Herts
England

John A. Kubincanek
Cuyahoga Community College
Western Campus, Fire Training Academy
Parma, Ohio

Glynn R. Lookabill, MAEd, EMT
PreMed Training Group
Enka, North Carolina

Jeffrey A. Magnifico, EMT-P, NPBO, FFI
Hazardous Materials Operations EMS Instructor
Valley Ambulance Authority
Lawrence County Department of Public Safety
Ellwood City, Pennsylvania

David Mather, AS, NREMT-P
Director of EMS
Amesbury Fire/Rescue
Amesbury, Massachusetts

Gregg Morris, PA-C
NSA Senior Steward
Emergency Department
Kent General Hospital
Dover, Delaware

Chief Rex Houston Prior, CFR-IT, BCLS-IT, CERT-IT
ECSI Training Center Coordinator
First Care Enterprises
Special Event Medical Services
Richmond, Kansas

Wright N. Randolph, Jr, CEP
Director of Emergency Medicine
Pima Community College
Tucson, Arizona

Scott Schaffer, EMT-P I/C
EMS Education Coordinator
MidMichigan Medical Center
Midland, Michigan

Stuart A. Smith
Senior Operations Manager
EMS Training Centre
Staffordshire
England

Kent R. Spitler, RN, NREMT-P, MSEd, CPP
Gaston College Department for EMS Education
Dallas, North Carolina

Michael Tarantino, BA, MAS, NREMT-B
EMT Coordinator
Bergen County EMS Training Center
Paramus, New Jersey

James K. Thompson, EMT-P
On Track EMS Supervisor
Darlington Raceway
Darlington, South Carolina

Stephen Traynor
London Ambulance Service
Clinical Education & Development Bromley
Bromley, Kent
England

Steven R. Vannatta, NREMT-P
Mercy College of Health Sciences
EMS Program
Des Moines, Iowa

Shelly B. Vaughan, EMT-P, EMS, I
North Central EMS Academy
Milan, Ohio

Robert S. Wales, BS, CCEMT-P
Upstate EMS Council, Inc.
Easley, South Carolina

Jim Wells, EMT-I, TO1
Lyndon, Kansas

Lt. Russell D. Wilson
Whitfield County Fire Department
Dalton, Georgia

Dedication

I'd like to dedicate this book to my grandmother, mom, and dad. Ajasage, my muse and best friend. BCFD Medic 7. I stand on the shoulders of giants.

—Clay Richmond

Photoshoot Acknowledgments

We would like to thank the following people and institutions for their assistance.

Damon Bailey
Baltimore, Maryland

Jaimie Burns
Silver Spring, Maryland

Michael C. Butler, NREMT-P
Baltimore, Maryland

FELD Motor Sports
Aurora, Illinois

Delaware Department of Transportation
Dover, Delaware

Dover International Speedway
Dover, Delaware

James F. Irons
Columbia, Maryland

Lt. David Mick
Kent County Department of Public Safety
Dover, Delaware

Sean Myers
Valley Lee, Maryland

Jonathan Noble
Preston, Maryland

Shariff Ruffin
Baltimore, Maryland

Lauren Schweizer
Baltimore, Maryland

Brian K. Slack
Baltimore, Maryland

CHAPTER

Foundation of SEMS

1

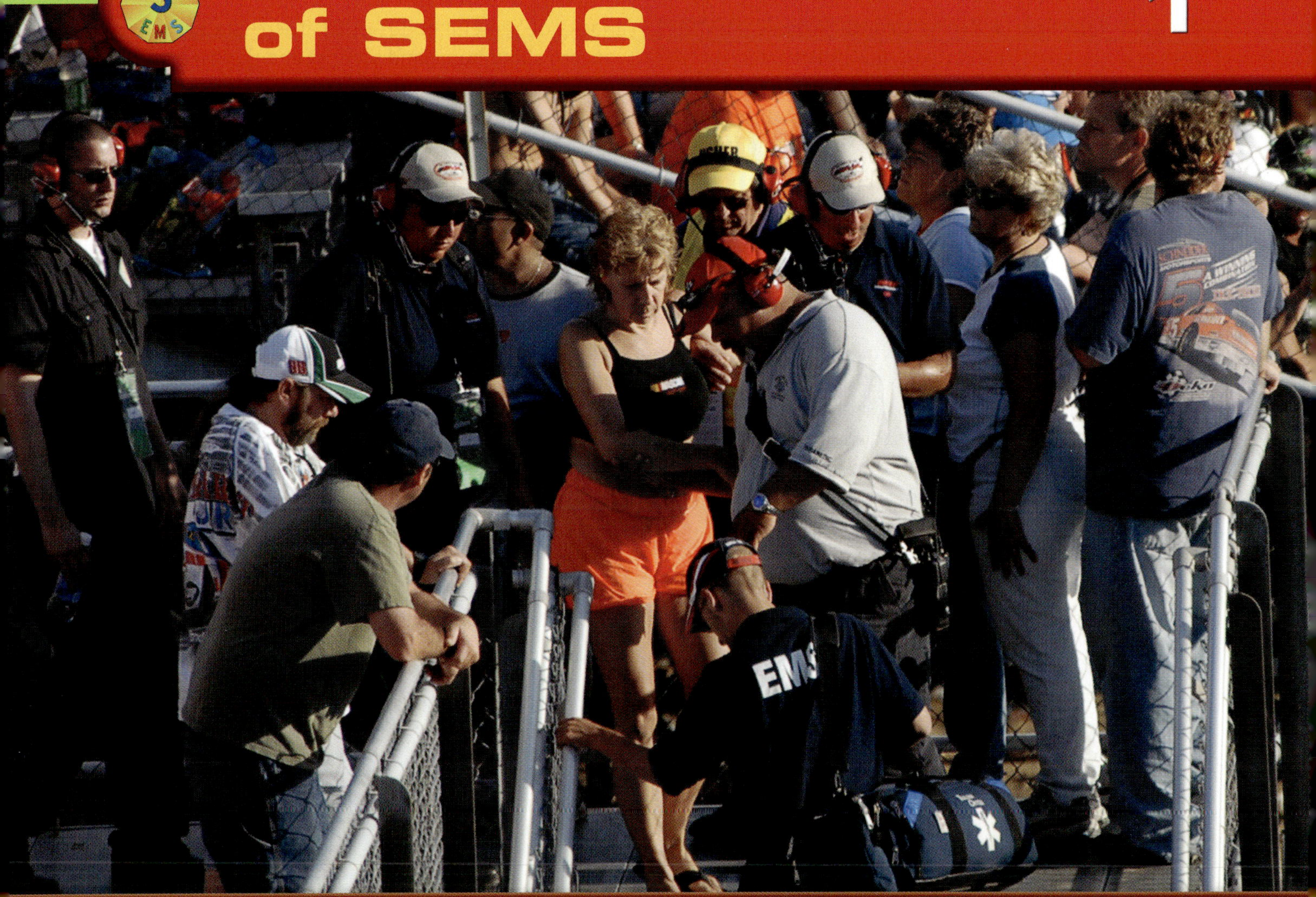

LEARNING OBJECTIVES

- Understand the importance of SEMS.
- List the SEMS 10.
- Understand the importance of preplanning.
- Learn the overall steps in planning a special event.
- Use the SEMS triangle.

Introduction to SEMS

The goal of the Special Events Medical Services (SEMS) course is to offer a standard method that clearly defines how to provide a comprehensive, reproducible emergency medical response plan that is tailored to the unique nature and challenging environment that accompanies the special event arena. Essentially, SEMS teaches emergency care providers and managers how to properly plan for, set up, and staff a special event.

When coordinating a special event, the event promoter will turn to the local emergency medical services (EMS) providers and agencies to provide emergency medical services at the event. Often, promoters and the general public assume that EMS providers know how to properly administer this type of service, but even the most seasoned medical providers can become perplexed by the immense number of considerations that go into properly preparing and executing a medical response in the special event setting. Until now, there has never been a standardized program like SEMS for the EMS provider.

Why is SEMS an emerging specialty? Since the attacks of September 11, 2001, there is a heightened concern about homeland security and the safety of large groups assembled in one location. The general public, public safety agencies, and the federal government have all become increasingly involved in ensuring that citizens are safe and well cared for in the event of a terrorist attack or natural disaster. This concentrated focus on public safety has driven the development of new specialties that improve the overall EMS industry.

Thus, properly providing medical services for **special events** and **mass gatherings** entails more than just showing up at the special event, being there all day, and getting a free meal or hat. EMS has evolved into a growing profession that values education and puts a premium on extensive training.

Today's EMS systems involve state of the art equipment and maintain a high standard of professionalism. EMS is

You Are the SEMS Provider

CASE 1

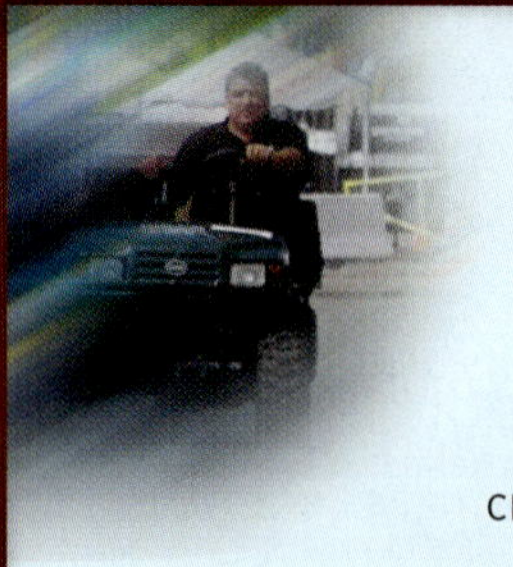

On a Friday afternoon, you receive a phone call that your service is needed to provide EMS coverage for an upcoming concert being held at a local park in late January. Thus, you need to formulate a strategy to warm pre-hypothermic patients, plan for supportive care for hypothermic patients, and arrange transport for later stage hypothermic patients.

Prior to the day of the event, your crew is scheduled to cover rehearsals that extend long into the night. The temperature has been predicted to drop to 7°F, and the rehearsals are scheduled to last until after midnight. As your standby progresses, one of the concert's crew members approaches you and states, "My hands really hurt and are red and swollen."

As you perform your initial assessment, you notice several other crew and band members are shivering and attempting to warm themselves around a small heater. You quickly evaluate for the signs and symptoms of mild hyperthermia and cold exposure: shivering and frostbite (noted with the red swollen hands). Then you observe that the band members are having trouble grasping their instruments.

Suddenly you realize you now have 16 patients who require warming for mild hypothermia and 1 patient requiring transport . . .

You immediately take the patients from the stage to the warming station located behind the structure. Fortunately, in the preplanning stage, your service had anticipated the need for warming stations. You also realized that, because the event is taking place at a national monument, you would have to work with the infrastructure and adapt accordingly. Thus, your service designated one of the "talent-holding" tents, or places where the performers relax offstage, as your rewarming station. The station is climate controlled, and your service stocked it earlier with emergency blankets, chairs, coffee, and hot chocolate. As the crew members and band settle into the rewarming station, you quickly take the patient who you suspect may have frostbite over to the transport unit so he can be fully diagnosed at the hospital. After half an hour of close monitoring, the patients who are still on site are fine and able to finish their work.

1. What information did you gather at your first meeting that led to your crew's success?
2. What did your preplanning include?

following the greater medical profession; 20 years ago, patients were cared for by a single physician for their entire lives. Now, to provide the most up-to-date care, physicians specialize in particular areas of medicine, and there are thousands of specialties. Likewise, EMS providers will be expected to provide more specialized care. The next rung on the EMS evolutionary ladder is a scientific methodology and standardization of such emerging specialties as flight paramedics, critical care transport providers, bariatric (obesity) prehospital medicine, and SEMS prehospital medicine.

The 10 Principles of SEMS

The "SEMS 10" is an icon that illustrates 10 important principles in providing emergency medical care at special events Figure 1-1. The 10 principles listed are often used in preparing for SEMS events:

1. Know your capabilities.
2. Be active.
3. Preplan, preplan, and then preplan.
4. More isn't better.
5. Mass gatherings are not mass-casualty incidents.
6. ALS (advanced life support) isn't always necessary.
7. Learn the language.
8. Stay in place.
9. Stock and staff for the max.
10. Do it right.

Know Your Capabilities

When planning an EMS response for a special event, SEMS personnel need to know their capabilities, expectations, and each individual's role Figure 1-2. In collaboration with the special event organizers, SEMS personnel should establish what is realistic and what is not when considering equipment, distances, and terrain.

SEMS personnel must gather information objectively: who, what, when, and why. They should then gather some subjective data and begin planning, always leaving personal bias out of the process while drawing on previous professional experiences to gauge the event. SEMS personnel should not mistake the event for better or worse than it is. They should just be honest in an assessment, making sure that they are using all available information during the planning process. This may include after action reports from previous events conducted by the organization, or even outside organizations, if these were created and are available Figure 1-3. An **after action report (AAR)** is a report consisting of a summary of lessons learned from an incident. The AAR should include recommendations for

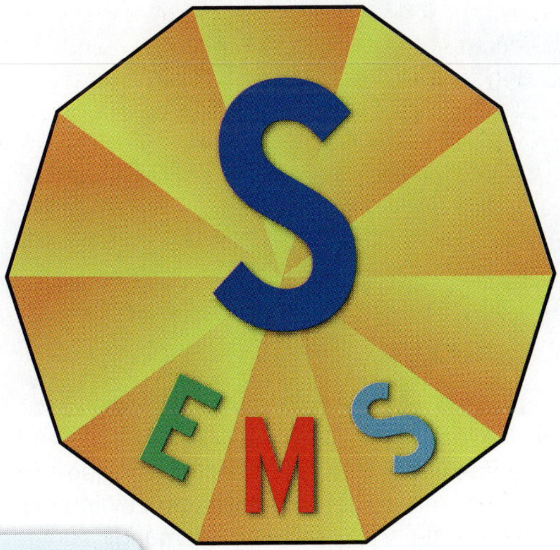

Figure 1-1

The SEMS 10.

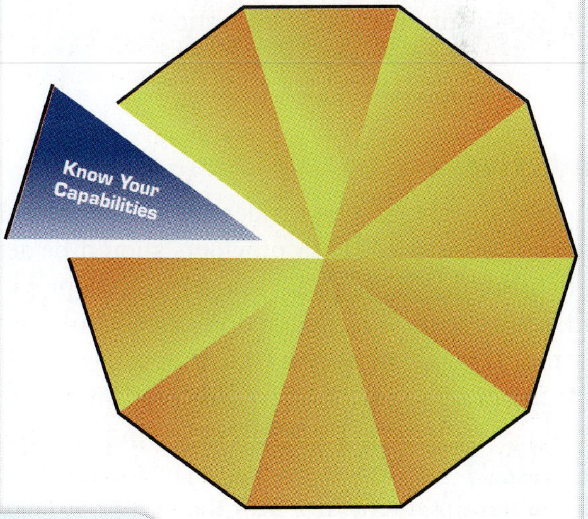

Figure 1-2

Know the capabilities, expectations, and roles of SEMS personnel.

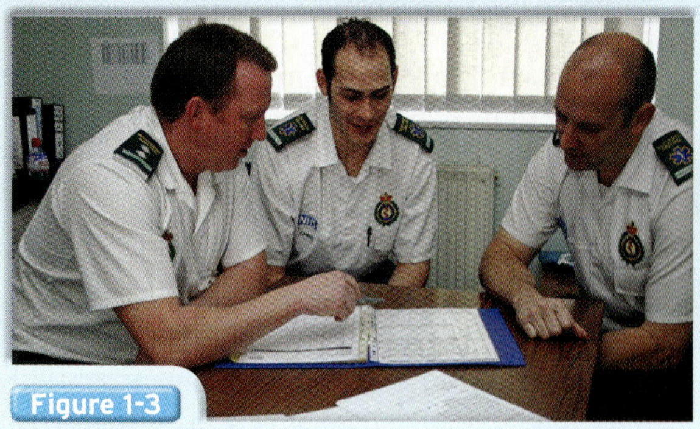

Figure 1-3

SEMS personnel must use all available information during the planning process. This may include AARs from previous events conducted by the organization or even outside organizations.

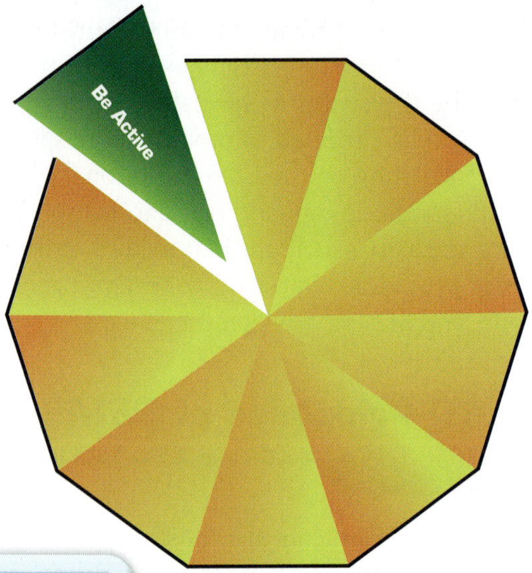

Figure 1-4

If you suspect trouble, engage the person in conversation and provide help.

improvements, and it is important for decision makers and agency personnel to consider and implement those recommendations quickly. Getting outside opinions will help eliminate personal bias from the process and will enable personnel to use the documented experiences of others as a basis for making decisions.

SEMS personnel must also consider subjective information:

- Recall a similar past event.
- Consider the reputation of the promoter.
- Examine the overall "gut feeling."
- Take the type of event into consideration:
  - A presidential inauguration
  - A heavy metal concert
  - A football game

Be Active

At a special event, SEMS providers should do more than respond to trouble. SEMS providers should be active participants Figure 1-4. Of course, if SEMS providers find that someone is having trouble, they should always be proactive and engage the patient in conversation.

Engaging a patient in conversation is called the **passive interaction interviewing** technique Figure 1-5. This technique enables providers to gather information by interacting with the event participants and thus gauge a potential patient's orientation to person, place, and time. In addition to asking questions,

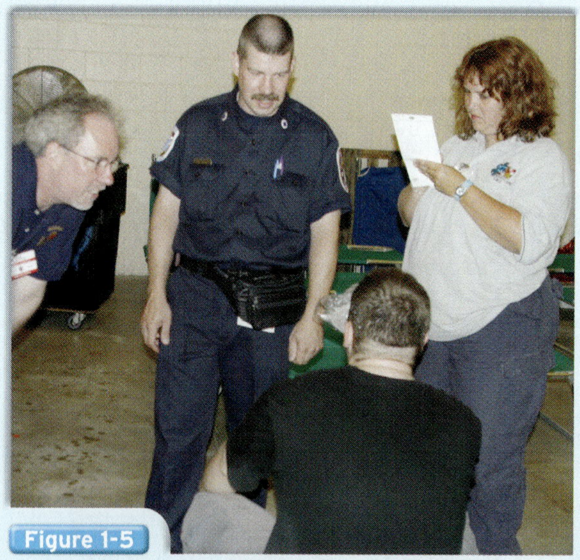

Figure 1-5

The passive interaction interviewing technique enables SEMS providers to gather information by interacting with the event participants and thus gauge a potential patient's orientation to person, place, and time.

the providers have an opportunity to obtain a general impression of the potential patient and even perform a primary assessment if necessary. Because the procedure takes about 15 to 30 seconds to complete and requires only eyes, fingers, and a watch, the provider can learn a lot about the patient's status through a simple conversation. Skin pallor, perspiration, respiration, orientation, the amount of time it takes the participant to answer a question, and the appropriateness of the responses can all provide indications of the individual's overall health.

While providers are evaluating them, participants will likely ask questions about the event and expect the SEMS staff to have the answers. In contrast to past EMS coverage of special events, today a trained SEMS provider is a part of the event. Generally, and just as important as ensuring that the event goes smoothly, the SEMS provider must also work to provide patrons with an enjoyable experience. This role is as vital as the roles of ushers or security personnel. To adequately answer questions and help to provide an enjoyable experience, staff members should arrive prior to the commencement of the special event and study the grounds to gain a working knowledge of the layout of the event. Every staff member should have a map. The staff should feel comfortable answering any questions, no matter the apparent relevancy. There are no dumb questions when preparing for and handling a special event.

Providers should honor the decorum of the special event. Each occasion will have a theme or accepted standard of behavior. The type of event will dictate the type of uniform and acceptable professional behavior. Sports events may be casual while inaugural balls will be more formal. SEMS personnel must always conduct themselves in a professional manner; they should be aware of their voice level and ensure that idle conversation topics are in keeping with what is appropriate for the decorum of the event. If providers are at a health-oriented event such as a marathon or triathlon, it is appropriate to refrain from smoking.

SEMS providers are constantly in the public eye. Most SEMS events attract large numbers of media personnel, and cell phone cameras are everywhere. To avoid being captured on camera, especially in difficult situations, the SEMS agency or organization should develop policies for dealing with the media. If the media requests to film or shoot pictures during an event, a point person must be assigned to secure all proceedings and communicate with the media. This measure helps to ensure that SEMS staff are shown properly. Be sure to inform the venue and event promoters about any media interviews that may occur with the point person. Not only is this a professional courtesy to the event promoter, but the promoter may also have policies regarding media interviews.

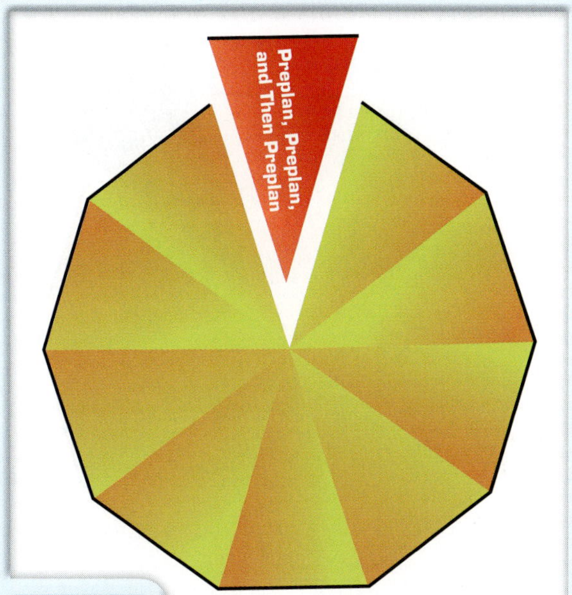

Figure 1-6

Preplanning is crucial to a successful SEMS operation.

Preplan, Preplan, and Then Preplan

Even the best medical setup and top quality responders cannot compensate for poor **preplanning** Figure 1-6. If the SEMS manager and personnel have not anticipated a situation prior to the special event, it is too late. For example, if providers have not designated a **comfort station** prior to the special event and it is unusually warm or an unexpected rain shower develops, providers will just have to make do. Dwight Eisenhower once stated, "Plans are nothing. Planning is everything."

More Isn't Better

Fire and EMS systems sometimes manage events by using any and all possible resources to solve a problem. This is not the best strategy for several reasons Figure 1-7.

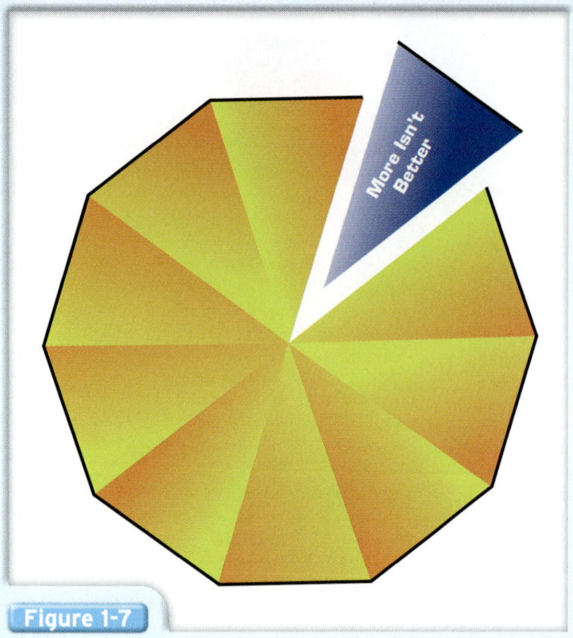

Figure 1-7

Plan so you know exactly what you need—no more and no less.

It is not always feasible to increase staff and equipment to deal with a problem. Even when it is feasible, it is not necessarily responsible or cost effective; departments will have to do more with less. Thus, when presented with an event, a service cannot arbitrarily assign ambulances and personnel. SEMS managers must be able to analyze an event's needs, devise a response plan, embrace new technology, and justify every resource and expense.

Nevertheless, EMS and fire services are professions that greatly value tradition and are sometimes slow to embrace new technology. SEMS is likely a new area of training for the providers studying it, and it may require more preplanning than a provider has engaged in previously. By analyzing formulas, collecting data, researching the event's needs, and crunching the numbers, solutions can be developed that provide maximum protection.

By the same token, not only do EMS and fire services need to embrace this new concept and technology, but managers need to educate the organizers of each special event and inform them of the appropriate response. The SEMS manager is responsible for formulating the appropriate plan, including the perfect amount of equipment and staff for each special event. A manager may be called upon to execute a plan on a constrained budget, with limited resources, and will have to plan accordingly.

Simultaneously, while there will be a shrinking resource pool, the public has been overly exposed to EMS as dramatized by television and will continue to expect more and more service. The military has learned that it is better to rely on small teams of highly motivated, highly trained operators known as special forces, and EMS is now experiencing that same paradigm shift. SEMS is one of the very first branches of the new special forces in EMS.

It is better to calculate the precise amount of resources needed. Instead of arbitrarily assigning 10 ALS units and 25 emergency medical technicians to the local fair or ball game, SEMS managers should analyze the weather, attendance, cycle rates, and all other factors that go into a good response. This research or preplanning stage will render the exact amount of resources needed to successfully staff and conduct an EMS operation at any event—no matter the scale.

Mass Gatherings Are Not Mass-Casualty Incidents

Federal Emergency Management Agency (FEMA) is the independent agency of the US government that provides a single point of accountability for all federal emergency preparedness and mitigation and response activities. FEMA defines public functions and mass gatherings as special events that are nonroutine activities within a community that bring together large numbers of people and result in extraordinary demands on public-safety sector services and the community's infrastructure.

However, this does not appear to be the consensus definition of a mass gathering Figure 1-8. Most researchers have defined mass gatherings in terms of the number of people attending the event. The general definition of a mass gathering is an event attended by more than 1,000 persons; other sources cite a minimum of over 25,000 attendees. Individual SEMS services and agencies should refer to their local definitions for additional figures.

The problem with using hard numbers is that such definitions focus on a single characteristic (ie, the number of people attending) rather than on a broader understanding of all the factors that come into play

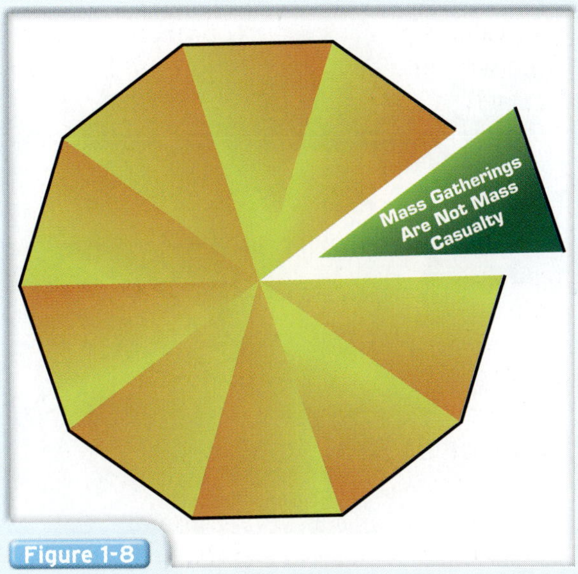

Figure 1-8

Remember that a mass gathering is not a mass-casualty incident. It could become one, but these are two distinct and separate concepts.

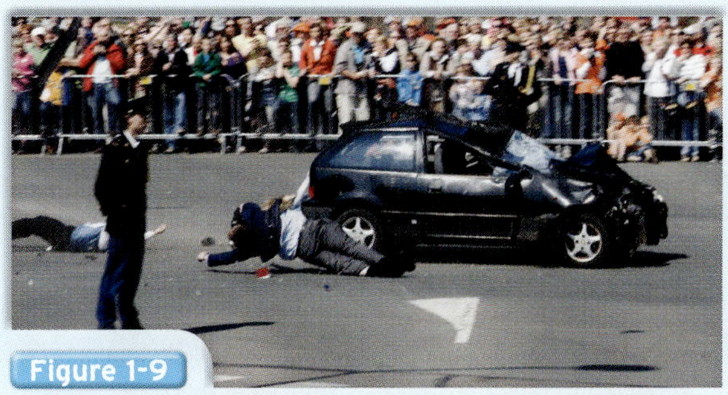

Figure 1-9

An MCI and a TOPL can appear to be the same, but the main distinctions are whether additional resources are required and whether the event can continue.

at a mass gathering. For example, a more appropriate definition of a mass gathering might be:

> A situation during which crowds gather and where there is the potential for a delayed response to emergencies because of limited access to patients, where attendee behavior may affect the types of emergencies that occur at the event, where types of emergencies will vary depending on whether the event is static or moving, or where other features of the environment and location will also affect the types of emergencies that occur.

This broader definition of a mass gathering may be useful for two reasons. First, it recognizes that planning for and delivering health services during mass gatherings is complicated by the context and situation in which the care will be provided. Second, it provides a definition that incorporates "nontraditional" mass gatherings as well as the more traditional large public events. Of course, there are other situations apart from public events in which crowds are gathered and access and management of emergencies are complicated by the environment and the crowd.

The average mass-gathering event will produce very few, if any, needs for medical treatment. Attending most mass-gathering events is not any more dangerous than attending any other event on an ordinary day. A special event of 10,000 participants will generally produce no more medical emergencies than does an average day in a small town with a population of 10,000 people. However, this is true only if there are no extenuating circumstances, such as excessive heat or cold, overly excited participants, use of alcohol or drugs, or a specific demographic such as advanced age of the attendees. Barring these circumstances, SEMS services and agencies can plan for the same amount and type of medical incidents that usually occur in a small town.

SEMS-trained companies and personnel understand the difference between a **mass-casualty incident (MCI)** and a **temporary overwhelming patient load (TOPL)** Figure 1-9. The accepted definition of an MCI is an event that overwhelms the internal and outside resources that are required to resolve the situation, resulting in an inability to resume the special event after the incident. The event must be cancelled due to the type and severity of the incident. An MCI is usually caused by a single incident such as a lightning strike, prolonged inclement weather, a fire, bleacher collapse, or a single catastrophic

TIP

Mass gatherings and special events should not be approached as mass-casualty incidents. These events can potentially produce a higher systemwide patient load, but a higher patient load is not the same as a mass-casualty event.

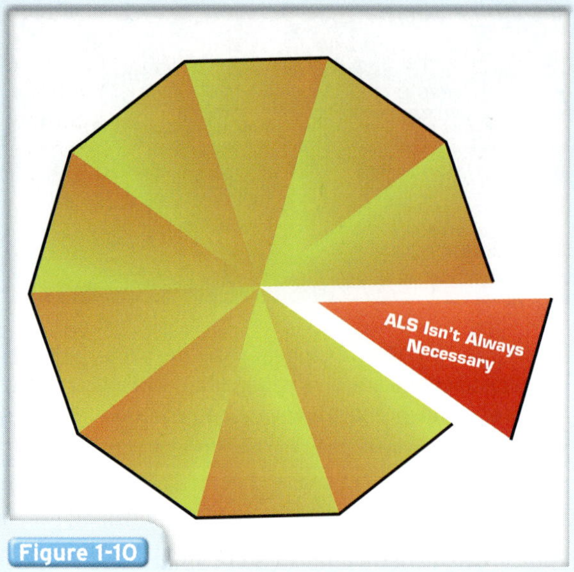

Figure 1-10

Remember to administer BLS when it is sufficient. ALS is not always necessary or appropriate.

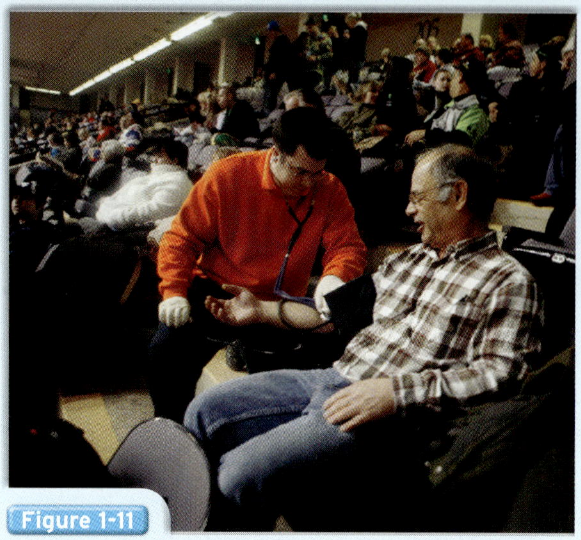

Figure 1-11

Instead of considering what type of support is generally best, providers should consider which type of support is most appropriate for a specific situation.

event that exceeds local logistic support capabilities. In contrast, a TOPL is a brief period during which there is a larger number of victims than the available resources can handle, but this does not prevent the event from continuing and subsides without external resources being required.

To the untrained provider, a TOPL may appear to be a mass casualty, yet there is one important distinction—the event can continue after the incident. Thus, although the planned resources are overwhelmed and additional assistance may be required, once the service works through the situation, the **patient load** will return to normal.

ALS (Advanced Life Support) Isn't Always Necessary

Sometimes, even experienced EMS managers and providers get caught up in the mindset that ALS equals better life support, rendering basic life support (BLS) strictly and unconditionally inferior to ALS Figure 1-10. Depending on the local statistics and systems, the percentage of BLS responses account for as much as 75% to 90% of all EMS responses. Rarely disputed by any respectable EMS authority, the bottom line is that the majority of EMS calls can be properly cared for with BLS. The same breakdown holds true for special events: the majority of calls for service are going to require BLS. Thus, instead of considering what type of support is generally best, providers should consider which type of support is most appropriate for a specific situation Figure 1-11. When staffing and planning for an event, providers should keep this in mind. The promoter should also be consulted when making these decisions. In some instances, ALS may be required as the minimum standard, such as for a standby at a boxing event. Local and state laws will also impact this decision. For example, in Pennsylvania, the state law requires one staffed and licensed ambulance vehicle per 5,000 to 25,000 attendees, two staffed and licensed ambulance vehicles for 25,000 to 55,000 attendees, and three staffed and licensed ambulance vehicles for any audience greater than 55,000 people.

SEMS-trained personnel strive to formulate a proper response to the specifics of each special event as well as ensure that the promoter understands that the best possible coverage will be provided.

Learn the Language

EMS providers should learn the language of the special event Figure 1-12. EMS has a language all its own: BLS,

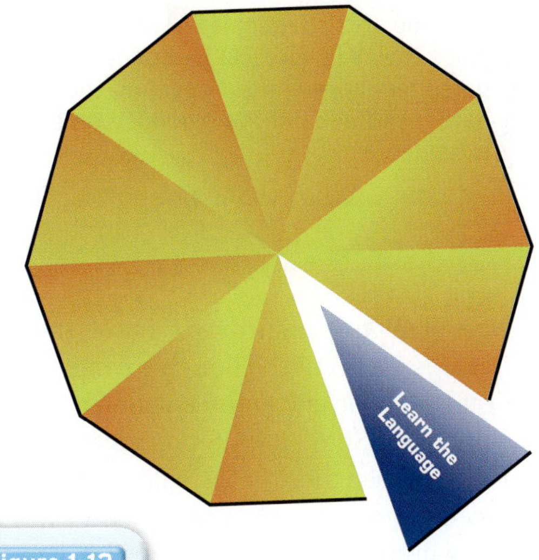

Figure 1-12

SEMS events have their own terminology. Become familiar with terms and concepts used at different types of events where you work.

ALS, SEMS, MCI, and the list goes on. To an outsider, this sounds like a foreign language. The same is true of different types of special events each type of event has its own language. These terms and languages may sound foreign to EMS providers, so it is imperative that they become multilingual to properly communicate at specific SEMS events.

Planning and executing a proper emergency response is already littered with pitfalls and variables that must be accounted for. The hidden danger of language barriers can be devastating. This danger comes in two forms. The first example is when individuals at a special event keep using a term that SEMS personnel are unfamiliar with and do not understand. When this occurs, the provider must be sure to find out what the word means. If a service is covering a steeplechase and the event announcer continuously refers to an "outrider," the provider should ask the event coordinator or a participant what this means. Asking for background information is especially important if the overall plan involves the unknown term in any way. In this case, outriders are like officials on the course. They are responsible for reporting fouls and gathering runaway horses. They are oftentimes the first to call for help when a rider is injured and will have direct communication with the medical team—an important link in SEMS management of the event.

TIP Beware of phrases and objects that have multiple meanings. For example, if you are providing SEMS at a historical or civil war reenactment, the participants may be yelling for help or acting injured even though they are not actually injured.

The best way to avoid confusion in all aspects of SEMS is by scheduling regular meetings with all groups involved in a special event. This group could be as small as the SEMS coordinator and the event promoter. **Mega-events**, which have an on-site attendance of more than 25,000 people, could have meetings that involve over 30 agency heads due to larger events needing multiple disciplines on site, such as police, hazmat, fire, security, and public health. No matter the size of the group, plans, policies, and required National Incident Management System (NIMS) forms should be agreed upon to eliminate as much confusion as possible and plan for potential emergencies at the event. NIMS will be discussed in greater detail in Chapter 6.

The second danger comes from terms, phrases, and objects that may have multiple meanings. Sometimes, terms and objects perform one function in the outside world but mean something very different at a special event. Everyday words, such as out, go, and unit, take on entirely different meanings in the context of a special event. It is the responsibility of the SEMS manager and personnel to learn this new language. They should also research the meaning behind any symbols or colors. Part of the information-gathering phase of the planned response is to gather this information. A safe and successful response depends on this step.

For example, during an off-road motorcycle event, when a rider goes down in a blind spot on the track, the flagger will wave a white flag with a red cross. If the SEMS personnel are not familiar with the meaning of this flag, and they assume that the flagger is calling for medical attention, they could be seriously injured by running onto the track. In fact, this flag simply means that riders may not jump any obstacles because another rider is down in a blind or dangerous position. It does not mean that the track is free for medical personnel to run to the potential injury.

Alternatively, during some steeplechases, the sign for medical help is waving a red coat in the air. Once a gate judge does this, he or she will immediately "close the gate," which, in steeplechase language, means that the jockeys should carefully guide their horses around any obstacles, especially if the medical team is working on a downed rider.

Stay in Place

EMS providers are action-oriented people, and people of action do not like sitting around. Inevitably, they fidget and start moving around. But it is very hard to hit a moving target; thus, it is best for SEMS providers to remain in one general area where they can be easily found by those who need them Figure 1-13. It is also important that SEMS providers be easily identifiable.

While it is important to move around a selected location and interact with the participants at a special event, the use of roving paramedics or patrols throughout an entire area is ineffective. Though roving patrol is a successful method for law enforcement, this model is not appropriate for SEMS. SEMS providers' duties and roles are different than those of law enforcement officers. Law enforcement officers are tasked with preventing and deterring crime, so they must patrol. Often SEMS providers cannot prevent someone from becoming sick or injured. Their duty is to respond after the fact as quickly and safely as possible. Shifting position can actually extend response time.

When someone becomes sick or injured, family and bystanders will come to his or her aid by returning to the last place they saw help. If SEMS providers are constantly on the move, help becomes a moving target. Inevitably, this will cause unnecessary stress in a critical situation because people become tense when they cannot find help in a timely fashion.

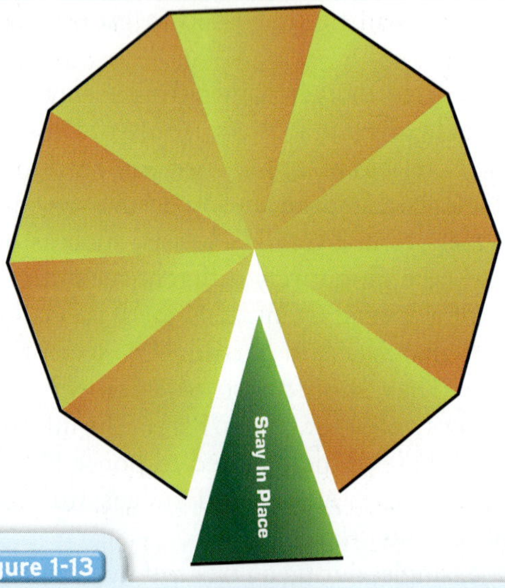

Figure 1-13

It is important to stay in one general area so that patients and event personnel can find you when needed.

TIP In a time of crisis, people will return to the last place they saw medical personnel. If medical personnel have shifted position, they will be harder to find, and the response time will be extended.

Stock and Staff for the Max

At first glance, the phrase "Stock and Staff for the Max" may seem to contradict "More Isn't Better." However, stocking and staffing for the max means having the right amount and type of equipment and staff for the expected maximum number of emergencies (the same message as "More Isn't Better"). Rather than using all possible resources, do a thorough analysis of the many different factors to determine an accurate expected number of emergencies, and then stock and staff for that number.

Later in this book, we will compare a **static attendance** to a **cyclical attendance** and go over the specifics of planning for each unique type of event. Static attendance involves a predetermined number of attendees, whereas cyclical attendance indicates that the number of attendees can rise and fall during the event. Ultimately, when staffing and stocking for an event, it is

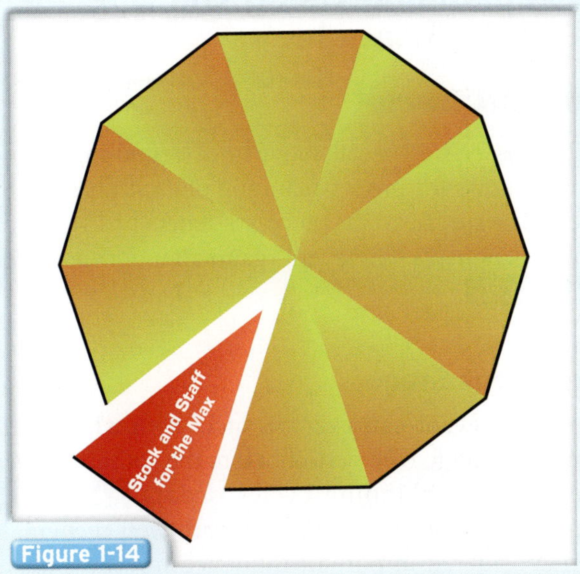

Figure 1-14

As a general rule, stock for half the total number of expected attendees. Staff for the maximum number of people expected at peak flow time.

important to consider the total amount of attendees as well as the total amount of attendees present at a single given time Figure 1-14.

For example, if 500,000 people are expected to attend a 3-day festival located in the parking lot of a local baseball team, the SEMS crew should stock supplies for 250,000 people. However, the crew should staff for the maximum number of people expected to attend at a peak flow time. In this case, the peak time for attendance will be on Saturday from 1 pm to 5 pm and on Sunday from 12 pm to 4 pm, with a maximum cycle rate of 15,000 attendees per hour. Considering no other factors at this time, SEMS would staff for 15,000 people. Again, the crew must remember to consult any protocols and local or state law for these issues. It also is crucial that all SEMS personnel are familiar with each piece of equipment.

Do It Right

As mentioned earlier, it is best to tailor plans and resources to each unique event. This is related to the concept of "more isn't better." By analyzing the needs of each specific event and planning based on these needs, SEMS providers will be planning correctly for the best outcome Figure 1-15.

Some situations may require planning with additional committees, depending on the size or scale of the event. In some cases, such as working with government organizations, an Emergency Action Planning Committee will perform the same function as the SEMS manager. The committee is designed to coordinate the efforts of several agencies that will be involved in the potential response to an incident on the site of the upcoming event. Large events such as a NASCAR race, Super Bowl, and large NCAA tournament commonly use this committee to plan their activities as they relate to emergency responses. The promoter and the event staff will have knowledge that providers may be lacking and that will be vital to success. At this stage, it is also important to include law enforcement in the planning if their services will be needed for the event.

You Are the SEMS Provider

CASE 2

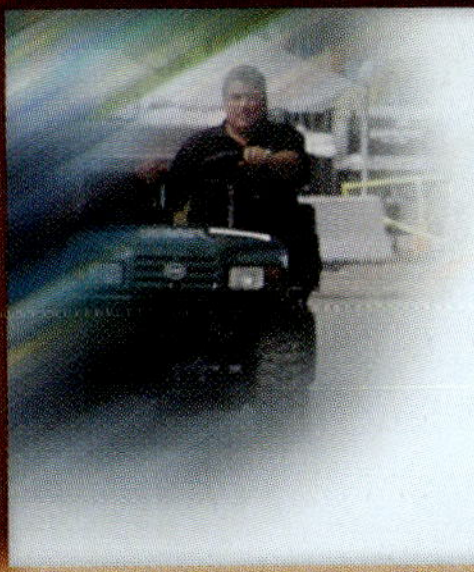

You are providing service for an event in the dead of winter. The event is expected to draw 15,000 people. The seating will be assigned, and the energy level is low to medium. After doing your calculations and research, you plan to have a single transport unit, five fully equipped medical personnel, one warming station, and one aid tent.

Suddenly, 4 days before Game Day, you discover that the promoter has permitted the attendance to expand to 35,000 people.

1. What should you do to cover the additional 20,000 people?

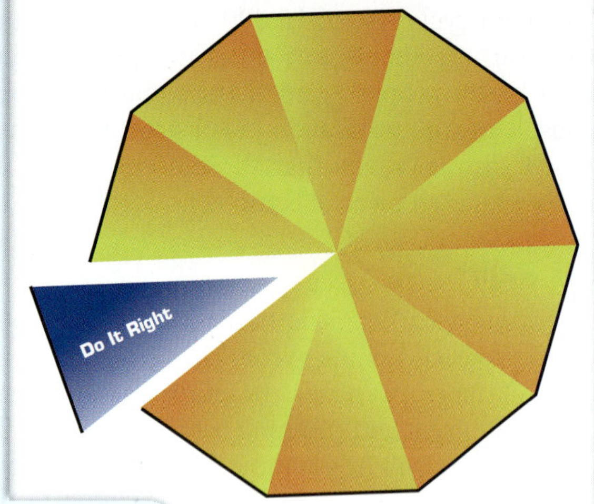

Figure 1-15

Plan for an event based on its specific needs.

Preplanning Using the Special Events Triangle

SEMS dissects a special event from beginning to end, which allows for proper planning of each phase of the event. The special events process is generally divided into three increments: pre-event, game day, and postevent Figure 1-16.

Pre-event Stage

No SEMS event can ever be successful without the pre-event stage (the period before the gathering when meeting and planning cycles occur) Figure 1-17. Key features of mass gatherings are well recognized and considered important influences on the demand for health care during such events. These key features include:

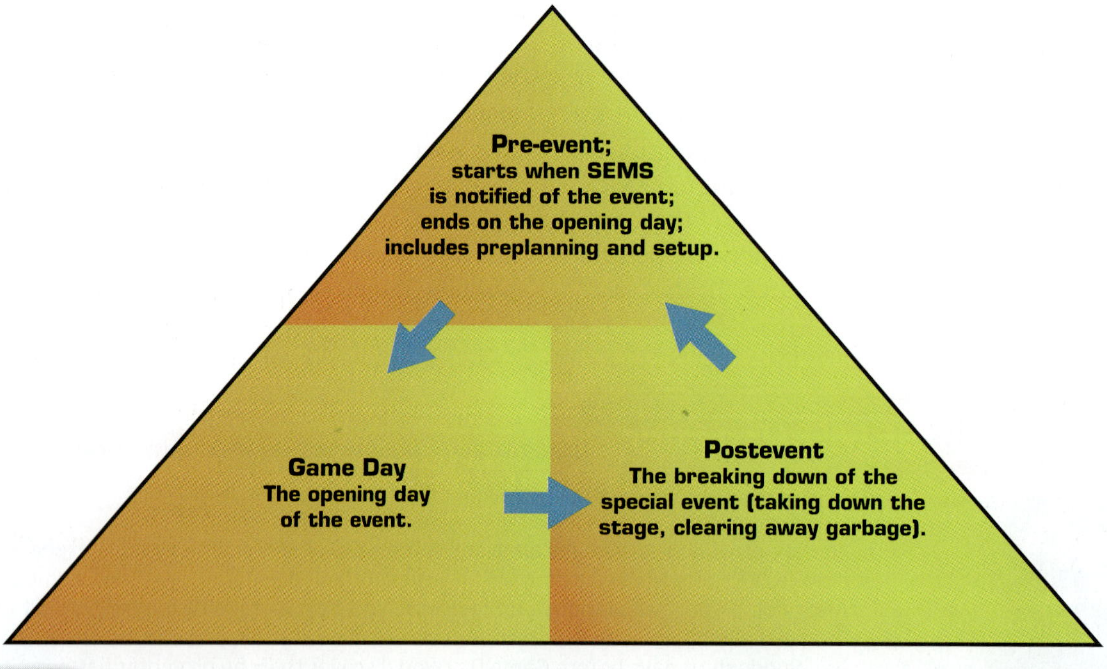

Figure 1-16

The special events triangle.

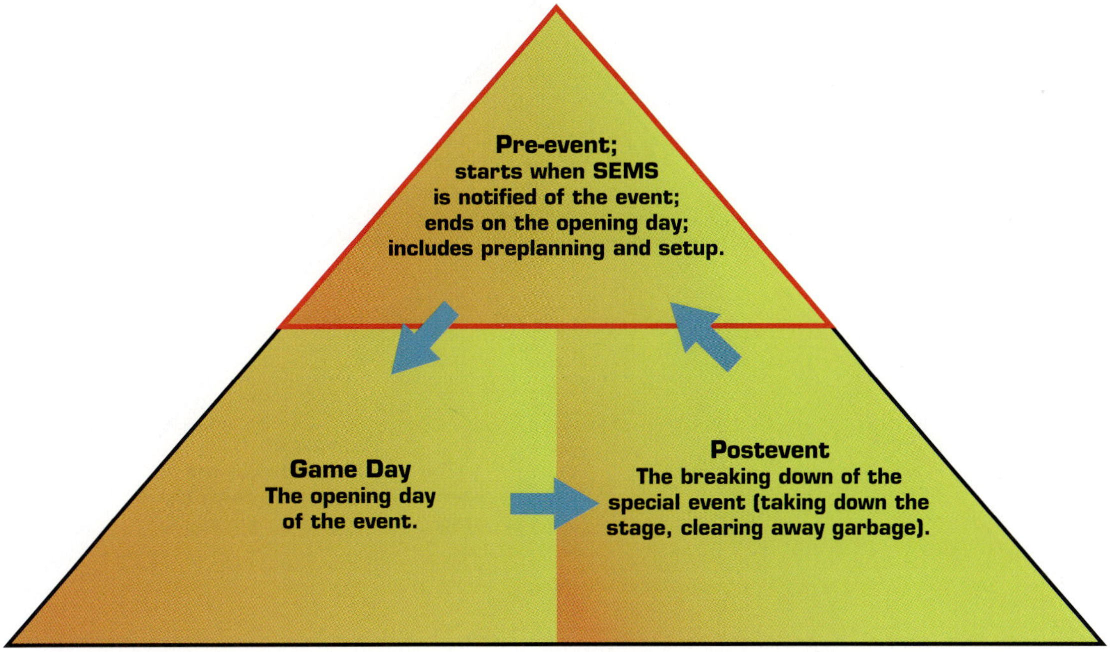

Figure 1-17

The pre-event stage begins when you learn you will be providing SEMS at an event, and includes preplanning, during which it is essential to consider every possibility of what could go wrong and to plan for it.

- The weather (temperature and humidity)
- Duration of the event
- Whether the event is predominantly outdoors or indoors
- Whether the crowd is predominantly seated or mobile within the venue
- If the event is contained (has defined perimeters, for example an enclosed area such as a stadium) or uncontained
- The type of event
- The mood of the crowd, availability of alcohol and drugs
- The crowd density, the geography of the venue (or terrain/locale)
- The average age of the crowd

Although this list of the characteristics of a mass gathering is not all-inclusive, it is a beginning point for most events.

Specific questions to consider are as follows:

- What level of care is SEMS to provide, and will SEMS treat participants as well as spectators?
- What type of injuries may occur, and how many injuries should be anticipated?
- What are the feasible levels of care?
- Where should aid stations be placed, and how should they be organized?
- How will medical personnel and patients find each other?
- What are the nominated receiving hospitals, and what are the arrangements for coordinating transport?

If your SEMS organization is a government organization, SEMS managers and personnel may need to set strategies that will provide the basis for tactical directions during the actual event. To create these, there are large amounts of information to gather. Sometimes,

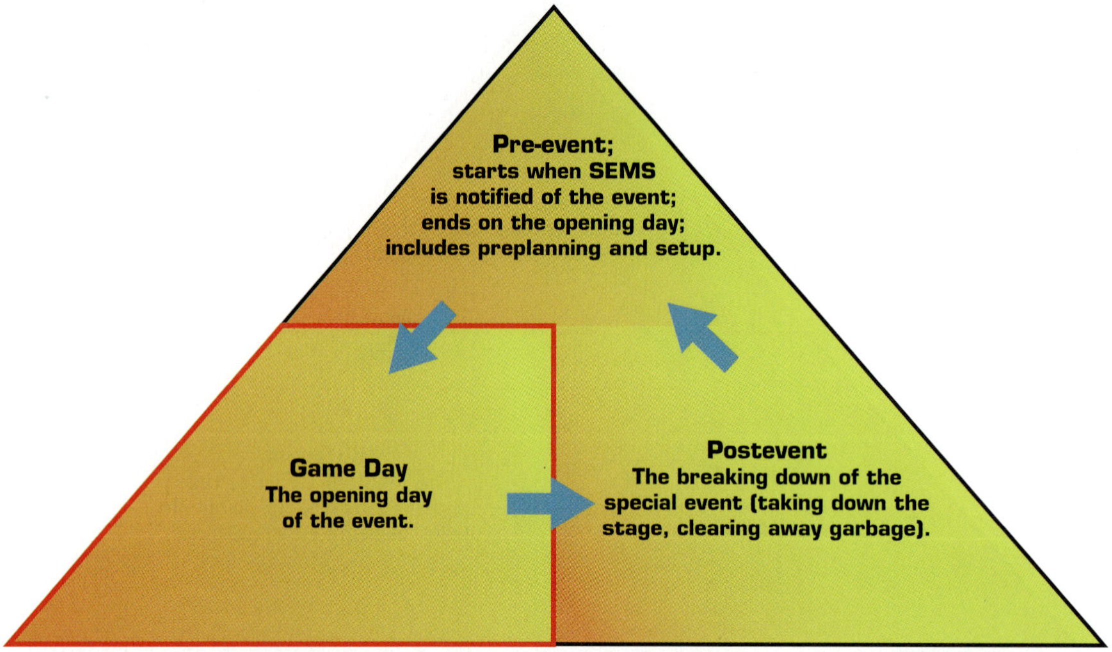

Figure 1-18

Game day is the day or days when the event takes place.

the research phase may take just a few minutes; in other cases, it can take up to 18 months and will require meeting with law enforcement, public health, fire services, venue and event personnel, and security. If the event is classified as an **Event of National Significance**, FBI, the Bureau of Alcohol, Tobacco, Firearms, and Explosives (ATF), and Homeland Security will all be stakeholders at this event and in the planning stages.

Months of planning must occur before the event day. On event day, preplanning is put to the test. When preparing for an event SEMS managers should ask:

- Have I taken into account all that can go wrong?
- Have I staffed the event properly?
- What will the day bring?

TIP When providing SEMS coverage at a special event, an EMS agency must still be able to meet all of the needs of the community.

No one can predict the answers to these questions. As previously discussed, preplanning for most contingencies will provide managers with the highest rate of success.

Game Day Stage

Events come in all shapes and sizes. Each type and size presents a unique set of challenges and circumstances to be faced and overcome. Covering game day at a NASCAR track event will require different tools and methods than a 4-H event at the local fairgrounds Figure 1-18. A crowd of 100,000 seated in a college football stadium will create different challenges than an outdoor festival of 8,000 participants roaming around the grounds. At this point, managers have to become flexible in their planning and adapt to the events that occur around them. They should consider:

- Are they experiencing normal patient volumes, or have they reached a TOPL?
- How are their resources managing these incidents?

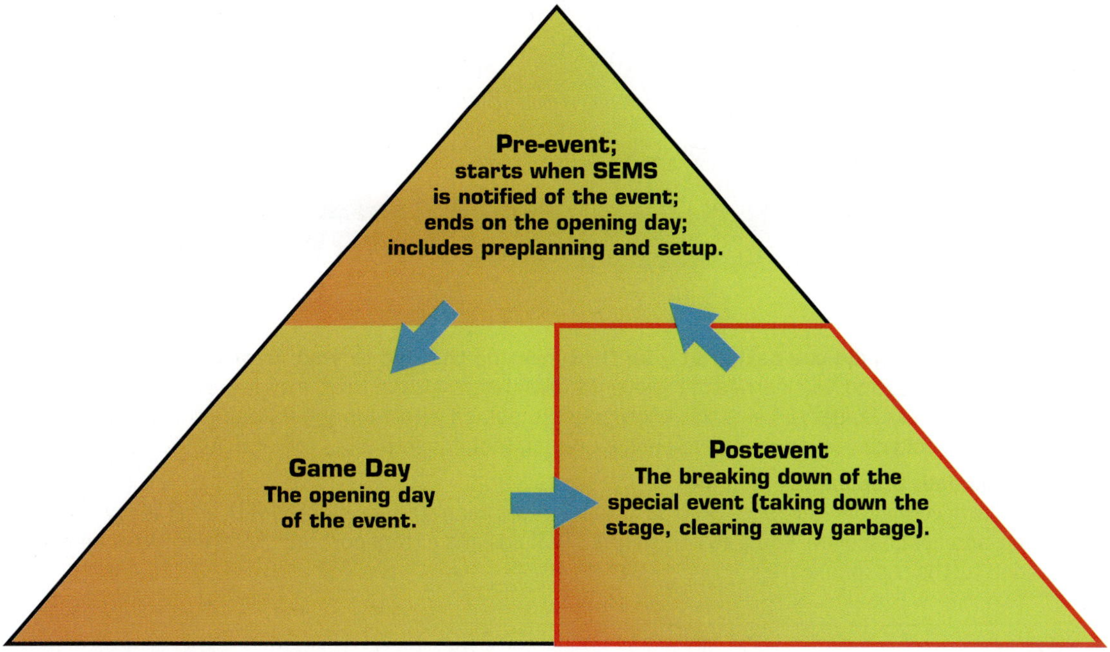

Figure 1-19

The postevent stage occurs after the event, when there are important tasks to complete, such as the AAR, if used by your organization.

TIP

Remember to wear comfortable, supportive shoes when providing medical services at a special event, as you will likely spend a large amount of time standing. This is especially important when you will be working at an event for several days in a row.

Postevent Stage

During the **postevent stage** Figure 1-19, managers need to analytically examine all aspects of the event coverage as soon as it has concluded. It is best to perform this step as soon as possible after the event so that each success and mistake is accurately recorded. This prompt reflection will aid in planning for future events at this venue as well as for similar events at any location.

Private SEMS organizations may have the flexibility to take care of any errors immediately as they occur during the event, and thus will, at this stage, record the problems and the resulting actions that were taken to resolve the issues.

Government organizations are likely to follow specified procedures, such as completing the AAR, mentioned earlier. This typed review should cover all aspects of the event and should be produced no later than 3 to 4 weeks after the event. When writing the report, keep in mind that several other parties will likely refer to it, including SEMS providers who covered the event, vendors and promoters of the event, and outside agencies.

A Comprehensive Strategy

Preplanning is vital to successfully provide care for the entirety of a special event—no matter the size, occasion, or geography. SEMS is 100% scalable and should always take into consideration the functional ability of the local EMS, hospitals, and surrounding entities.

In today's world, mass gatherings are increasingly frequent and growing larger. We, as EMS providers, must develop methods to provide care and transportation to the participants, while not impacting the resources needed to provide coverage to the residents and visitors of that same geographic area. Using the SEMS 10 will help the SEMS manager develop staffing requirements and equipment needs. Addressing key steps in each portion of the SEMS triangle will allow for a successful special event and help improve future events.

You Are the SEMS Provider

SUMMARY

CASE 1

1. **What information did you gather at your first meeting that led to your crew's success?**
   In your initial meeting, you learned of the event's parameters, including time of day (evening), location (outside), and time of year (January). Using this knowledge, combined with your understanding of what emergencies an exposure to cold can cause, you developed a preplan that covered all of the anticipated needs.
2. **What did your preplanning include?**
   Armed with your knowledge, your preplan included rewarming stations stocked with emergency blankets, chairs, coffee, and hot chocolate. You also had warmed IV fluids and a transport unit to care for the one member who needed further hospital care.

CASE 2

1. **What should you do to cover the additional 20,000 people?**
   Adjust your SEMS 10, and, by considering your calculations, simply scale up the existing response plan. In this case, the original number of attendees expected was 15,000, and you had planned to have a single transport unit, five fully equipped medical personnel, one warming station, and one aid tent. The number of expected attendees has increased to 35,000, which is more than double the original expected 15,000. Therefore, you would need to increase your resources to 10 fully equipped medical personnel, two warming stations, and two aid tents. You do not need to arrange for an additional ambulance because one ambulance can typically handle a 35,000-person event. These increased resources will enable you to remain in control and provide the same level of quality care.

Ready for Review

- The goal of the SEMS course is to offer a standard method that clearly defines how to provide a comprehensive, reproducible emergency medical response plan.
- The SEMS 10 provides specific guidelines for personnel to follow before, during, and after an event.
- When planning an EMS response for a special event, SEMS personnel need to be honest about their capabilities, expectations, and each individual's role.
- If SEMS personnel find that someone is having trouble, they should always be proactive and engage him or her in conversation.
- Even the best medical setup and top quality responders cannot compensate for poor preplanning.
- In today's climate, SEMS managers must be able to analyze an event's needs, devise a response plan, embrace the new technology, and justify every resource and expense. ALS is not always necessary.
- When staffing and planning for an event, instead of considering what type of support is generally best, providers should consider what type of support is most appropriate for a specific situation.
- SEMS-trained companies and personnel understand the difference between an MCI and a TOPL. An MCI overwhelms internal and outside resources, and the special event cannot resume. A TOPL is a brief period during which there is a larger number of victims than the available resources can handle (though additional resources may need to be brought in), but this excess demand eventually subsides. Remember that ALS is not always better life support. In the majority of situations, BLS is sufficient to treat the patient.
- SEMS providers should learn the language of the special event.
- The SEMS response model is based on a rapid response after someone has become sick. It is not based on roving providers, who can be hard to find when an injury occurs.
- When staffing and stocking for an event, it is important to consider the total amount of attendees as well as the total amount of attendees present at a given time.
- The special events process is generally divided into three stages: pre-event, game day, and postevent.
- Preplanning is vital to successfully provide care for the entirety of a special event—regardless of size, occasion, or geography.

Vital Vocabulary

after action report (AAR) A report consisting of a summary of lessons learned from an incident; it should include recommendations for improvements for decision makers and agency personnel to consider.

comfort station A station that is designated for rehabilitation, cooling, or warming of staff and patients, as needed; for example, this station may be air conditioned or heated, if needed, and is ideally indoors.

cyclical attendance The number of attendees as it rises and falls during an event's operational period.

Event of National Significance An event classification assigned by the US government, which means that FBI, ATF, and Homeland Security will be stakeholders in the event and in the planning stages.

Federal Emergency Management Agency (FEMA) An independent agency of the US government that provides a single point of accountability for all federal emergency preparedness and mitigation and response activities.

mass-casualty incident (MCI) An event in which a large number of casualties are produced in a relatively short period, exceeding local logistic support capabilities. MCIs are usually the result of a single incident such as a military aircraft accident, hurricane, flood, earthquake, or armed attack.

mass gathering A situation (event) during which crowds gather and where there is the potential for a delayed response to emergencies because of limited access to patients or other features of the environment and location.

mega-event An event that has an on-site attendance of over 55,000 people at any given time.

passive interaction interviewing A technique used to interview a potential patient using everyday questions that reveal key patient data, such as mental status.

patient load The number of patients who require care at a given time.

postevent stage Analysis stage that allows all involved parties to assess the performance of resources and plans that were developed to cover the event.

pre-event stage A period before a gathering when meetings and planning cycles occur.

preplanning A process that involves all interested parties and develops event response plans and needs.

special event A gathering of people for a specific reason, such as music, sports, or politics.

static attendance The term used to describe a predetermined number of attendees that cannot change, such as attendees at a preticket sales–only event.

temporary overwhelming patient load (TOPL) A brief period during which there is a larger number of victims than the available resources can handle (though additional resources may need to be brought in), but this does not prevent the event from continuing and subsides without external resources being required.

CHAPTER

Preplanning Step By Step

2

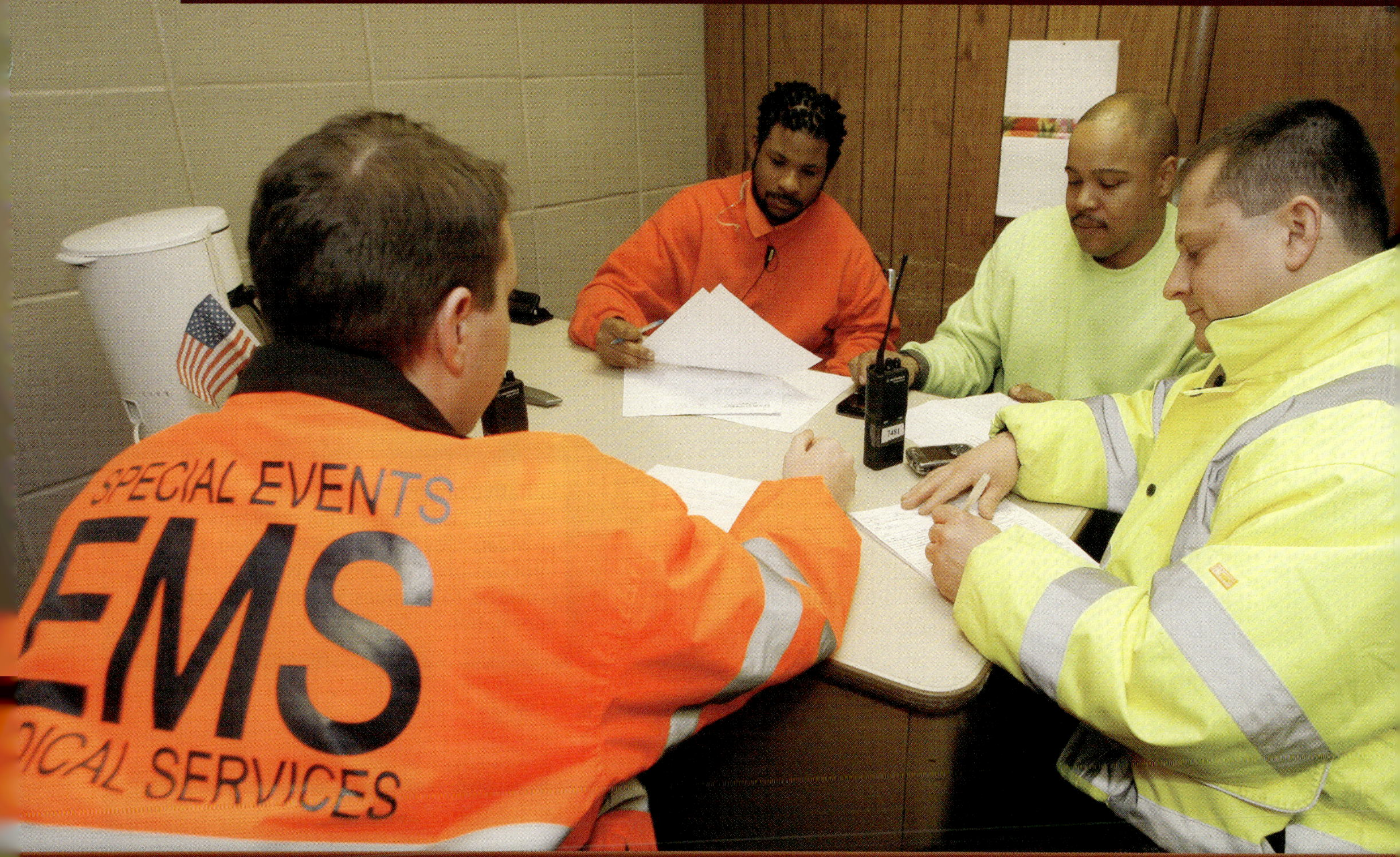

LEARNING OBJECTIVES

- List factors to consider during the preplanning process for a special event.
- Describe objective and subjective factors, and list which ones to consider during preplanning.
- Discuss weather and environmental considerations and how to preplan for an outdoor event.
- Explain the potential emergencies to expect for a seated audience versus a mobile audience.
- Describe how the number of attendees affects preplanning for special events medical services (SEMS) coverage.
- Discuss how crowd demographics factor into preplanning.
- Discuss considerations for planning access and egress routes for SEMS providers and ambulances.
- Understand the importance for SEMS providers, event staff, and attendees of having maps that denote the location of first aid stations, medical facilities, structures, and choke points.
- Describe the process of the theoretical walk-through and the physical walk-through.
- Explain the importance of communicating with event vendors and other involved parties.
- Discuss the importance of preplanning for major emergencies at a special event and the creation of an evacuation plan.

Step One: Research

To accurately assess the needs of a particular special event, a systematic, scientific approach must be used. This process begins by defining the parameters of the special event and then by placing the event into a specific category. The categories are based on both objective and subjective factors. By asking your event contact for information and performing an Internet search, you can gather objective background information on the type of event, the history of the promoter, the types of attendees, and other necessary information to help formulate an organized plan.

Objective factors are the proven, unbiased facts about the event. They include:

- Event type
- The weather (temperature and humidity)
- Duration of the event
- Night events
- Indoor versus outdoor events
- Seated or mobile audience
- Event boundaries
- Crowd size
- Venue geography and terrain, including access (egress, ingress, and traffic flows)
- Crowd demographics

Subjective information is derived from what other people perceive about the special event. Consulting former participants, attendees, organizers, and outside services that previously covered the same special event can provide valuable information.

The subjective factors refer to details that people may impart that are not provable facts. They can include the following:

- Attendability
- Gut instinct
- Crowd mentality
- Previous experiences with a particular event
- Intelligence reports (police and security)

Objective Factors

Event Type

When planning for an event, the type of activity is going to dictate all aspects of preparation and touch upon each

TIP

Initiative on the part of SEMS providers and managers is crucial during preplanning. Event providers may not give SEMS providers all the information they need. It is up to the SEMS providers to ask questions and obtain needed information.

You Are the SEMS Provider

CASE 1

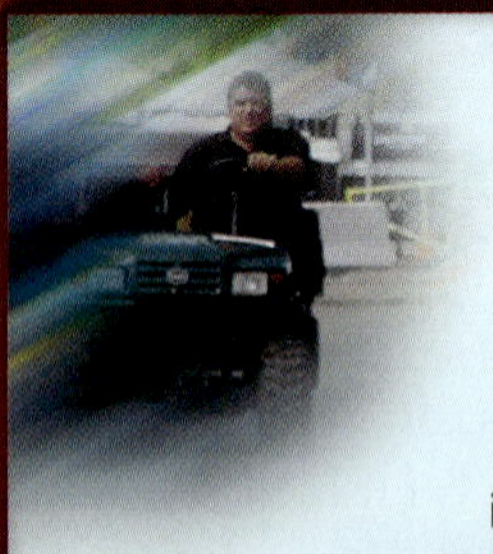

Your service is signed up to provide coverage for a music festival for the second year in a row. You meet with your primary contact, the festival promoter, 2 months after your first festival to go over the logistics for next year.

Overall, during the event in the first year, you counted 248 patient contacts and 38 transports to the hospital; this means about 15% of patient contacts (38 divided by 248) were transported. On average, you treated one patient every 10 minutes for 24 hours. The local volunteer fire department was responsible for all transports and was the second-level incident response inside the venue when you became overwhelmed. Their assistance was required several times throughout the weekend. You determine that the fire department handled 10% to 15% of the patient load responsibilities. You know that their role is incredibly important because once you turn a patient over to them, your personnel are free to resume coverage at the event. Without the fire department, your people would be required to remain out of service longer, thus creating more opportunity for the remaining unit to be overwhelmed.

Three days before the event, the fire chief calls to alert you that they will not be supporting the event this year. You have 72 hours to Game Day.

1. What additional resources can you draw on at this point to ensure that you are not overwhelmed on Game Day?
2. Taking your answer to the first question into consideration, by what percentage should you increase your staff?

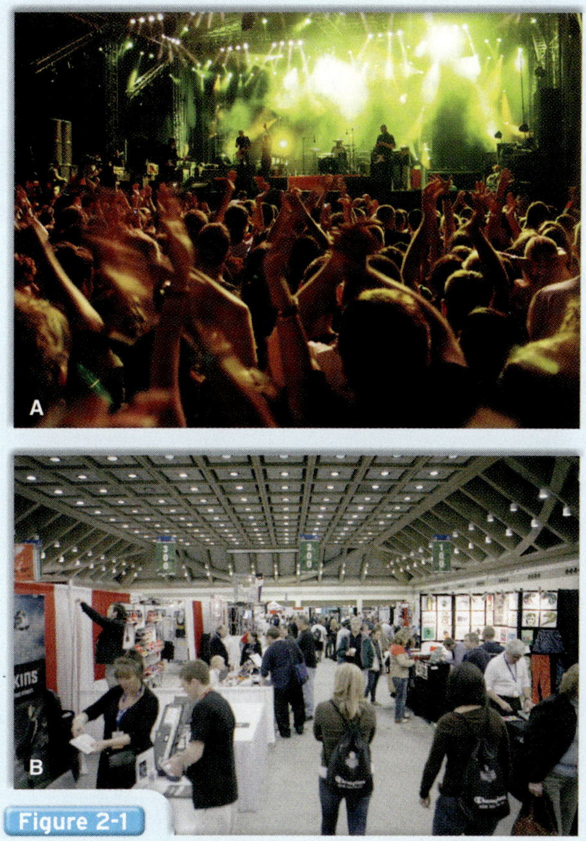

Figure 2-1

When planning for an event, consider the vast difference between a heavy metal concert (**A**) and a convention (**B**).

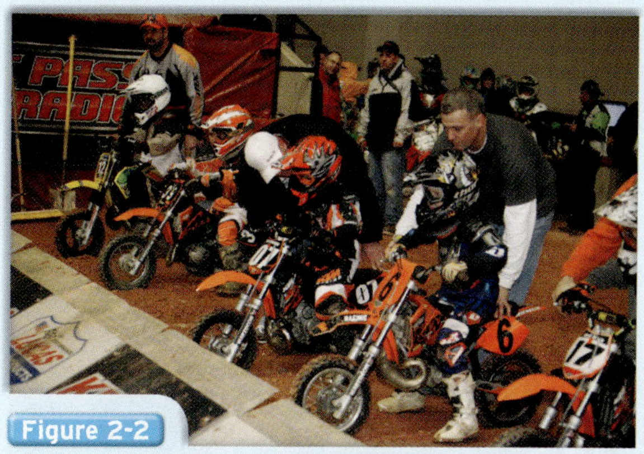

Figure 2-2

Note whether children or older people will be participating or attending, which could affect your preplanning because they may experience different types of emergencies and may require different equipment.

TIP Find out how many SEMS providers and transport units are required by law and what is required by the event promoter. Also find out if the SEMS providers must have a specific certification level.

factor involved in the SEMS evaluation (Figure 2-1 and Figure 2-2). Consider the vast differences among the following events:

- A football game
- A local fair
- A heavy metal concert
- A scientific conference

Defining the event type is the starting point when planning SEMS coverage. Specific types of events are discussed in detail in Chapters 7 through 10.

Duration of the Event

Especially for outdoor events, it is imperative to be aware of the event schedule and the role of SEMS personnel. Important questions to cover with the event manager about the duration of the event include:

- What time will the event start?
- What is the expected arrival time of the SEMS staff?
- How long is the event, or what time will it end?
- When will the SEMS staff be released?
- Will more than one shift of people be needed to cover the duration of the special event?

Venue Considerations

Important questions to pose about the venue and the event manager's expectations include:

- Where will the SEMS staff be operating?
- How will they operate and communicate?
- Are there any time or environmental concerns?
- Are there any safety concerns for the crews?
- How will a patient be moved within the venue? Are there stairs to traverse? Is the venue equipped with an escalator or elevator and if so, is it wide enough to fit a cot in the supine position, plus the accompanying SEMS providers?
- Does the venue have good lighting?
- Will the event provide lighting?
- Where are the parking lots?

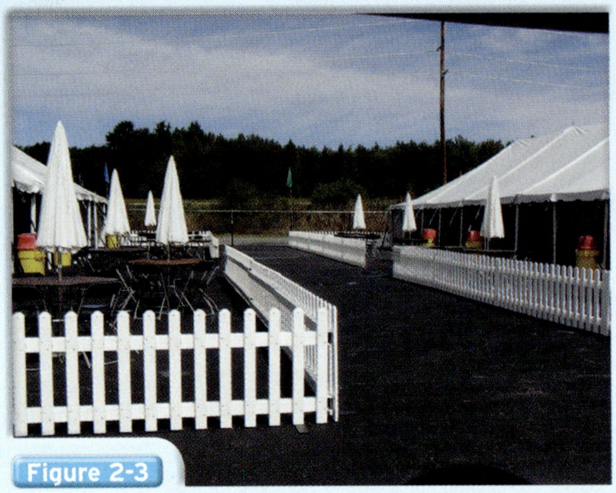

Figure 2-3

Choke points are places where obstructions prohibit the crowd from moving freely and could also limit access for SEMS providers. Fenced-in areas could become choke points during the event.

- What will be going on in the nonpublic areas?
  - Does the public enter or cross any of these areas?
  - Who does have access?
  - How can the emergency medical services (EMS) team gain access if needed?
  - Is the area secure or unsecure?
- Will the event be moving equipment, and if so, how will the event move equipment?
- Are there bleachers, chairs, or dedicated seating areas?
  - Are they permanent or temporary?
  - Where are they located? In the sun or shade?
- Is there a **mosh pit** (an area, usually in front of a stage, where members of the audience flail and smash into each other)?
  - Where are the access points?
  - Where are the **choke points**, or places where obstructions prohibit the crowd from moving freely that could also limit access for SEMS crews Figure 2-3?
  - How will injured people be identified?
  - What safety arrangements are in place for your crew?
  - Who will remove the patients?
  - Will the event use barricades, and if so, is the security staff trained in barricade operations or how to manage these areas?
- If the event is a festival, is this a routine use for the grounds? What and where are the permanent and temporary structures?

TIP

If security is inadequate, the number of patients may increase, for example, if a violent situation escalates. If the information is available during preplanning, consider the amount and type of security personnel versus the type of event.

Indoor Versus Outdoor Events

Is the location indoors or outdoors? Location makes a big difference; special considerations for outdoor events are covered in detail in Chapter 7. Indoor operations may differ in many ways from outdoor operations. From the obvious differences in exposure to the elements to differences in ingress and egress, this factor can change resource needs dramatically. For indoor events, providers should consider the type of venue:

- Stadium
- Arena
- Sports complex
- Banquet hall
- Hotel
- Private home

For outdoor events, too, the type of venue should be considered:

- Park
- Closed-off street
- Waterfront
- Mountain
- Downtown
- Private land
- Farm
- Amphitheater
- Parking lot

While the venue is being considered, it is also imperative for the SEMS manager to go over all gathered data in order to consider all potential emergencies. The discovery of a possible emergency could drastically affect how resources are distributed.

The Weather

Weather and environmental factors are very important to consider if the event, or any portion of the event, will occur outdoors. Weather and outdoor events are covered in detail in Chapter 7.

Night Events

Nighttime operations create new safety concerns. If SEMS crews are working in parking lots that are not well lit, this is a real concern. In the dark, it is easier to lose track of partners and patients. Operating under the rule of three is especially important at night

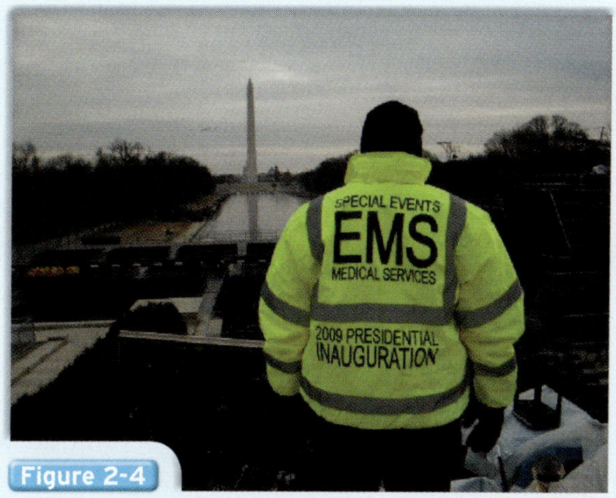

Figure 2-4

SEMS providers who wear flashing beacons or reflective gear are much easier to locate. Visibility increases both provider safety and response times.

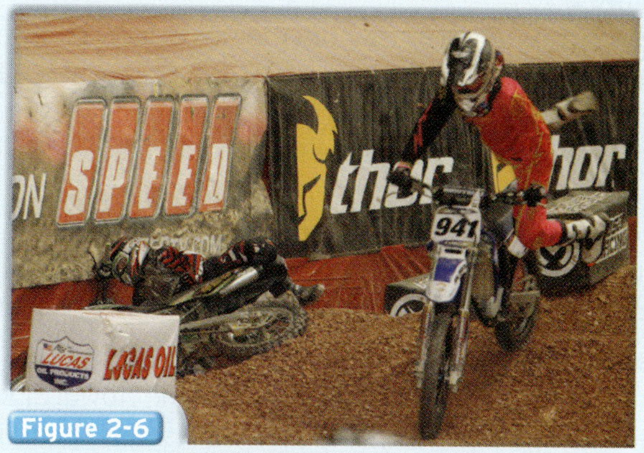

Figure 2-6

Each special event presents its own set of challenges. For example, in preplanning, establish whether you are expected to access patients such as this motocross rider (at left), or whether the patient will be brought to you by other event personnel.

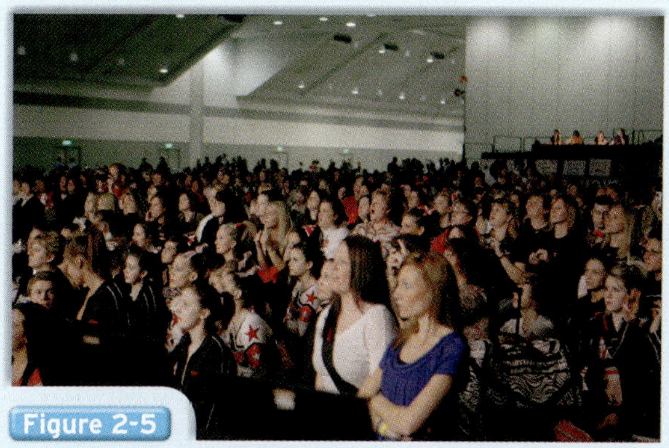

Figure 2-5

Seated groups are less likely to be injured, but they are harder to access.

events. The rule of three is discussed in detail later in this chapter, and means that three SEMS providers should be together at all times, especially if any roving is required. Although roving teams can present problems under any conditions, roving is especially dangerous at night. For all nighttime special events, crews must be equipped with reflective clothing and flashlights. Flashing beacons, such as those used on life jackets, are especially effective at making it easy to spot SEMS providers at night for both safety and response reasons Figure 2-4.

Seated or Mobile Audience

The difference between a seated and mobile audience will have a significant impact on staffing requirements as well as equipment needs. Seated groups are less likely to be injured, but they are harder to access Figure 2-5. Mobile crowds are harder to move through and may require SEMS personnel to be more mobile and require an increase in the number of first aid stations.

For a seated crowd, SEMS personnel must consider the following:

- What are the numbers of seats and rows?
- Will personnel have access to each row?
- Are the aisles wide enough for a stretcher?

For a mobile crowd, personnel must consider the following:

- What is the size of the general area?
- What is the potential number of visitors per area or section?
- Will SEMS personnel have trouble accessing areas around choke points where the crowd will encounter obstructions?
- Will different events attract different types of crowds?

Event Boundaries

A **bound event** is a special event held within set perimeters, like walls, fences, or natural barriers such as lakes or ponds. With a contained area, it is easy to calculate the actual square footage that has to be covered. An **unbound event**, such as a road race, marathon, charity walk, or outdoor festival, may have no, or very few, structured boundaries. Each type of special event presents its own set of challenges with crowd movement, vehicle movement, patient extraction, medical insertion (including medical personnel into the situation), and action strategies Figure 2-6.

Crowd Size

SEMS providers must consider two factors when considering size: the crowd and the venue. To determine the size of the crowds, a reliable news source and previous event data are useful. Crowd size will directly affect SEMS response. Although the size of the venue will affect response, knowing the number of attendees will help SEMS providers determine how to best move around the venue and how to move patients.

Venue Geography and Terrain

In close relation to studying the size of the crowd, SEMS providers should ask the following questions about the physical space and the terrain of the special event:

- What type of facility is it?
- What is the layout of the entire facility?
- Where are the entrance and exit points?
- Is the structure temporary or permanent?
- What is the type of surface:
  - Grass
  - Loose gravel
  - Asphalt
  - Concrete
  - Temporary flooring
- What is the condition of the surface?
- Is the surface even or uneven?
- Are there any fences, walls, or obstacles, either at the event boundaries or within the venue?
- Are there areas that cannot be easily viewed?
- Where is the best vantage point?
- Where are the spectators located?
- How are the spectators contained?

Access/Egress Routes

Another important consideration is the access and egress routes for ambulances during the event. You may need assistance from the venue staff in establishing access routes if the event will be over a large area and/or have a large number of attendees. Sharing the information about these routes with all parties involved is vital to ensure these routes remain open and are not used for parking, display areas, etc. Consider the provision of suitable "sterile" routes for your exclusive use or "rapid-clearing routes" for incoming and outgoing emergency vehicles. These routes are usually used only at very high-profile events, but for any event, an emergency plan with routes in mind is an excellent idea. If a mass-casualty incident occurs, this route will be needed.

A good example of route use is the SEMS coverage of the 2009 presidential inauguration. There was a sterile route on the inner secure perimeter, which meant that no vehicles were allowed to use this route; it was kept clear to allow for quick access/egress of an ambulance should one be needed Figure 2-7. There was also a stationary staging area for the ambulance, so patients could be brought to the ambulance. The routes were known by all parties, and the ambulance always started from the same predetermined point. Paths were well defined and clearly marked. Because not every patient could be brought to the starting point of the sterile route, the other option was to rapidly clear routes. These routes were used when a different ambulance starting point was needed. In this case, when the ambulance would leave a staging area to respond to an emergency, a route would be cleared to exit the venue.

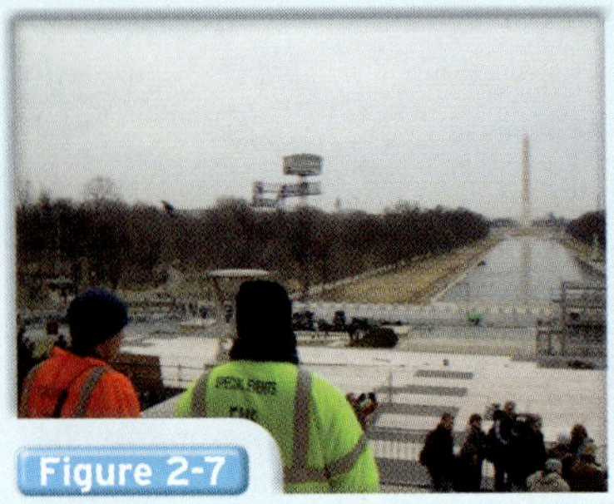

Figure 2-7

Some events may require an inner secure perimeter that remains clear for ambulances and other crucial vehicles.

Maps and Plans

The locations of first aid facilities must be available to all attendees. Provide adequate signage, and clearly mark the location on maps. These maps must be created in the preplanning stage. Consider suggesting to event personnel that they print the location of first aid facilities on the tickets. In addition, all ushers and security staff should be aware of the location of the first aid station and how to contact the medical staff.

Maps are also important for SEMS providers to have before the special event so they can consider the specific layout and its features during preplanning. As always, detailed maps or plans of the site must show the position of medical facilities and should also include the surrounding roads and access routes.

One useful technique may be for the map to include a grid, as shown in Figure 2-8. A grid may be especially useful at a large venue, allowing staff to know details about the venue layout beforehand. Moreover, the grid is useful during the event because it allows SEMS providers and event personnel to quickly identify the area where an incident occurred by naming the corresponding

TIP You may wish to use a laminated plastic sleeve to protect maps and forms from outside elements.

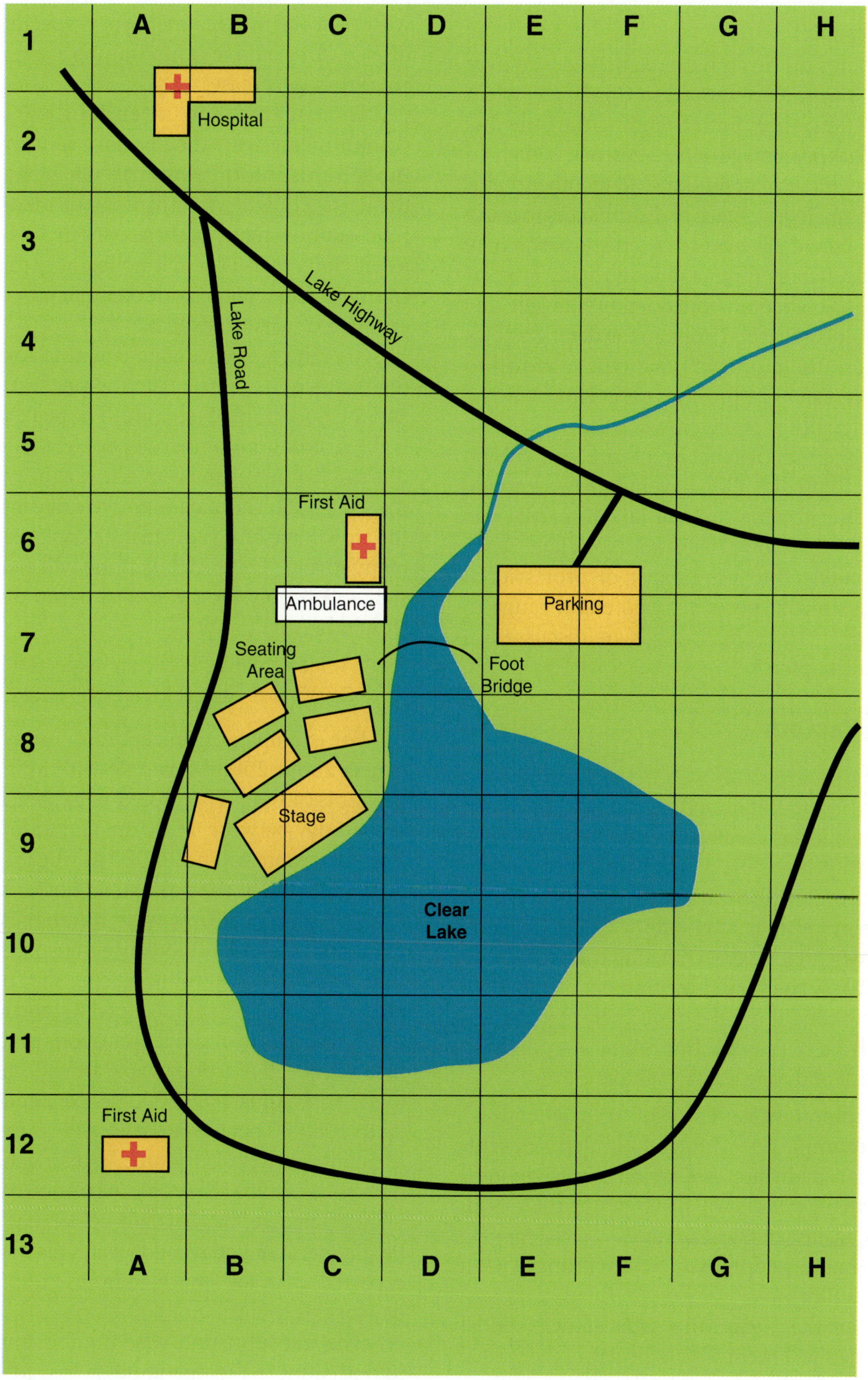

Figure 2-8

A map with a grid overlay can be a useful tool for SEMS providers and event managers.

portion of the grid. Dispatch could communicate, for example, that the incident is in area D10.

Crowd Demographics

The demographics of the crowd take precedence over the size of the event. As discussed in Chapter 1, when analyzing the attendance, understanding the crowd is paramount. What percentage of the audience is likely to have preexisting medical conditions? Remember that it may take only a small percentage of disturbances to cause a problem in a crowd. The cause of a disturbance may be nonmedical, such as trauma among rowdy fans, or medical, such as a diabetic attendee acting strangely due to a low blood glucose level. To obtain the demographics of the crowd, ask the promoter what type of crowd to expect. Again, research the previous events to obtain the potential demographics of the crowd.

The demographics of some events are well known and thus easier to predict. Other events are less known. For example, the growing sport of mixed martial arts seems to be drawing a crowd that is hard to define. SEMS managers are advised to use boxing or professional wrestling, two similar sports, as a potential gauge to help plan for such an event. Crowds are discussed in more detail in Chapter 5.

Subjective Factors

Attendability

Attendability is the likelihood that sick people will attend an event, and it is usually related to the importance of the event to a person's life. For example, people who are ill are usually more likely to attend a graduation than a sporting event. Why is attendability so important? This factor is essential when estimating the probability of injury or illness. The greater the number of attendees with preexisting conditions, the more likely that medical treatment will be necessary. Important attendability questions to ask and to research include:

- How important is this event to the attendees? (For example, is it a once-in-a-lifetime event, such as a graduation or a swearing-in ceremony?)
- How many people will be attending the special event against medical advice?
- How many people will be attending with a serious illness?
- What are the chances that some of the potential attendees will become sick the day of the special event and will not attend the special event?

It is not uncommon for people to leave hospitals after surgery to attend a grandchild's graduation. The attendability for this type of event is high because it is a once-in-a-lifetime event. Also, SEMS providers may cover events where the known attendance and potential patient population is constructed of persons dealing with or receiving treatment for a specific condition or disease (for example, a fundraising event relating to that condition or disease).

To research the attendability of an event, communicate with the special event organizers and, though this information may not be available, ask if there are known participants with medical problems. Find out how many of these participants have attended in previous years. There is no real way to determine the exact numbers, but historic data can provide a very good estimate of what to expect.

After the subjective attendability factor is determined, the next step is to calculate the **peak attendance rate** and the **maximum cycle rate**. The peak attendance rate is the maximum number of people attending in a span of a single hour of an event—ie, the peak of attendance Figure 2-9. The maximum cycle rate is the turnover of the crowd, meaning how many people leave versus how many arrive. These calculations will help to properly staff and supply for the special event. SEMS providers should be sure to ask:

1. How many people are expected in total?
2. What is the cycle rate per hour?

For example, organizers for a 3-day special event expect about 250,000 people with an average hourly cycle of 15,000. The crowd is expected to peak the second day between 11:00 am and 4:00 pm. The peak attendance rate will be 25,000 during this time. Always plan and staff for the peak attendance rate.

The **transport unit-wise number** is the expected number of potential ambulance transports for the event. This number is determined using the total number of people, the expected number of days, and the assumption that on average, there are 1.5 transports per 50,000 people. For example, if 250,000 people are expected over 3 days, this is approximately 83,000 people per day. Round this up to 100,000 people per day for the purposes of simple and conservative calculations. Assuming that there are 1.5 transports per 50,000 people, when you calculate that for 100,000 people, there would be 3 expected transports. Finally, because you should always plan for more than is expected, plan for anywhere from 3 to 6 transports per day for this event.

The transport unit-wise number should also take into account the temperature, access to water sources, comfort provisions, age of the attendees, and the health of the attendees because these factors can increase the expected number of emergencies and transports.

If event calculations suggest 1.5 transports per 50,000 people, but the event involves an older crowd

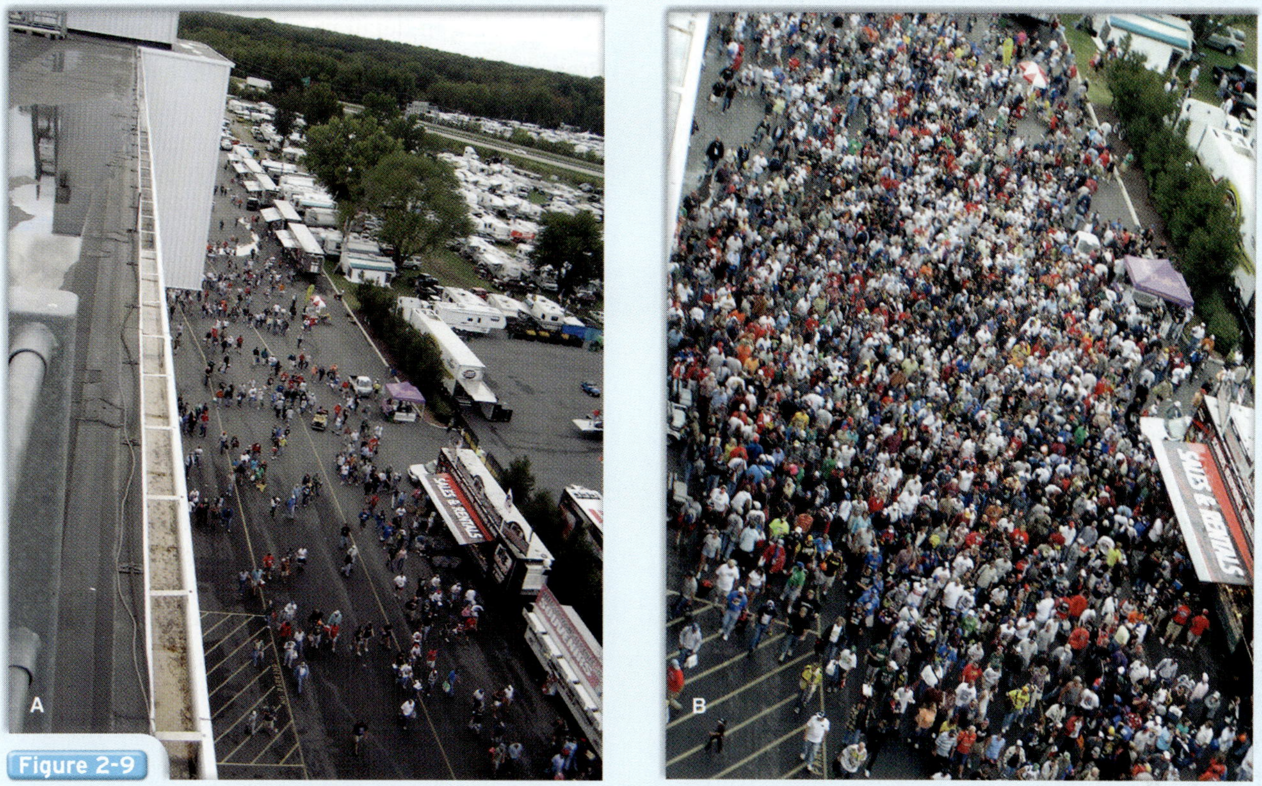

Figure 2-9

Attendance can fluctuate significantly during an event, as pictured here at the main walkway of a NASCAR event. **A.** Taken the morning of the event. **B.** Taken in the late afternoon.

and the consumption of alcohol, as a rule, estimates should be increased to 2.5 per 50,000. Hospital distance must also be considered. If the hospital is more than 30 to 45 minutes from the event, a single ambulance will be gone for over 2 hours; this time needs to be factored into the calculations.

The following are general steps for calculating daily expected transports:

1. Using all available research, determine the total number of people estimated to attend over the total number of days (for example, 50,000 people over 3 days).
2. Estimate the total number of transports (for example, 1.5 transports per 50,000 people).
3. Consider the weather. Adjust the number of transports up or down for weather warmer than 90°F or colder than 32°F. Transports should increase by 10% to 15% if the temperature is in either of these ranges (for example, 15% of 1.5 transports equals 0.225. This added to the initial 1.5 totals 1.725 transports, which should be rounded to 2, meaning that 2 transports are expected). As a general rule, if there are factors that will increase the number of emergencies, assume 2.5 transports per 50,000 people.
4. Consider the availability of water. If a water source is present, anticipate a 30% decrease in medical emergencies.
5. Consider the availability of shelter. If shelter is available for participants and attendees to rest, cool off, and rehydrate, anticipate an additional 30% decrease in medical emergencies.
6. Consider the age of the attendees. If the majority of attendees are expected to be older than 60 years or within the age range of 13 to 24 years, expect an increase in medical emergencies by 30%. (Older attendees are more susceptible to environmental factors, whereas young people have a higher likelihood of engaging in risky behavior that could lead to trauma.)
7. Consider the health of the attendees. If the majority of attendees are expected to have existing health conditions, expect an increase in medical emergencies by 30%.
8. Consider the distance to the nearest hospital. If the hospital is more than 45 minutes away or if a complete turnaround (transport to the hospital and return to the event) will average more than 2 hours, consider adding additional units.

9. To calculate the expected number of attendees per day, divide total number of expected attendance by the number of days (or duration of the event). For example, 50,000 people divided by 3 days equals 16,666 people per day.
10. Finally, calculate the expected number of transports per day, assuming that as a rule, there are 1.5 transports per 50,000 people. For example, if 1.5 transports are expected per 50,000 people over 3 days, then 0.5 transport would be expected per 16,666 people in one day. Round up to 1 transport because you cannot transport 0.5 people! Remember, you will need to increase the expected number of transports to take into account the factors described above.

Gut Instinct

Gut instinct is hard to define and place into subjective or objective terms. It is best defined as an "inner voice" that speaks up when something seems wrong or slightly out of place. EMS training teaches providers to pay attention to signals that are not directly or consciously recognizable. In reaching for a door handle, if an inner voice suggests that there may be trouble on the other side, providers are taught to listen and plan accordingly.

The same concept applies to SEMS. If a SEMS manager senses that a particular event will attract violence, such as in the form of rival gangs, it is imperative to listen to that inner feeling and be prepared for the most extreme possibility. SEMS providers should pay attention to gut instinct.

Crowd Mentality

Despite best efforts, judging the crowd's mentality drifts into the realm of subjective factors. Similar to listening to gut instinct, gauging the overall mentality of the crowd can facilitate planning. Crowd mentality can differ dramatically from one event to another and can change during the course of an event. A football game, for example, will present significantly different challenges than a heavy metal concert. Also, by looking at previous NASCAR events, the SEMS manager can surmise that alcohol will be present and play a role in the overall mentality of the crowd. By considering the fights that broke out at the last event, which may or may not have been related to alcohol consumption, the manager should prepare for similar occurrences and resulting patient loads.

Likewise, when covering a sporting event, providers should find out through Internet and news research if the teams and their fans are engaged in an extreme rivalry. Heated exchanges between teams or fans can lead to fights both on and off the playing field. Crowds are discussed in detail in Chapter 5.

Previous Experience and Intelligence Reports

Experiences from previous events are integral to the research process. At larger events, specific intelligence gathering is a must. While the SEMS manager may do the bulk of the research, it is wise for SEMS providers to do their own research and ensure that they are informed in advance. When gathering these experiences from personal memories and the files recorded by the service, providers should consult other services that have covered the same or similar events elsewhere. Of course, when talking with individual providers and consulting databases, the perceptions of others may be biased and are subjective.

For more factual or objective information, as listed previously, providers should research news articles at the local library or on the Internet. These sources will likely provide a less biased account of the event. They can also establish patterns of past significant incidents for an event.

A preplanning checklist should be filled out, identifying all objective and subjective factors. This document can serve as a useful guide throughout the preplanning process and during the event. A master checklist is shown in Figure 2-10. Some of the items in this list, such as communications and weather, will be covered in more detail in later chapters.

Step Two: Theoretical Walk-through

After completing the research stage, SEMS managers and staff must perform a mental or theoretical walk-through of the entire event. The purpose of this procedure is to locate any components of preparation that may have been overlooked thus far.

Roles and Responsibilities

It is important to define roles and responsibilities for every event. The SEMS manager should ask the special event organizers what they expect the role of SEMS to be at the event. After they share their expectations, the manager can explain to them what can reasonably be provided.

During the past decade, the American viewing public has been bombarded with portrayals of EMS services. Some are flattering and others are not. The result is a population with a distorted view of what

Part I: BASIC INFORMATION

1. Estimated attendance
   - ❑ Fewer than 5,000
   - ❑ 5,001-10,000
   - ❑ 10,001-25,000
   - ❑ 25,001 or more
2. Type of event (check all that apply)
   - ❑ Outdoor
   - ❑ Indoor
   - ❑ Concert
   - ❑ Festival
   - ❑ Stadium
   - ❑ Sport
   - ❑ Extreme sport
   - ❑ Combat sport
   - ❑ Equestrian
   - ❑ Rodeo
   - ❑ Event involving water
   - ❑ Political
   - ❑ Other: ______________________
3. Nature of event
   - ❑ High profile
   - ❑ Potentially violent
   - ❑ High likelihood of drug/alcohol use
   - ❑ Event of national significance
   - ❑ Other: ______________________
4. Location(s) of event

   Name of facility: ______________________

   Address: ______________________

   City: ____________ State: ______ Zip: ______
5. Organizational information

   Name of organization: ______________________

   Address: ______________________

   City: ____________ State: ______ Zip: ______

   Contact person: ______________________

   Telephone:

   Work: ______________________

   Cell: ______________________

   Other: ______________________

   E-mail address: ______________________

Part II: RESOURCE NEEDS

6. Resources needed

	Type	Number
Personnel	❑ First responder	❑ ____
	❑ BLS	❑ ____
	❑ ALS	❑ ____
	❑ Registered nurse	❑ ____
	❑ Physician	❑ ____
	❑ Other: ______________	❑ ____
Vehicles	❑ Carts	❑ ____
	❑ Other: ______________	❑ ____
Medical Equipment	❑ Gloves	❑ ____
	❑ AED	❑ ____
	❑ Stretcher	❑ ____
	❑ Other: ______________	❑ ____
	❑ Other: ______________	❑ ____
First Aid Stations	❑ On-site	❑ ____
	❑ Tent	❑ ____
	❑ Other: ______________	❑ ____

Figure 2-10

Preplanning form.

(continues)

7. Description of on-site first aid facilities

____

____

____

____

8. Copies of maps and schematics of facility and any other special areas (list areas here and check off once maps have been obtained and distributed to all personnel)
   - ❑ Facility
   - ❑ Parking areas
   - ❑ Access/egress routes
   - ❑ Surrounding streets
   - ❑ Other: ________________________________

9. Description of patient transfer protocols and agreements that will be used

____

____

____

____

10. Communication needs and capabilities (indicate which type of communications matrix will be used and which channel each party will use)

____

____

____

____

Part III: RESEARCH AND ACTIONS TAKEN

11. Measures that have been or will be taken to coordinate SEMS for the event with local EMS and public safety agencies, such as ambulance, police, fire, rescue, and hospital agencies or organizations (if not yet taken, state actions to be taken and target dates for these to be accomplished)

    Action: ________________________________

    Target date: ____________

    Action: ________________________________

    Target date: ____________

    Action: ________________________________

    Target date: ____________

12. Security concerns and plans for addressing these:

____

____

____

____

Figure 2-10

Preplanning form.

13. Weather history (consult 2-3 sources and list results here)

Source: ______________________________

Information: ______________________________

Source: ______________________________

Information: ______________________________

Source: ______________________________

Information: ______________________________

14. Possible inclement weather

- ❑ Rain
- ❑ Snow
- ❑ Lightning
- ❑ Tornado
- ❑ Hurricane
- ❑ Other: ______________________________

Preplanning measures taken:

Action: ______________________________

Target date: ______________

15. Surface considerations

Type of surface:

- ❑ Grass
- ❑ Loose gravel
- ❑ Dirt
- ❑ Asphalt
- ❑ Concrete
- ❑ Temporary flooring
- ❑ Other: ______________________________

Condition of surface:

- ❑ Smooth
- ❑ Rough
- ❑ Slippery
- ❑ Other: ______________________________

Levelness:

- ❑ Even
- ❑ Uneven

Preplanning measures taken:

Action: ______________________________

Target date: ______________

16. Credentialing process

Describe the event's credentialing process:

____

____

Do SEMS providers need to bring a photo ID to be used for creating a badge?

- ❑ Yes
- ❑ No

Figure 2-10

Preplanning form.

(continues)

17. Security clearance

Will security clearance be needed?

❑ Yes

❑ No

If so, how far in advance of the event is it needed?

____

Preplanning measures taken:

Action: ______________________________

Target date: ______________

Part IV: SPECIAL CONSIDERATIONS

18. Special concerns and considerations (describe what you know about the following factors)

Communication:

____

____

Attendees:

____

____

Demographics:

____

____

Where are the spectators located?

____

____

How are the spectators contained?

____

____

Access/egress:

____

____

Are there areas that cannot be easily viewed?

____

____

Where is the best vantage point?

____

____

Treatment issues:

____

____

Transportation:

____

____

Other considerations:

____

____

Figure 2-10

Preplanning form.

real EMS can realistically do. The public is likely to gauge every action and reaction using the television programs as distorted yardsticks. In a time of crisis, these views can become a hindrance if the crowd decides that EMS personnel are not behaving like the "doctors on TV." In the special events arena, every move is scrutinized. This is one reason why it is essential to establish beforehand with the special event organizers what is realistic regarding equipment, distances, and the terrain being covered. The SEMS manager must be honest about what could happen and what it will look like if something catastrophic happens. It is imperative for a successful emergency response to establish a dialogue as early as possible and for the discussion to be on realistic terms. If multiple agencies are involved, it will also be important to preplan the roles and responsibilities of each agency.

At some events, especially with attendance lower than 5,000, SEMS providers may be volunteers who have a dual role. Nonmedical tasks that would fall to such providers include keeping aisles clear and providing proactive seating assistance. Also, at the event it is a good idea to note the location of handicapped, elderly, or unstable attendees and perform periodic checks of these areas at intermissions and the end of the performance.

Staffing

Even the most seasoned EMS provider may have questions about how many SEMS providers are needed for a special event. This number will vary depending on the event, but Table 2-1 lists five general categories that could be used to gauge the needs of a particular special event. Note that an event will probably not fit exactly into any one category, and these are general guidelines. SEMS providers will need to consider a multitude of factors unique to the event and plan for them.

An event that generally fits into category 1 would need relatively minimal staffing and equipment, while an event in category 5 would need extensive resources. The higher the category number, the more emergencies the SEMS provider should expect.

The number of SEMS providers and first aid stations will vary depending on the type of event. Table 2-2 is a general guideline for determining the number of SEMS providers and first aid stations to have at a special event. As shown in the table, one first aid station will usually suffice if event attendance is fewer than 5,000 people, but if there are 25,000 people or more in attendance, more first aid stations will be needed. As mentioned, the number of SEMS providers and first aid stations will need to be adjusted to take into account special characteristics of the event that could result in more injuries and emergencies.

The certification level required of the SEMS staff will depend on the types of emergencies expected at the event (and whether they will require ALS care), as well as state and local protocols. An event may require only BLS providers, or a combination of BLS and ALS providers. The definition of an ALS response varies from state to state; in some states, an ALS response may be defined as having one paramedic present in a group of BLS providers, whereas in other states an ALS response may be defined as having one ALS provider for every BLS provider. In general, events with more than 30,000 attendees may require ALS capabilities.

When planning the number of SEMS providers for an event, consider the **rule of three** Figure 2-11, which states that three SEMS providers should respond to and handle each emergency at an event. This helps ensure provider safety but also provides needed manpower. With this model, two providers directly handle patient assessment and management, and the third provider is responsible for the following:

- Ensuring provider safety and requesting security backup if needed
- Retrieving needed equipment
- Activating needed medical resources, such as requesting an ambulance for transport
- If applicable, alerting the command center of the exact location, nature, and needs of an incident
- Controlling crowd incursion into the situation
- Addressing bystanders' questions
- Meeting and directing incoming transport units/personnel to the scene
- When applicable, locking and unlocking areas as needed to provide emergency care. Note that if this situation applies to your event, the third SEMS provider should have keys and combinations for locks that may need to be opened to provide emergency care.

While preplanning the event, it will be necessary to specify who can assess and treat patients, as well as make decisions should any disputes arise regarding patient care, transport, and refusal of care. This may vary depending on the established protocols in your area and the number and type of providers covering the event.

TABLE 2-1 Categories for Assessing Special Event Needs

Category	Attendance	Activity Level	Attendabilty	Weather	Other
1	Low	Low	Low	Fall/spring	One of the following: ❑ History of event suggests many emergencies ❑ Drug/alcohol use expected ❑ Outdoor event ❑ Extreme or combat sports ❑ Other
2	Low/medium	Medium	Medium	Fall/spring	Two of the following: ❑ History of event suggests many emergencies ❑ Drug/alcohol use expected ❑ Outdoor event ❑ Extreme or combat sports ❑ Other
3	Medium/high	Medium/ high	Medium	Summer/winter	Three of the following: ❑ History of event suggests many emergencies ❑ Drug/alcohol use expected ❑ Outdoor event ❑ Extreme or combat sports ❑ Other
4	High	High	High	Summer/winter	Four of the following: ❑ History of event suggests many emergencies ❑ Drug/alcohol use expected ❑ Outdoor event ❑ Extreme or combat sports ❑ Other
5	Mega-event	Varies	Varies	Summer/winter	All of the following: ❑ History of event suggests many emergencies ❑ Drug/alcohol use expected ❑ Outdoor event ❑ Extreme or combat sports ❑ Other

The larger the event and the more providers, the more important it becomes to ensure that everyone is assigned a specific role and understands that role.

Overall provision of medical, ambulance, and first aid resources should be based on all activities taking place within the venue. At special events attended by a very young audience or at street carnivals, the number of SEMS providers may need to be significantly increased, or the ratio of SEMS providers to transport personnel, nurses, and physicians may need to be altered.

Guidelines for determining the number of ambulances needed at an event are discussed in Chapter 8 because these most often apply at stadium and mega-events.

Staff Comfort Considerations

EMS personnel work in all weather conditions, and a special event is no exception. The SEMS manager must be mindful of the type of responses needed for each event. The manager must ensure that all personnel have the clothing and equipment needed to function in adverse weather conditions. Suggested equipment includes:

- Knit cap
- Extra socks
- Extra gloves
- Rain gear
- Sunglasses

TABLE 2-2 Guidelines for Determining the Number of SEMS Providers and First Aid Stations*

Number of Attendees	Number of SEMS Providers	Numbers of First Aid Stations
Fewer than 5,000	1-2	1
5,001-10,000	2-3	1
10,001-25,000	2-4	1-2
More than 25,000	≥ 4	≥ 2

*Note that these numbers can widely vary based on factors other than attendance, such as demographics and geography. Adjust these numbers as needed to take all event factors into account.

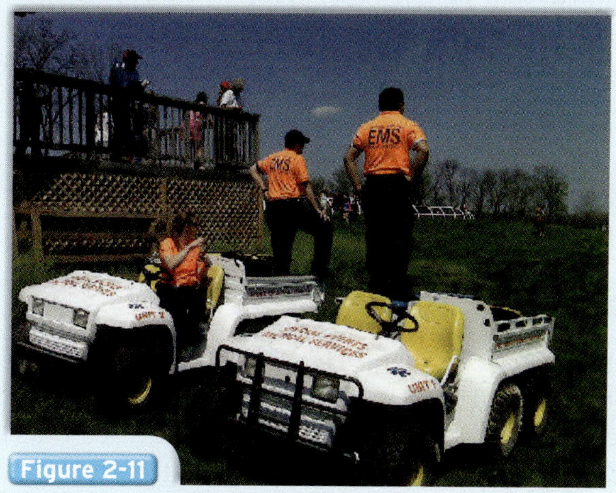

Figure 2-11

Consider using the rule of three when planning staffing for an event.

- Sunscreen
- Baseball hat
- Wide-brimmed hat
- Water bottle
- Change of clothes

With extreme temperatures, the manager must give SEMS personnel a rotation schedule and create cooling and warming stations when appropriate. During cold weather, each provider should have an aid kit, emergency blanket, and appropriate heat packs. For extreme heat, the manager should provide cooling stations, misting tents, ice, and cold packs, not only for participants, but also for providers.

In hot weather, patient loads increase, but personnel are also subjected to the same environmental conditions as the participants of the event. The SEMS manager should consider issuing a summer uniform made of light-colored and lightweight material. There are specially designed materials that fit these requirements.

Water has to be readily available and SEMS personnel should be regularly encouraged to drink water. As a general rule, providers should be consuming enough fluids to urinate once every hour. Of course, this is only a general guideline and varies from person to person. If SEMS providers cannot be stationed in a cool, air-conditioned environment, the manager should rotate staff frequently from a hot environment to a more comfortable environment, and the frequency of the rotation should increase with the increase in temperature Table 2-3. Be sure to allow for down time with rotation schedules.

In large special events that are sustained for more than several hours, one provider should be assigned the job of monitoring personnel for heat-related illnesses. This provider should be familiar with the signs and symptoms of heat-related illnesses, such as slurred speech, confusion, lack of sweating, and an unsteady gait; these findings precede seizures, coma, and even death. He or she should be given the authority to remove and treat staff as warranted. If the special event does not have a comfort area—and many will not—the manager should consider supplying one or designate the back of an ambulance as a cooling comfort station.

TABLE 2-3 Provider Rotation Schedule Based on Temperature

Temperature (°F)	Rotation Schedule
Below 75	No rotation is required.
75-80	Monitor staff and rotate when needed.
81-85	Rotate staff every 2.5 to 3 hours. Monitor staff for heat effects.
86-90	Rotate staff every 1.5 to 2 hours. Monitor staff for heat effects.
91-95	Rotate staff every 45 minutes to 1 hour. Monitor staff for heat effects.
96-100	Rotate staff every 45 minutes. Double the available staff. Monitor all staff for heat effects.
Over 100	No one works for longer than 45 minutes a day. Double the available staff. Monitor all staff for heat effects.

The cold weather will decrease the staff's ability to work outside. Many of the same rules for hot weather apply to cold weather operations. The manager should rotate and warm personnel frequently, and he or she should ensure that all personnel are dressed for the weather.

Step Three: Identifying and Communicating Specific Needs

Once the SEMS manager has preplanned each step, mentally reviewed the entire event, and checked all mathematical figures, it is time to alert each outside vendor and the assisting services of the items that will be required to ensure the success of the event. These parties include the local emergency room, the venue's security services, the local police department, the fire marshal, and other applicable agencies. Personnel should dictate the time and efforts spent on this contact by gauging the size of the event and the depth of coverage. For a 2-hour, 5-kilometer footrace or a 3-day music event requiring no substantial outside assistance, a phone conversation may suffice, but it is always best to schedule a face-to-face meeting. For more in-depth or complex responses, such as for a presidential inauguration, NASCAR event, or papal visit, a face-to-face preplanning meeting is required with all relevant parties.

The SEMS manager must secure receipts and signed contracts! This crucial step is often overlooked but is vitally important and should be done in a timely manner. These contracts should contain the budgets, necessary resources, expectations, and requirements from all involved parties, but most importantly between the covering service and event planners. There is nothing worse than, in the middle of an event, discovering that both parties assumed the other was providing a vital resource. Contracts and agreements help ensure that no details fall through the cracks, no matter how small they may seem during the planning stages.

Event Credentialing and Security Clearance

Some event venues will have a credentialing procedure for staff who will be working at the event. This process varies for each event, depending on the event organizers. Establish the process with event organizers prior to the event. For example, SEMS providers may need to report to the event office, sign in, obtain a badge (possibly with a photo that they must bring with them), and obtain a wristband or other type of identification.

At certain events, including events of national significance, some or all event staff including SEMS

You Are the SEMS Provider

CASE 2

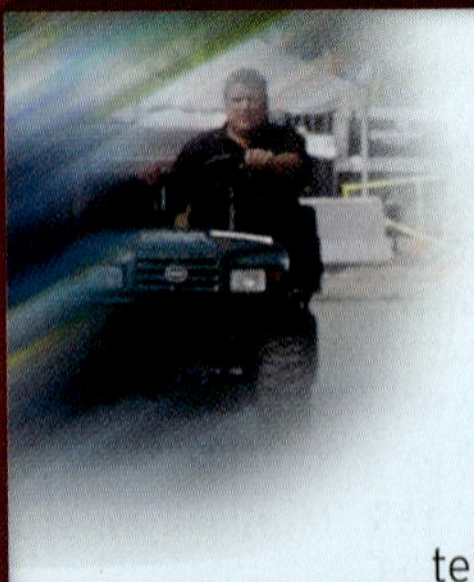

You are covering a bike jam, which is a 1-day professional bike race. The venue is a 1-mile track with 12 heats (or races) and 3 professional heats. In your preplanning meeting, you and your team carefully show the organizer on the map where to put your aid station and where to park the ambulance. You leave the meeting in good spirits and are confident that this event will be successfully covered.

On the day before the event, during your second-to-last scheduled walk-through, you discover that your first aid tent has been moved to a fenced area inside the course. Unfortunately, someone within the racing organization overrode your placement, but the new tent and ambulance location has only one egress route. To make matters worse, you discover that this egress route involves maneuvering through throngs of people to get to an exit.

1. How do you address this reversal of your directions for where to place the first aid station and ambulance?
2. What can you do to ensure that this problem does not occur again at this event as well as at future events?

providers and ambulance crews may need to obtain security clearance. Prescreening may begin as early as 6 months before the event. Before the event, find out what measures will be taken, and take all of the necessary steps to ensure that you and other SEMS staff are cleared for working at the event. Once at the event, staff may need to undergo further screening. Security personnel may take additional measures such as searching equipment bags and ambulances. Consider how this will affect your coverage. For example, SEMS providers may need to arrive early to allow time for obtaining security clearance.

Equipment

Prior to Game Day, equipment needs must be planned. In addition to determining the type of equipment that will be needed, it is also important to determine whether SEMS providers will be expected to provide emergency response for spectators, event performers, or both. If SEMS providers will cover all event emergencies, they must determine whether a dedicated cart and ambulance are needed for event performers.

All necessary emergency equipment should be at the site by Game Day and should be quickly accessible. The equipment needs must be communicated to all involved parties, which should include the rental companies for any equipment the service does not own, such as transport carts, first aid station trailers, radios, tents, caterers, and ice. Needs must also be communicated if pick-up and delivery of equipment has to be done by an outside service. Likewise, a backup system that addresses immediate repair or replacement of equipment needs to be established, just in case any item breaks down. This system is especially crucial for events that span multiple days.

Personnel should be familiar with the function and operation of each type of emergency equipment, whether it is owned by the service or rented from outside vendors. Service-owned equipment should be in good operating condition, and personnel must be trained in advance to use it properly. Emergency equipment should be checked on a regular basis, and emergency personnel should rehearse with the equipment as well. The emergency equipment available should be appropriate for the level of training for the emergency medical providers. In addition, it is important to know the proper way to care for and store the equipment. Equipment should be stored in a clean and environmentally controlled area. See Chapter 3 for more information on equipment.

TIP

Communication with each agency is imperative. Remember to communicate with all parties involved—responding agencies, the event coordinator, the event supervisors, the system supervisors, and anyone else who may have dealings with the event.

Communications

It is necessary to preplan how staff and security will contact SEMS providers. At large events, a separate medical radio channel may be needed to allow ambulance services to communicate with medical personnel and security personnel. Small special events may only need one radio channel, but larger special events may need a more complex communication matrix. A communications plan should be created, detailing medical communications links (ie, which channels medical personnel should use for communication). This communications plan should then be posted at the first aid station and the incident command post. A phone list should include all necessary numbers, such as the local emergency department, local EMS command post, and cell phone numbers for all event staff. These items need to be addressed in the preplanning stage. Communications are discussed in detail in Chapter 4.

Documentation

During the special event, a **special event log**, which is a record of the patient interactions that occur at a particular event, should be maintained and should include any actions or decisions taken by the manager of the medical provisions and the reasons for those actions Figure 2-12. Special event logs, report forms, and records completed at a special event may be required at a later date to assist in the reporting of incidents and injuries. Be sure to bring an appropriate log form to the event, and ensure that you have enough copies for all SEMS providers. Also note whether there are any specific forms required by your state. Finally, it is a good idea for

Patient name: ______________________________

Time: ______________________________

Complaint: ______________________________

SEMS action:

- ❑ Transported
- ❑ Provided treatment and released

Treatment provided:

- ❑ Ice
- ❑ Band-aid
- ❑ Other: ______________________________

Event grid location (for statistical purposes, denote the map grid area where the emergency occurred): ______________________________

Figure 2-12

A sample special event log.

the SEMS manager to discuss HIPAA regulations with SEMS providers to refresh their knowledge of how these may affect documentation of emergencies at the event.

Preplanning for a Major Incident

During your preplanning stage, list possible emergency threats to the facility, such as a ride collapse at a local fair, a threat of violence from a gang, or a terrorist threat because of a visiting dignitary. Train your providers to identify these threats, and teach them how to respond. The decision for planning should be guided by the Homeland Security mantra of "high risk, high probability," which means that you should plan for any emergency that is likely to happen and has the potential to cause either severe injuries or a large number of casualties. For example, a sudden thunderstorm with lightning should be included in this list for a summer outdoor event (high risk, high probability), but bleacher sabotage (an act of terrorism affecting the bleacher mechanism) is rather unlikely (high risk, low probability) and need not be included in the preplanning list. Having said that, SEMS personnel can never be overprepared for an emergency, no matter the probability of the event occurring. An all-hazards approach, which considers assets (eg, staging patient care supplies, extra personnel, and vehicles), should be part of any preplanning effort.

Incidents that could involve a multiple-agency or multiple-jurisdiction response will need a **unified command system**. In this case, plans must be drawn up in advance by all cooperating agencies that assume a shared responsibility for decision making and cooperation. The response plan should designate the lead and support agencies in several kinds of MCIs. Agencies bordering each other should practice often with each other to ensure that a unified command system will function well and that communication among the people involved is well established before a real incident occurs.

Evacuation Planning

Evacuation plans are imperative and are an important part of any preplanning effort. **Evacuation plans** are created for safety in the event of an emergency. It is essential to have a clearly documented evacuation plan and outline to implement the plan in a timely manner (safety and security procedures should be direct and easy to follow during an emergency). These plans must consider all aspects of the facility, such as the structural design, the number of entrances and exits, spatial limitations, and location. Who creates these plans depends on the event—the venue may already have an evacuation plan in place, or SEMS providers may work with a committee to create an evacuation plan for a specific event.

SEMS providers should be assigned to particular duties during a crisis situation. However, in case a certain individual is not present during the event, an alternate person should be trained and ready to respond in that role. It may be useful to appoint an emergency control officer to designate who is in charge of procedures during an emergency to alleviate stress for all people involved in deciding when and how to use an evacuation plan.

Likewise, when preplanning for a catastrophic incident, you can use the National Incident Management System (NIMS) incident command system (ICS) structure to ensure that all public safety organizations that may be involved in managing such an incident are coordinated with each other. The ICS structure will provide you with the roles that will need to be filled without having to designate a person's actual name until the catastrophic incident occurs. This way you can insert people trained in certain areas and utilize their skills and abilities to help mitigate a catastrophic incident successfully.

In addition to ensuring that staff are familiar with an emergency or evacuation plan, you must communicate the plan to the spectators; after all, they are the ones that you need to evacuate or keep safe. Consider how people will be informed of an emergency (eg, radio, telephone, sirens) and how SEMS providers and staff will know that the catastrophic incident plan has been enacted. These procedures must be thoroughly understood and practiced through repetitive training and spontaneous drills.

You must also know how SEMS providers are to communicate in the event of a major incident. For example, if you are engaged in an event that is using a single-channel radio and an emergency occurs, how would you clear the radio air to transmit your evacuation plan? By using training and preplanning drills, the SEMS coordinator should go over how this situation would be handled. One approach is to break in with the word "urgent." Upon hearing this key word, all personnel would be trained to stop all other radio traffic until the situation is resolved; thus, the radio would be cleared and those communicating about the urgent event would be able to do so uninterrupted.

Evaluating the plan and design will identify any flaws. Examine the techniques and procedures, and try to solve any possible conflicts that could arise. In addition, ensure that the evacuation plan is approved by the fire marshal, and aim to create a liaison with fire fighters, police officers, and other personnel you may be working with at a catastrophic incident.

TIP

During preplanning, ensure that you establish subdivision names for large, unmarked parking lots. This will help quickly find a patient in the parking lot should an emergency occur there. Work with event management to ensure that signs are posted with the lot's naming/numbering system.

Step Four: Physical Walk-through

Planning the Walk-through

To complete the physical walk-through, SEMS managers must arrange with the venue manager for the SEMS team to evaluate the physical space of the event. For most events, multiple walk-throughs should be performed in collaboration with the promoter as well as by the agency on its own.

The parameters of the physical walk-through will depend upon the size and complexity of the event. For a simple event that will last only a few hours, the SEMS team will most likely decide to perform the walk-through upon arriving at the location on Game Day. However, only for very small events should the SEMS personnel perform the walk-through on the day of the event; for longer and more extreme events, it is best to perform several walk-throughs. As other components of the event set up, such as vendors or performers, the landscape of the event will change. If SEMS personnel perform a walk-through 3 months prior to a large festival, for example, and then do not return until Game Day, they may find that the region that had been reserved for the first aid tent now contains an amusement park ride, large waste receptacles, or other equipment that cannot be moved. Thus, it is always best to evaluate an event several times when planning the walk-through process.

For example, when SEMS personnel were assigned to cover the Virgin Festival 2007 at the Pimlico race course, they performed their first walk-through at the 3-month mark to gain a feel for the size and scope of the infield of the Pimlico race course. They walked through again at 6 weeks prior to the event at the preplanning meeting. Throughout the following weeks, SEMS personnel walked through numerous times as they set up to note changes to egress routes, stage locations, vendor placement, and comfort stations. Forty-eight hours prior to Game Day, they had all staff perform a final walk-through to familiarize themselves with the layout.

Walk-through Personnel

Although the SEMS manager provides a vital role in planning the walk-through, it is essential that each member of the staff engage in as many of the walk-throughs as possible. Although the manager will supervise the event, the SEMS personnel must be knowledgeable about every aspect of the venue because they will likely be called upon to use this information during the emergencies that occur during the event.

During the Walk-through

For some large events, a site map will be provided to the SEMS team **Figure 2-13**. If this tool is available, it is a great starting point, and SEMS personnel should cover the entire grounds while familiarizing themselves with the land and where features are in relation to the map.

This luxury is not usually available for events. Even in the absence of this helpful tool, it is essential that SEMS personnel comb every inch of the venue, and even create their own map if possible.

When a venue is evaluated, additional tools include knowledge gained by previous experience, gut instinct, and common sense. Personnel should look for the following and label them on a map (if available):

- Choke points
- Any potential hazards (such as sharp corners, steep drops, areas with low visibility)
- First aid tent placement
- Access (egress and ingress routes)
- Entrances and exits

During this juncture, try to anticipate factors that may come into play during preplanning and Game Day. Such factors could include an egress route that becomes blocked by a vendor's tent or a locked gate. If it seems that any complications have the slightest chance of occurring, the SEMS team must have a backup plan in place, such as a secondary egress route and extra staff.

Tips for Best Results

Again, when performing the walk-through, examine every part of the venue. SEMS personnel should look at the site through the eyes of a sick or confused patron.

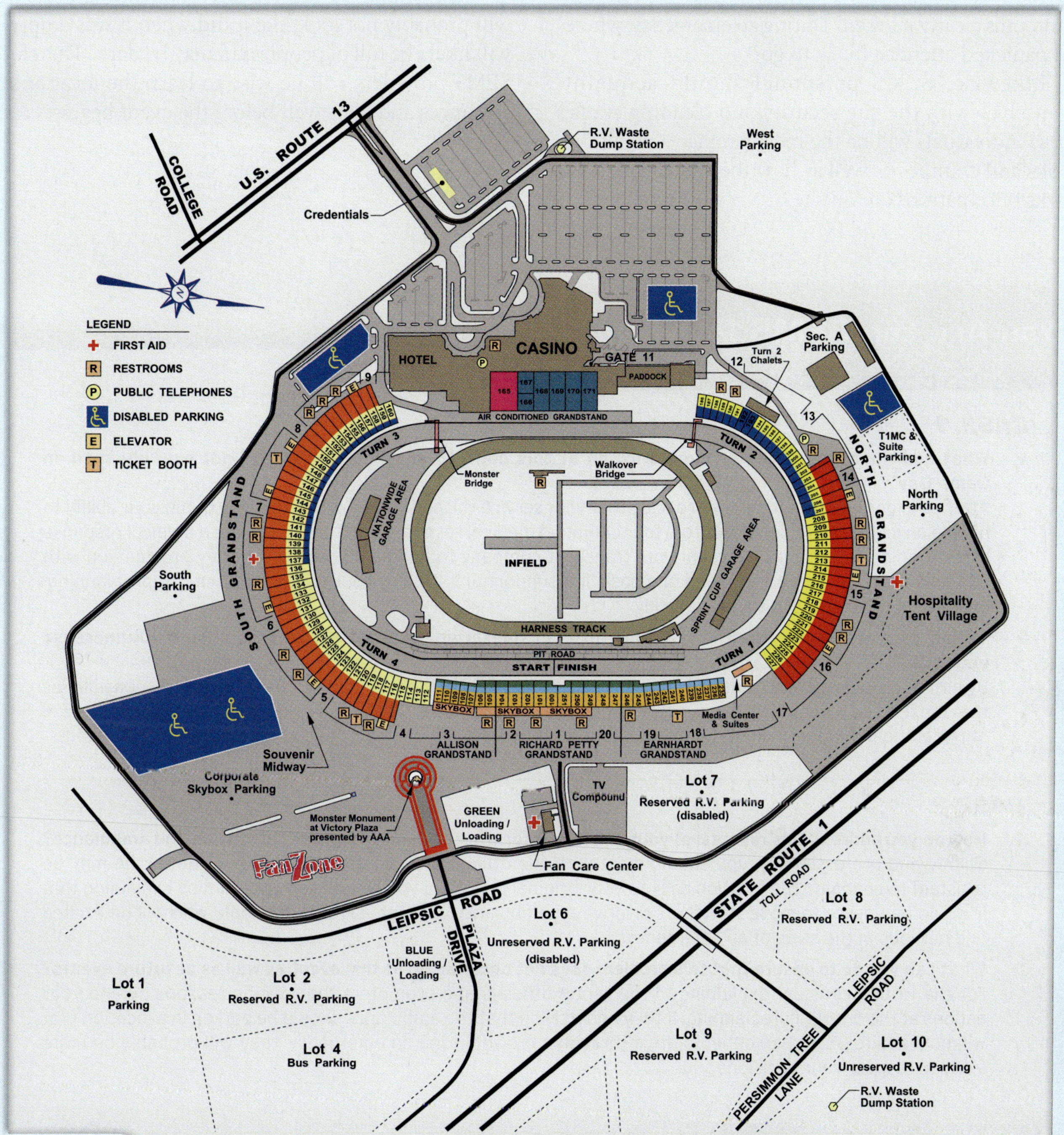

Figure 2-13

For some large events, a site map will be provided to the SEMS team.

Are the exits obvious to a person in distress? Are the bathrooms clearly marked? During an emergency, where is a panicked attendee likely to go?

Likewise, SEMS personnel should acquaint themselves with the site security and cleaning staffs. These individuals will be the most familiar with all the nooks and crannies as well as how the venue generally works once patrons are on site.

Remember, during the last walk-through the area will probably not look like it did when it was empty. It will likely be full of people and may be dark. Therefore, SEMS providers will be wise to learn the locations of entrances and exits well before the event begins.

You Are the SEMS Provider

SUMMARY

CASE 1

1. **What additional resources can you draw on at this point to ensure that you are not overwhelmed on Game Day?**
   After considering the numbers, you decide that your service will add enough resources to expand your ability to handle an increased patient load from four equipped medical response carts to six equipped medical response carts. You locate and hire a local private transport company to handle all transports; they provide you with one advanced life support unit and one basic life support unit. Due to your scalable system for preplanning, everything is executed easily and quickly.
2. **Taking your answer to the first question into consideration, by what percentage should you increase your staff?**
   By hiring the local private transport company, you have already compensated for the transport responsibilities that the fire department would have provided. Since you estimated that they would ultimately also handle 15% of patient load responsibilities, increasing your staff by 20% should more than compensate for staff needs.

CASE 2

1. **How do you address this reversal of your directions for where to place the first aid station and ambulance?**
   Calmly and professionally, you should meet with the official who dictated the move. Although he may be resistant to changing the location back to your original direction, you should convince him by explaining that it would be unwise to move stretchers or drive an ambulance through a crowd of people who will be excited and nervous in the state of an emergency.
2. **What can you do to ensure that this problem does not occur again at this event as well as at future events?**
   For the future, consider explaining to the venue officials and promoters the specific reasons behind your actions at the onset of preplanning. If they understand that the ambulance should be parked in a location that will not require SEMS personnel to drive through a crowd during an emergency, they will probably be more likely to respect your decisions.

Ready for Review

- To accurately assess the needs of a particular special event, a systematic, scientific approach must be employed.
- Objective factors are the proven unbiased facts about the event.
- Subjective information is derived from what other people perceive about the special event.
- When planning for an event, the type of activity occurring at the event will directly relate to the expected emergencies and, therefore, is a factor to be considered during preplanning.
- Weather and environmental factors constitute a major influence on the patient load.
- Especially for outdoor special events, it is imperative to be aware of the event schedule and the role of SEMS personnel.
- Indoor operations may differ in many ways from outdoor operations.
- The difference between a seated and mobile audience will have a significant impact on staffing requirements as well as equipment needs.
- Each type of special event, bound or unbound, presents its own set of challenges with crowd movement, vehicle movement, patient extraction, medical insertion (including medical personnel into the situation), and action strategies.
- While the size of the venue will affect SEMS response, knowing the number of attendees will help providers determine how to move around the venue and how to move patients.
- The demographics of the crowd take precedence over the size of the event.
- The greater the number of attendees with preexisting conditions, the more likely that medical treatment will be necessary.
- Consider access and egress routes for ambulances when preplanning. Specific routes may need to be preplanned and kept free of crowds and other vehicles. Consider creating a "sterile" route and also using the "rapid clearing routes" method.
- Maps indicating the location of first aid facilities are important for attendees, event staff, and SEMS personnel. These maps must be created in the preplanning stage. It may be useful for the map to include a grid.
- After completing the research stage, SEMS managers and staff must perform a mental or theoretical walk-through of the entire event.
- When planning the number of SEMS providers to staff at an event, a multitude of factors unique to the event will need to be considered.
- Five general categories that can be used to gauge the needs of a particular special event are attendance, activity, attendability, weather, and other factors (ie, history of the event, drug/alcohol use, if the event is occurring outdoors, and if the event involves extreme sports or combat sports).
- The number of SEMS providers and first aid stations will vary depending on the type of event. The number of SEMS providers and first aid stations will need to be adjusted to take into account special characteristics of the event that could result in more injuries and emergencies.
- A general guideline for determining the number of first aid stations is that one first aid station will suffice for an event that has fewer than 5,000 attendees.
- The rule of three states that three SEMS providers should respond to and handle each emergency at an event. Two providers directly handle patient assessment and management, and the third provider is responsible for other aspects such as ensuring provider safety and retrieving needed equipment.
- Once the SEMS manager has preplanned each step, mentally reviewed the entire event, and checked all mathematical figures, it is time to alert each outside vendor and assisting parties of the items that will be required to ensure the success of the event.
- It is important to determine during preplanning which channels medical personnel should use to communicate. This information and a phone list of all necessary numbers should be posted at the first aid station and the incident command post.
- Bring a special event log to each event. This is a record of the patient interactions that occurred at a particular event and should include any actions taken by the manager of the medical provisions and the reasons for those actions.
- During preplanning, SEMS providers must consider possible major emergency threats and plan for them. They should consider all possible hazards.

- Incidents that could involve multiple-agency or multiple-jurisdiction response will need a unified command system. Plans must be drawn up in advance to designate the lead and support agencies in several kinds of MCIs.
- Preplanning must also cover how evacuation will occur, should a major incident make it necessary. Create an evacuation plan with clear safety and security procedures to follow during an emergency. These plans must consider all aspects of the facility. You may need to use the NIMS ICS structure. There must also be a plan for how information will be communicated to event attendees should a major incident occur.
- To complete the physical walk-through, SEMS managers must arrange with the venue manager a time for the SEMS team to evaluate the physical space of the event.

Vital Vocabulary

attendability The likelihood that sick people will attend an event, usually related to the importance of the event to a person's life.

bound event A special event that is contained within set perimeters, such as walls, fences, or natural barriers such as lakes or ponds.

choke point Any area that prohibits the crowd from moving freely and can cause a pedestrian backup, such as doorways, riot gates, or places where people naturally stop to talk, blocking the pathway of others.

evacuation plan Plan created during the preplanning stage that outlines the method of evacuating the entire crowd from an event in an emergency situation.

maximum cycle rate The turnover of the crowd, meaning how many people leave versus how many arrive.

mosh pit An area, usually in front of a stage, where members of the audience flail and smash into each other.

objective factors Proven, unbiased facts about the event, such as the type of event, duration, and crowd size.

peak attendance rate The maximum number of people attending in a span of a single hour of an event.

rule of three A policy that three SEMS providers should respond to and handle each emergency at an event.

special event log A record of patient interactions that occur at a particular event.

subjective factors Information that is not made up of provable facts; examples include crowd mentality and memories from previous experience.

transport unit-wise number The estimated number of transports expected per day, determined using the total number of people, the expected number of days, and additional factors that could affect the number of emergencies, such as temperature, comfort provisions, age of attendees, and health of attendees.

unbound event A special event that has no or very few structured perimeters, such as road races, marathons, charity walks, and outdoor festivals.

unified command system A command system used in larger incidents in which there is a multiagency response or multiple jurisdictions are involved.

walk-through The opportunity for the SEMS team to evaluate the physical space where an event will take place; it can be theoretical or actual (physical).

CHAPTER

First Aid Station and Equipment

3

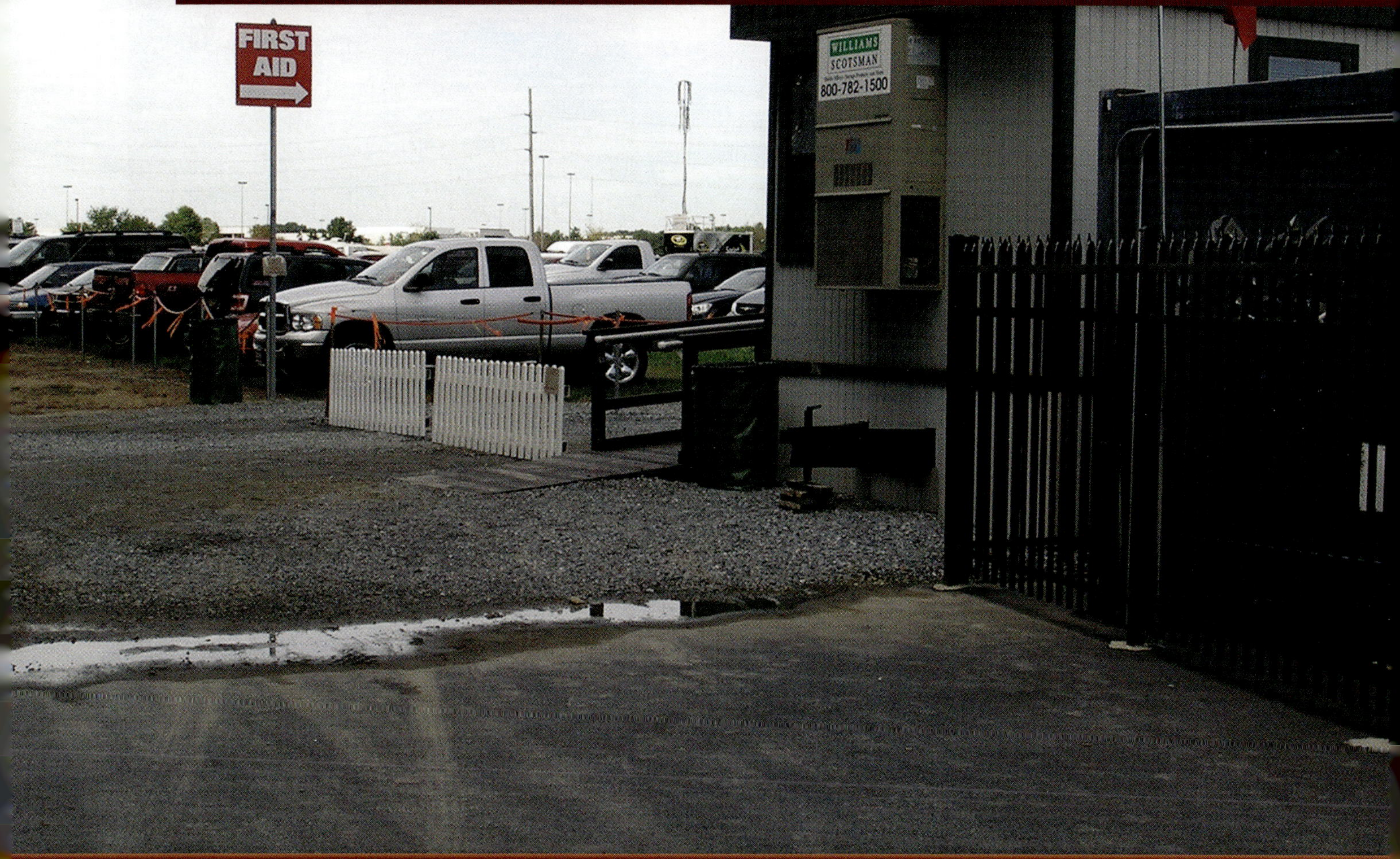

LEARNING OBJECTIVES

- Describe the purpose of the first aid station.
- Discuss the importance of the first aid station location.
- Discuss why adequate signage for the first aid station is important.
- Describe the equipment that should be included in a first aid station and the factors to consider when designing its layout.
- Explain situations when a first aid tent should be used.
- Describe a mobile aid station and when it might be used.
- Describe a multilevel emergent care facility and when it might be used.
- Discuss possible staffing configurations for a first aid station.
- Describe other types of first aid stations, including comfort stations and misting stations.
- List the standard equipment that should be stocked at a special event.
- List the vehicles that may be used at a special event, and safety considerations for each vehicle.

First Aid Stations

No matter the type and size of event, the most common issue special events medical services (SEMS) providers will deal with is minor first aid requiring only basic life support (BLS) care. Attendees will inevitably wear sandals to walk for miles or consume large amounts of cotton candy and soda before jumping onto every carnival ride in the park. Providers will need to tend to the resulting blisters and nausea, as well as people in need of water, cooling or warming, bandages, or ice who will present at the **first aid station** Figure 3-1.

A first aid station is a place that is dedicated to the medical aid of attendees and comes in many different forms, from tents to 32-foot mobile homes. While one of the most commonly used tools when providing SEMS at an outdoor special event, the importance of the first aid station is frequently overlooked.

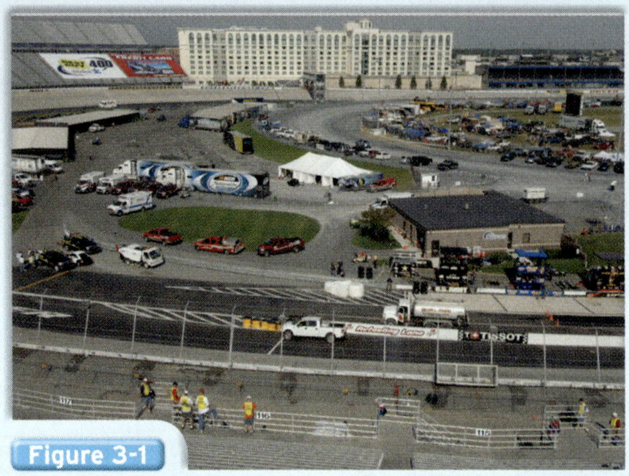

Figure 3-1

A first aid station tent.

Location

When planning the first aid station, there is much more to consider than just the size of the facility. The configuration of the site and the location are also vitally important for the efficient dispensing of medical services. SEMS professionals may want to be in the center of the special event for easy access. However, being in the "center of the action" could be one of the worst places to be located. If providers need to transport a patient to the hospital, they may encounter any number of obstacles and pitfalls. They should be centrally located, but not the center of attention.

Much time and consideration should be given to the placement of aid stations, and their importance should not be taken lightly. Locate an area where the station can be easily accessible but will not impair the patrons' ability to participate in the event or obstruct their view. Patient transport may be necessary, so if there is not an easy ingress and egress from the aid station, other plans will have to be made that will allow for the extrication of patients to a designated transport rendezvous location. Ensure that units responding to these rendezvous areas are aware of their location and are provided with a marked map of the area Figure 3-2.

You Are the SEMS Provider

CASE 1

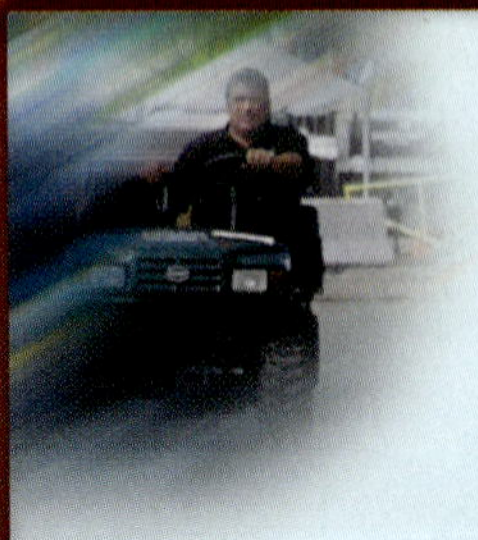

Forty-five days prior to a BMX event, you meet with the special event organizer and learn that the facility is 100 acres in total. The track is divided into two parts: the main track (about 1.5 miles around) and a secondary track, which the event refers to as the "back 40" (an additional 1 mile). The event's planners provide you with maps that show the track area, crowd area, roads, and parking. They are expecting a crowd of 12,000 people and have a sponsorship agreement with the local medical center. They provide you with the contact information for the person who is the point of contact. They show you where they are planning to have a separate medical tent (in addition to the first aid station). You walk through the facility, discover the best line of site, and determine there are three ways to exit the course. The terrain is very even but hilly. The event will be using a rented radio system.

The event is hosting eight races. The secondary track will be used during some races; in other races, the primary track will be used. The weather at this time of the year averages 76°F. There are two entrance/exit points for the facility.

1. What types of equipment will you designate when preplanning for this event?

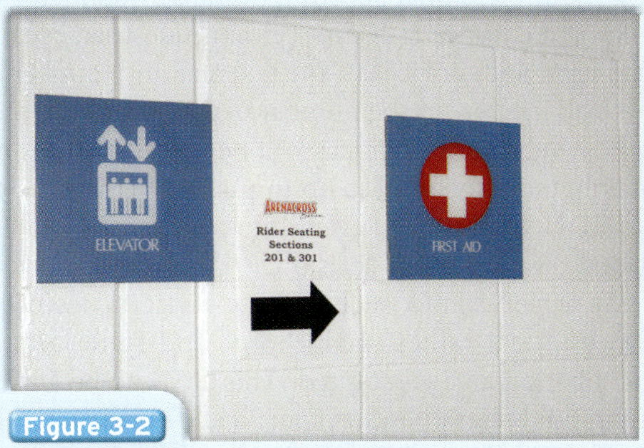

Figure 3-2

The location of the first aid station should be clearly marked.

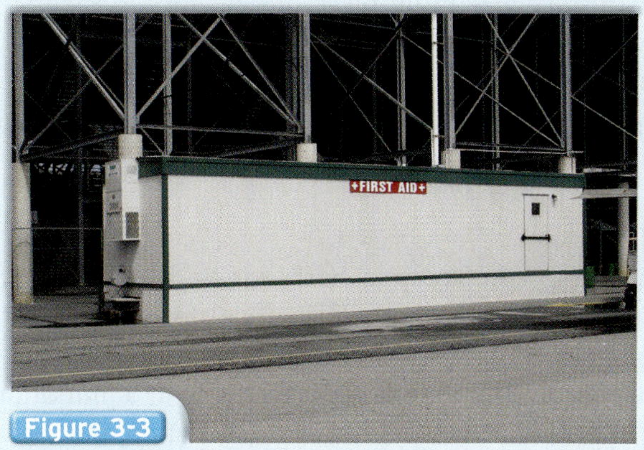

Figure 3-3

The first aid station should be clearly marked by color coding or signage.

Providers should try to place the station near entrance and exit areas or on paths. Preferably, this should take place during preplanning when looking at the maps, but nothing can be confirmed until providers visually inspect the appropriateness of the chosen site. Such placement may not always be an option, and providers may not get to view the area until the day of the event. Thus, they should be prepared to adjust quickly and improvise when needed. The area where the first aid station is placed needs to be large enough to contain at least two examination couches (or cots) and an ambulance stretcher. It needs to have adequate space to walk around. To determine this space, providers should be able to walk around the station two abreast with enough room to easily and comfortably move equipment. They must be mindful of hazards, especially tripping hazards, such as tent poles, pegs, pallets, vendors' wares, and other obstructions.

The first aid station must be placed in an area that will facilitate a clean and hygienic condition and must be designated as a no smoking area. There must be adequate heating, shade, lighting, and ventilation. The location of the first aid station is crucial to successfully covering an event and must be considered with care.

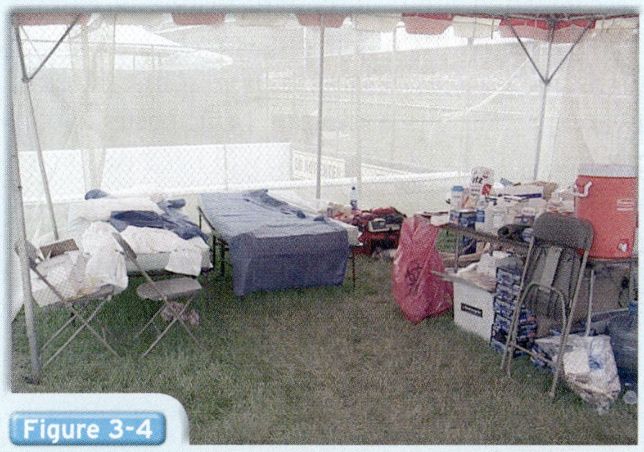

Figure 3-4

The inside of a first aid station.

TIP

Location names can be confusing. If you name your first aid stations "North," "South," etc, be sure that event management is not calling those stations something different. Try to establish consistent names for first aid station locations prior to the event.

Signage

The location of the first aid station should be clearly marked either by color coding or by signage **Figure 3-3**. Any maps or signs created by the special event operators should clearly mark where the first aid station is in case of emergency. The SEMS manager should ensure that the other staff members who are working the event, such as security and gate personnel, know where the aid station is located. They will likely be the first people that come in contact with patrons needing care.

Accessibility

The first aid station needs to be readily accessible for the admission of casualties and ambulance crews. This means it should be seen and identified as the aid station. There should be nothing impeding the flow of traffic to and from the station. The doorway needs to be large enough to allow the access of an ambulance stretcher or a wheelchair.

The first aid station needs to have an area for the treatment of sitting casualties **Figure 3-4**. To prepare for this space, simply place one person on each side of the stretcher and practice entering and exiting the station. With fixed aid stations, this may not be possible, but ensure that if the stretcher fits into the area, it can also exit the area when fully loaded with a patient.

Size

The station can vary in both size and function. For smaller events, a tent will suffice; for large events, especially those with large venues, providers may need multiple aid stations in fixed facilities. It is important to understand each type of first aid station and which station best facilitates each type of event.

The first aid station needs to be the adequate size for the anticipated number of casualties. There is no hard-and-fast rule, but, generally, it should be able to comfortably handle the peak patient load. Once you have calculated the peak patient load, you will need to consider how many patients each of your first aid stations will hold. For example, if your first aid station can hold 8 patients and your peak patient load is expected to be 14 patients, you will need two first aid stations.

You will also need to decide how to best configure your first aid station. For example, if you expect the majority of the injuries to require only minor first aid, you may arrange for your first aid station to have 2 beds and 6 chairs.

Privacy

The configuration of the first aid station must account for patient privacy. The first aid station should have as much privacy as can be reasonably expected under the circumstances. Privacy walls are available for most 10-foot × 10-foot pop tents and can be joined to make a 10-foot × 20-foot tent if needed.

Types of Stations

The First Aid Tent

The general rule is that most special events, at a minimum, require a 10-foot × 10-foot tent. This small tent will provide a basic treatment area for patients and can be as simple as a few chairs, a cooler, and some water. Typical events that usually need only the basic first aid station include block parties, small festivals, local nonprofessional sporting events, 5-kilometer to 10-kilometer running events, certain equestrian events, small fairs, and movie sets.The tent size and number of tents will increase as the number of attendees increases (events with more attendees will need larger tents and possibly more tents). It is up to the SEMS manager to take all the factors of an event into consideration when making the aid station decision.

At bigger events, such as large concerts, festivals, large political rallies, marathons, and state fairs, a rehabilitation area is required. This area can be within the first aid station and is specifically constructed to provide attendees (and providers) with a place to rest and rehydrate. It must be a climate-controlled area. At bigger events, the area will likely need to accommodate cots, which may require a 20-foot × 20-foot tent.

Whether the SEMS manager determines a large or small tent is needed for the event, providers will need a method for controlling access at both an entrance and exit. These access points need to be clearly marked and, if possible, used only by patients and staff, which will preserve privacy. A means of controlling access can be as simple as a flap on a tent that acts as a doorway. The entrance must be unimpeded, easily identifiable, and accessible to patients and staff.

Mobile Aid Stations

In most cases, a tent will suffice for a first aid station at an outdoor special event, but with a tent, SEMS managers need to plan for protection from extreme temperatures. If an agency only occasionally covers special events, a tent will do quite nicely. A local tenting service can supply heating and cooling equipment systems for the tent.

If an agency is involved in outdoor special events more frequently, the SEMS manager may consider purchasing a **mobile aid station** as a replacement for the tent. Mobile stations can range from very simple and inexpensive to massive and expensive Figure 3-5.

To determine the appropriate mobile station for a specific agency, examine historic data. It is very important to consider the size of the mobile aid station. Outdoor special events have a very limited space, which can make setup difficult. Although agencies may want and can afford a large mobile station, the outdoor special events may not have the space for a 52-foot motor home, for example. The SEMS manager must let common sense prevail. The largest vehicle should be no greater than 32 feet long Figure 3-6. A trailer that can be towed may also be an option Figure 3-7.

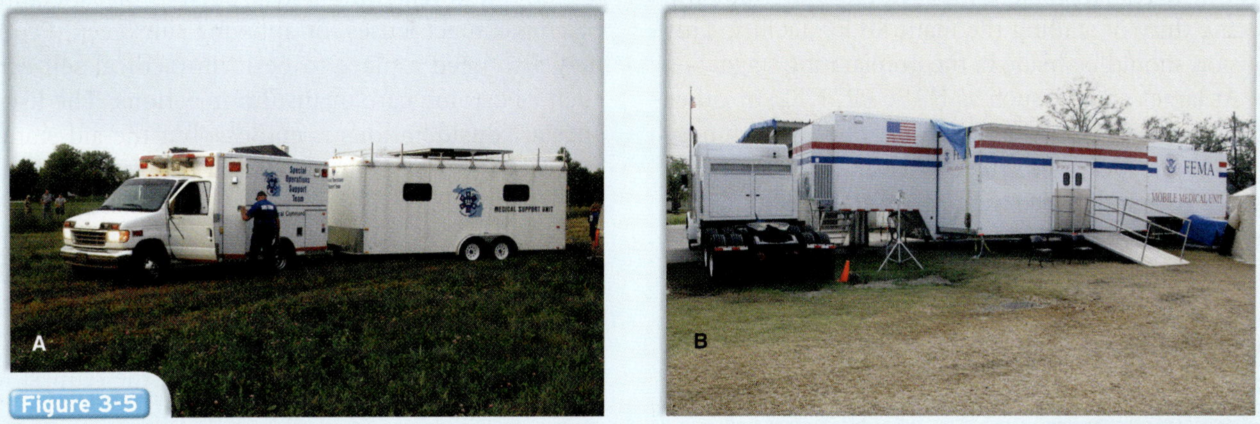

Figure 3-5

A. A basic mobile aid station. **B**. A massive mobile aid station.

Multilevel Emergent Care Facilities

Multilevel emergent care (MLEC) facilities are staffed and equipped with additional equipment and supplies as well as the minimum equipment required for the first aid station Figure 3-8. MLEC facilities may care for patients requiring longer-term management on site, such as patients requiring observation or rehydration. MLEC facilities also help prevent the special event from overloading local emergency departments or emergency medical services (EMS) resources.

Staffing of an MLEC may include physicians, nurses, paramedics, and professional sports technicians who have the ability to administer some emergent care on site, including stitches, headache medication, and other minor procedures. If nurses and physicians are to be a

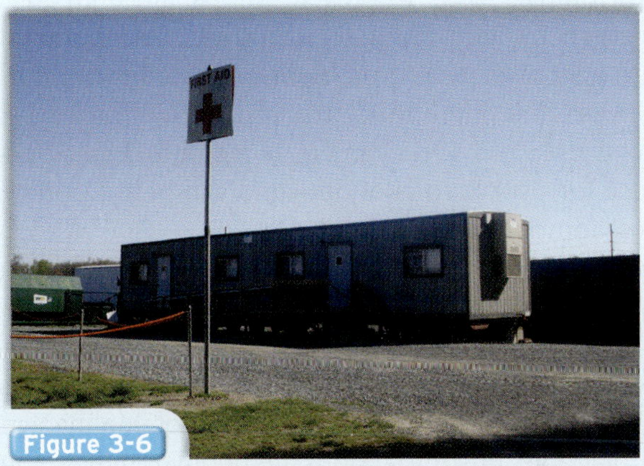

Figure 3-6

A motor home can be converted into a mobile aid station.

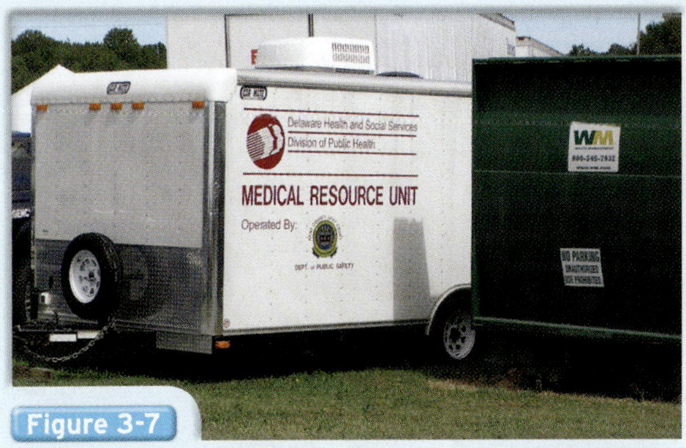

Figure 3-7

A tow trailer can also be converted into a mobile aid station.

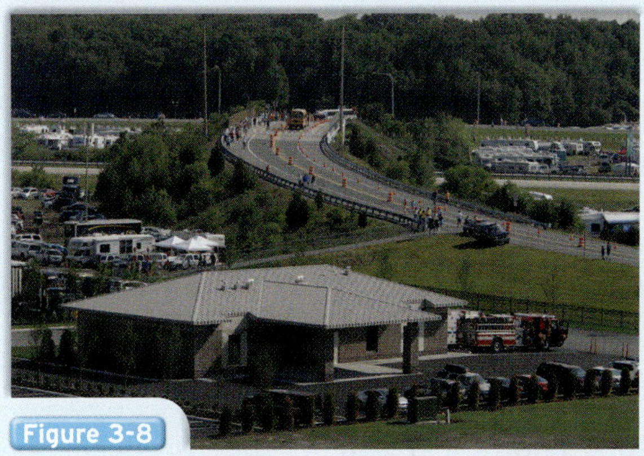

Figure 3-8

An MLEC facility.

part of the response plan, they should undertake the specific duty of staffing the main MLEC facility. This decision should be made in the preplanning stage.

At larger events, such as NASCAR, NFL, or other more permanent fixed sites, MLEC facilities are common. Some event locations, such as NASCAR tracks, are located such a distance from the nearest hospital that the venues have established on-site walk-in care centers for all visitors.

Station Staff

The first aid station must be staffed at all times. It is essential to discuss who supplies the first aid station and who will work with the special event organizers to set up the station before the big day. Providers should aim to be accessible but not intrusive.

First Aid Station With a Nurse

A first aid station with a nurse is staffed by at least one registered nurse (RN) or medical professional with higher-level training. These stations are usually used at mega-events, such as sporting events, or at the organizer's request. It is preferred that the nurse be experienced in emergency medical care and triage of seriously ill or injured patients at higher levels of care. The SEMS manager must clearly define the roles and responsibilities of the RNs and gauge their comfort level with working in the field.

First Aid Station With a Physician

A first aid station with a physician is staffed by at least one physician. It is preferred that the physician be experienced in emergency medical care and triage of seriously ill or injured patients at higher levels of care. Again, the SEMS manager should clearly define the roles and responsibilities of the physicians and gauge their comfort level with working in the field.

Additional Functions of a First Aid Station

More Than First Aid

Many times, the first aid station has the shared responsibility of being an all-purpose aid station—a place where people can seek relief for what ails them. Often, people just need a place to rest, to cool down, to warm up, or to rehydrate. People may need a place to attend to non–life-threatening issues, such as breastfeeding, placing contact lenses, or applying sunscreen. People may also need a place to perform medical self-care, such as ostomy care or insulin injections. The list of special considerations is endless, but the aid station represents a place of refuge and answers. First aid stations ideally have an area specially designated to address these nonemergencies, and all aid stations and providers should prepare for these situations. For the most part, no special equipment needs to be provided for nonemergencies. The challenge may come in balancing the privacy of patients with the request for nonemergency uses of the aid station.

Cool Comfort

In most parts of the country, the bulk of outdoor special events are held in the summer. It is the mission of SEMS professionals to try to prevent illness and injury. Heat emergencies are preventable ailments. Heat combined with age, prior health problems, or alcohol drastically increases the likelihood that injuries will arise at an event. EMS providers can create a **comfort station**—a place for people to cool off—and can help to prevent these injuries from occurring Figure 3-9. Water must be made available for people who need to rest, as well as a chair and an ice pack. Every outdoor special event should have ice available. A **misting station** is a place that includes sprinkler-like equipment that provides a gentle water vapor with the intention of cooling event participants. Misting stations are popular with younger crowds, and they go a long way toward maintaining good health Figure 3-10. They can be very expensive to purchase; rentals from a local company may be a viable alternative.

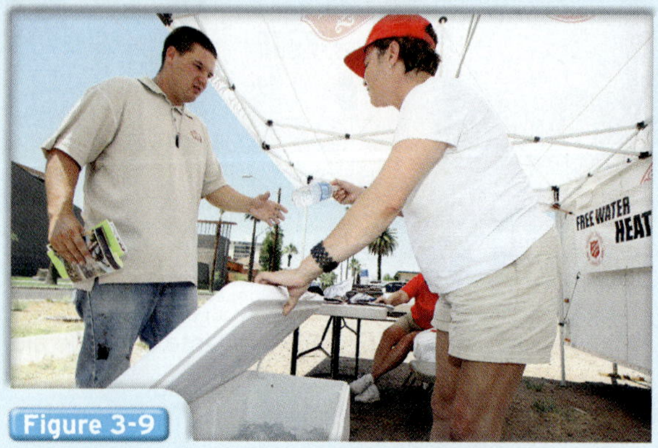

Figure 3-9

A comfort station at the first aid station.

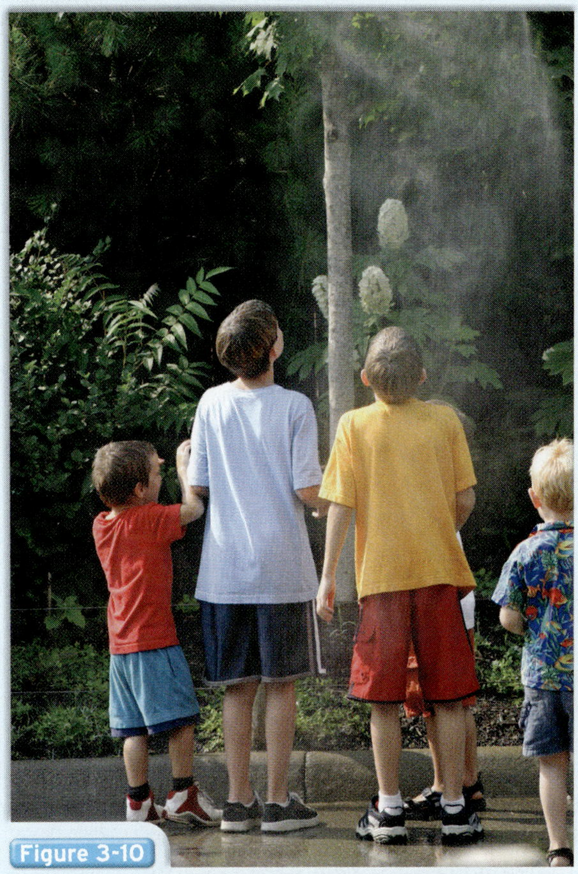

Figure 3-10

A misting station.

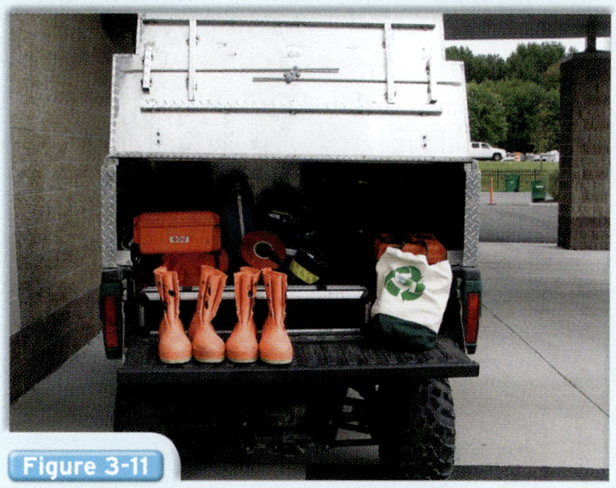

Figure 3-11

Equipment should be at the site and quickly accessible.

TIP Ice and water quantities should be discussed with the event coordinator prior to the event to ensure they are adequate. These must be available and must be able to be dropped off to the first aid station routinely. Have the event coordinator's contact information in case the supply line of these items breaks down.

Equipment Overview

This section briefly discusses the minimum equipment and supplies necessary to stock a first aid tent to SEMS standards. The SEMS manager must refer to the minimum standards set by the state or the event's jurisdiction.

Emergency Equipment

All necessary emergency equipment should be at the site and quickly accessible Figure 3-11. Personnel should be familiar with the function and operation of each type of emergency equipment. Equipment should be in good operating condition, and personnel must be trained in advance to use it properly. Emergency equipment should be checked on a regular basis and rehearsed with by emergency personnel.

The emergency equipment available should be appropriate for the level of training for the emergency medical providers and should also include items that may be needed per local protocol, such as certain advanced airway devices. This means that if an agency is staffed at a basic life support (BLS) level, the providers should have all the minimum equipment required by the state for that level and for acceptable practices performed at that level. Likewise, it is important to know the proper way to care for and store the equipment. Providers must follow their organization's accepted protocol for care and cleaning of equipment. If they still have any questions or concerns about care for any equipment, the manufacturer should be able to provide specific instructions.

Equipment should be stored in a clean and environmentally controlled area. The following equipment list is the SEMS suggested minimum for a BLS aid station:

- Cots (stretchers)
- Blankets
- Chairs
- Lightweight portable plastic storage cabinet
- Refrigerator or cooler
- Oral fluid for hydration (water, sports drinks)
- Stethoscope
- Oxygen with flow meter
- Oxygen-delivery devices

- Bag-mask device/pocket masks/CPR barrier shields
- Oral/nasal airways
- Automated external defibrillator
- Flashlight
- Blood pressure cuff
- Tongue blades
- Safety pins
- Alcohol swabs
- Wound cleaner
- Ice packs or bags
- Scissors
- Bandage strips
- Eye patch pads
- Cotton tip applicators
- Exam gloves (various sizes)
- Sling or triangular bandage
- Kling bandages, various sizes
- Triangular bandages
- Splints
- Emesis bags
- Plastic bags (with sealable top)
- Moist towelettes (individual)
- Paper
- Pen
- Coins (for children who need to call their parents)
- Red bag
- Sharps box

BLS Backpack

As a rule, it is better to carry as little as possible; a small bag is better than a big one. A backpack is ideal because the provider's hands remain free. For BLS equipment, providers should try to stock a backpack with the following:

- 4-inch × 4-inch gauze pads (20)
- 3-inch Kling bandages (10)
- Ice pack (2)
- Blood pressure cuff
- Stethoscope
- Sterile water or saline solution
- Latex gloves (10 pairs)
- Roll of 2-inch tape (2)
- Roll of 1-inch tape (2)
- Pen light
- Shears
- Bag-mask device
- Suction device
- Cervical collars
- Any other minimum supplies and devices required by the event's jurisdiction

ALS Equipment

If SEMS is providing advanced life support (ALS) for an event, the tent must have the minimum equipment required by the state for that provider level. The SEMS minimum list consists of:

- Electrocardiogram monitor with pacing
- Oxygen
- Intravenous (IV) fluids
- IV administration kit
- All required drugs
- Endotracheal intubation kit
- Any other minimum supplies and devices required by the event's jurisdiction

You Are the SEMS Provider

CASE 2

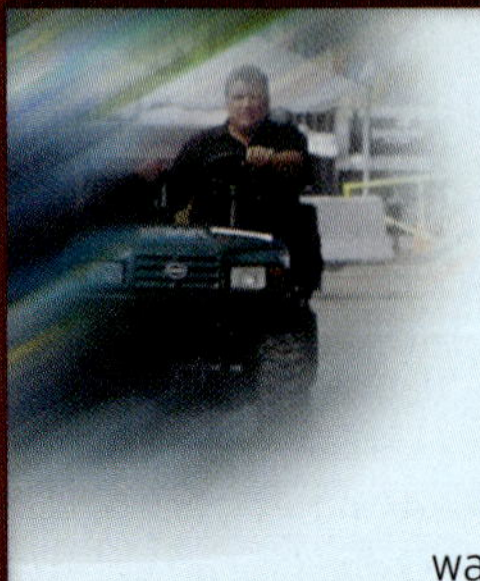

Your service is providing SEMS at a three-day festival. On the second night, you are dispatched for a woman with an injured leg. The woman is located in an area of the venue that is difficult to access, at the top of a high hill to the left of the concert area.

You and a fellow SEMS provider begin your response in a cart but are forced to abandon the vehicle and proceed on foot, due to the size of the crowd and the steep grade of the hill.

When you reach the patient, she is in obvious pain. Your quick assessment reveals deformity of the lower left leg, which you suspect is a fracture. The woman states that there was an accident, in which a large man fell on her leg after jumping off of the shoulders of a friend.

You stabilize the leg with splints, position the patient on a long backboard, and spider straps, and then realize there is no easy way to extract her from this location.

1. How will you proceed with moving the patient from this location to the ambulance?
2. What other personnel can you request and how can they assist with removing this patient?

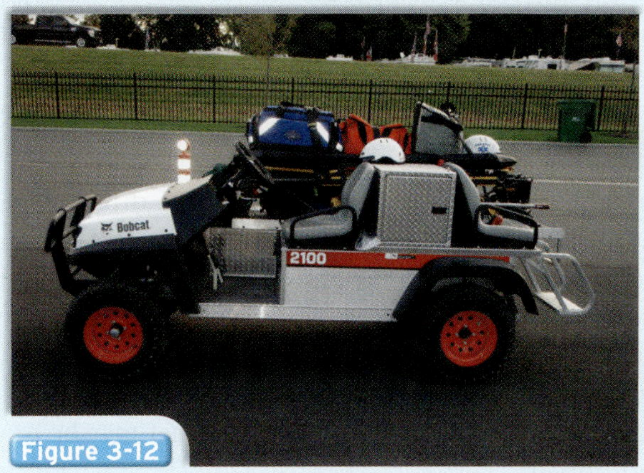

Figure 3-12

A type of cart that can be used at a SEMS event.

Vehicles

Carts

Depending on the size and the situation, carts can be the best way to operate in the special event environment. Specific carts can be used at a SEMS event Figure 3-12. Carts are useful in some environments, but not all. No matter the location, discretion and prudence should be used at all times while operating a motorized cart. SEMS professionals should avoid operating carts of any sort in large groups of people because of the unpredictable nature of crowds, though if a vehicle must be used, a cart is the preferred vehicle (rather than a bicycle). If operating in a crowd, providers should avoid aggressive, high-speed operations, and they should not overload the cart. If you must use a cart in a crowd, consider having someone walk in front of the cart to clear the path.

Ensure that the special event can support the cart or multiple carts. Make certain that an electric cart will be fully charged or that there will be opportunities to recharge throughout the special event. Because an outlet for an electrical cart can be difficult to find at times, gasoline- or diesel-powered carts may be the best alternative. However, refueling is an issue, as are exhaust fumes. For both electrical and gasoline-powered carts, spare parts, tires, and batteries will inevitably be needed. If an agency owns a cart, routine maintenance should be performed on it, just like any other vehicle in the fleet.

Vehicle Safety

Certain precautions need to be taken when using carts at special events. Is the special event going to take place at night? If so, the cart will need headlights. In addition, emergency lights should be affixed to the cart. Caution should be used with certain carts that utilize mounted stretchers Figure 3-13. When fully loaded, these carts become top-heavy and unstable. When operated in an aggressive fashion, they tend to roll over (and aggressive driving is never safe with any vehicle).

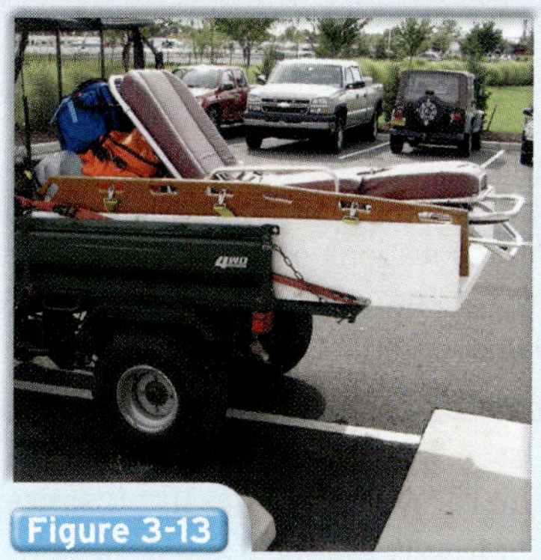

Figure 3-13

A mounted stretcher could be dangerous for the patient; be sure the patient is properly secured.

Bicycles

Since the early 1990s, mountain biking has been very popular. Police departments put mountain bikes to frequent use, and EMS initiated bike-mounted providers. However, in the SEMS environment, there are many important drawbacks to using bicycles. They are best used only on a very limited scale in road events such as 5-kilometer or 10-kilometer races, or when responding at events that include campsites. Even in marathons, they are not as beneficial as perceived because there is too much ground to cover.

Using mountain bikes within crowds can be extremely dangerous to both the crowd and rider. The unpredictable nature of crowd movement is always a challenge regardless of the vehicle being used; however, using a bicycle creates additional problems. In a crowd, it is nearly impossible to safely operate a bicycle. Warning devices, such as bells, are necessary but can startle people and trigger unpredictable actions. Even worse, paramedics on bicycles have a higher rate of collisions with civilians in a crowd.

Another drawback of bike-mounted providers is that they do not make a response more efficient. A bicycle can carry very limited supplies, which can lead to problems. For example, if a bike team is dispatched, reaches the patient before the providers who are racing on foot, and initiates care, they will be unable to transport the patient to the ambulance. Instead, they will have to wait for the stretcher to arrive. Additional complications created by the use of bicycles include:

- Bicycles and equipment attached to bicycles are more easily stolen. When equipment has been

> **TIP** If your event will have a command center, it will ideally not be located with or too close to any first aid station. However, the location of the command center will depend on the event. At certain events, a location near a first aid station is the only option. The command center location should always be preplanned.

strapped to the bicycle, it can easily disappear within a large crowd.

- Responders need to be able to operate the bicycles at top performance. If responders are not in good enough shape, they will have difficulty responding quickly, guiding the bicycle with precision, and avoiding obstacles.
- Finally, bicycles do not operate well on loose, wet, or steep terrain.

If a SEMS provider does opt to use a bicycle despite all of these drawbacks, the rider must be trained in the use of a bicycle and how to provide care from a bicycle.

Instead of using bicycles, it is best to use specially designed medical carts. They can carry all the equipment for a response and possess the ability to transport patients safely from the site of the incident to the waiting transport units.

Ambulances

Some services will be able to dictate a different size ambulance for each event. If possible, it is ideal to match the ambulance size to the physical space available at the event location. For example, if an event does not have much space to spare, a van may be most appropriate. On the other hand, if the unit will also function as an aid station, the medium-duty freight liner may be more appropriate.

> **TIP** EMS services may wish to use four-wheelers at events, but there are some negatives associated with this. The speed cannot be controlled as easily as with carts. Four-wheelers cannot carry larger equipment such as backboards, and cannot transport backboarded patients, meaning that other vehicles are needed. Finally, four-wheelers require experienced drivers.

You Are the SEMS Provider SUMMARY

CASE 1

1. **What types of equipment will you designate when preplanning for this event?**
   While there is a wide range of answers to this question, specifics can include the following. Because there will be a separate medical tent, you should have an event radio for the supervisor and physician at the medical tent. You should also have an independent radio system for providers. Based on the guidelines in Chapter 2, a crowd of 12,000 requires two to four SEMS providers. Ideally at least two carts would be used. Because of the hilly terrain and the size of the tracks, you will need a spotter in the tower at the highest point on the track to act as incident command and give the initial go/no-go orders. Finally, as with all events, you will need a schedule of the event, maps, and on-site reconnaissance.

CASE 2

1. **How will you proceed with moving the patient from this location to the ambulance?**
   The goal is to move the patient with as little pain as possible. At this point, it is advisable to request assistance, for example from the fire department to assist with removing the patient. Together you can devise a viable extraction plan. For example, the fire department may be able to provide a specialized all-terrain-vehicle (ATV) that can maneuver steep slopes. In this case, once at the top of the hill, the ATV could be placed as close to the fence as possible, so that the crowd would only be on one side of the vehicle.
2. **What other personnel can you request and how can they assist with removing this patient?**
   Fire department personnel and other personnel, such as security, can provide manpower to carry the patient and can assist with asking attendees to clear a path. If an ATV is used as discussed above, these personnel can ask attendees to clear the fence area, allowing the ATV to travel to the site of the ambulance. These additional personnel should walk in front of the SEMS providers (or ATV) to ensure a clear path.

Ready for Review

- No matter the type and size of event, the most common issue SEMS providers will deal with is some type of minor first aid.
- A first aid station is a specific enclosure that is dedicated to the medical aid of attendees and comes in many different forms, from tents to 32-foot mobile homes. Most special events require a 10-foot × 10-foot tent at a minimum.
- The location of the first aid station is important. It should be centrally located but not the center of attention. The station should be accessible, without impairing patrons' ability to participate in the event. It should have easy ingress and egress, or other plans must be made regarding extrication and transport. There must be adequate heating, shade, lighting, and ventilation.
- The location of the first aid station should be clearly marked either by color coding or by signage. Maps or signs created by the special event operators should clearly mark where the first aid station is in case of emergency.
- The first aid station needs to be readily accessible for the admission of casualties and ambulance crews; therefore it should be visually obvious and identifiable as a first aid station.
- The station can vary in both size and function, depending on the size of the event. It needs to be the adequate size for the anticipated number of casualties. Providers should consider peak patient load when planning the size of the first aid station.
- The first aid station must provide a level of privacy for patients. Privacy walls are available for most tents.
- In most cases, a tent will suffice for a first aid station at an outdoor special event, but with a tent, SEMS managers need to plan for protection from extreme temperatures.
- Multilevel emergent care (MLEC) facilities are staffed and equipped with additional equipment and supplies as well as the minimum equipment required for the first aid station.
- The first aid station must be staffed at all times.
- A first aid station may be staffed with a nurse or physician in addition to the SEMS providers.
- The first aid station has additional functions beyond providing medical care. It also serves as an all-purpose aid station—a place that people use for nonemergency situations such as breastfeeding and applying sunscreen.
- In most parts of the country, the bulk of outdoor special events are held in the summer. It is important to have cooling measures available, such as water, ice, and misting stations.
- All necessary emergency equipment should be at the site and quickly accessible. Personnel should be familiar with the equipment. It should be in good operating condition and should be properly cleaned and stored.
- The emergency equipment available should be appropriate for the level of training for the emergency medical providers. It should include the minimum equipment required by state for that level and for acceptable practices performed at that level.
- It is best to carry as small an equipment bag as possible, but it is even better for providers to have their hands free, so a backpack is best.
- Depending on the size and the situation, carts can be the best way to operate in the special event environment.
- With any type of vehicle, certain precautions need to be taken at special events.
- Mountain bikes used within crowds are extremely dangerous to both the crowd and rider.
- Ambulances may also be used at an event if the event is large enough to accommodate them.

Vital Vocabulary

comfort station A station that is designated for rehabilitation, cooling, or warming of staff and patients, if needed; for example, this station may be air conditioned or heated if needed, and is ideally indoors.

first aid station A specific enclosure that is dedicated to the medical aid of attendees and comes in many different forms, ranging from tents to 32-foot mobile homes.

misting station A place that includes sprinkler-like equipment that provides a gentle water vapor with the intention of cooling event participants.

mobile aid station A specific enclosure that is dedicated to the medical aid of attendees and has the ability to move around the event.

multilevel emergent care (MLEC) facility A more permanent type of medical care station generally used at a mega-event, whose staffing may include physicians, nurses, paramedics, and professional sports technicians.

CHAPTER

Communication 4

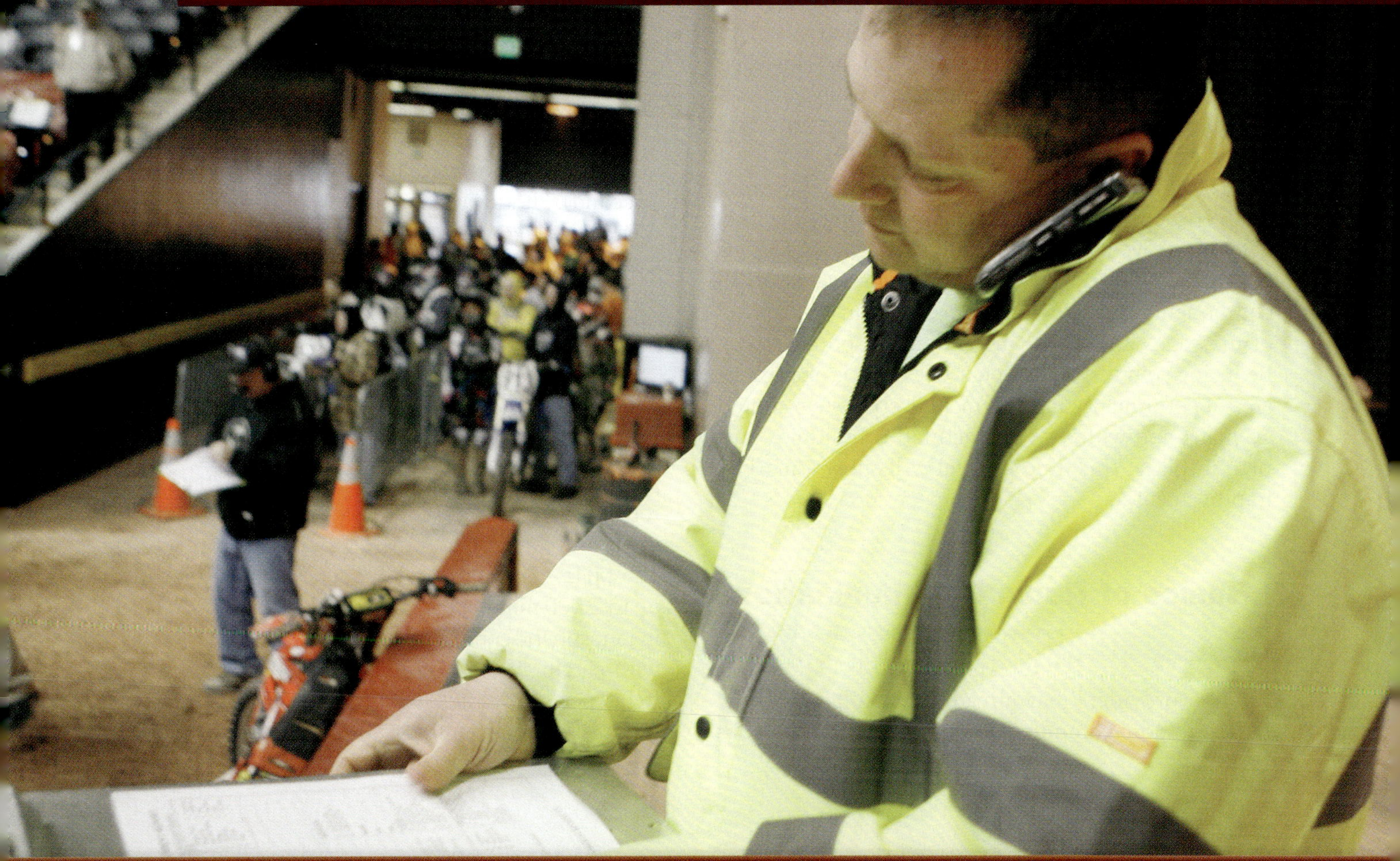

LEARNING OBJECTIVES

- Review the basic principles of radio communication systems and how they apply at a special events medical services (SEMS) event.
- Describe several potential configurations for a communications matrix.
- Correlate different communications matrix configurations with the types of events where they would likely be used.
- Discuss the importance of determining communication procedures for SEMS providers at a special event.
- Discuss the role that dispatch may have at a special event.
- Discuss the importance of dispatch when working with offsite public safety agencies.
- Describe proper radio etiquette.

Communication

From speaking face-to-face to communicating over great distances, effective and comprehensible communication is a vital key to success in any facet of emergency medical services (EMS). Preparing the communications plan and equipment for a SEMS event is no different. However, communication for SEMS events requires specific and careful consideration—even outside of the systems EMS uses everyday.

The efficiency of the EMS response at a SEMS event is largely dependent on the communication of the EMS network. A well-planned, integrated communications network with direct radio and/or landline access to all components will provide the most rapid transmittal of messages and result in minimal response times. Reducing your dispatch to on-scene times is one crucial area of performance improvement every system should evaluate, and with a well-structured communications plan in place, this time interval will show a marked improvement.

Basics of Radio Communication

Though providers may already be familiar with the basics of radio communication, this section provides a review of this subject because communications systems are such an important part of properly setting up SEMS events.

Even though the digital revolution is improving communications, most EMS communications systems today are still based on the use of radios. Radio transmits signals by electromagnetic waves. When energy is emitted in the form of waves, the energy can be characterized by the length of the waves it produces. Radio wavelengths are used for tuning by adjusting the radio to the proper **frequency**, a term that refers to how frequently the wave recurs in a given time (usually 1 second). Short wavelengths are repeated more often—with higher frequency—than longer wavelengths. Radio frequencies are designated by their cycles per second, or **hertz (Hz)**. Radios that operate at 800 megahertz (MHz) are common in EMS systems.

Frequency bands are portions of the radio frequency spectrum assigned for specific uses. The most commonly used bands for medical communications are the **very high frequency (VHF) band** and the **ultrahigh frequency (UHF) band**. The VHF band extends from roughly 30 to 175 MHz and has been arbitrarily divided into a low band (30 to 50 MHz) and a high band (150 to 175 MHz). The low-band frequencies may have ranges up to 2,000 miles but are unpredictable because changes in ionospheric conditions may cause "skip interference," with patchy losses in communication. The high-band frequencies are almost wholly free of skip interference, but at a price—a much shorter transmission range.

You Are the SEMS Provider

CASE 1

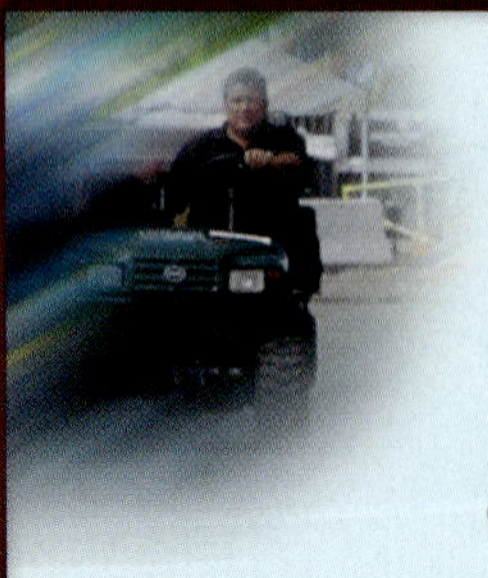

You and your agency are hired to cover a 3-day outdoor festival held in the mountains of West Virginia. With such rugged and steep terrain, you know that successful communication is going to be much more complicated to achieve than at past events held in stadiums, concert halls, and, put simply, on flat ground. The festival promoter has already attempted to piece together a radio system, which involved borrowing a repeater from the county and using rented repeaters where necessary. The plan is that the repeaters will pick up any communications and remit them at a higher and stronger frequency, thus creating a stronger signal for the difficult terrain.

For the first 2 days of the festival, radio communications work perfectly. On the third day, just after the sun sets, a call comes in from one of the far corners of the event. You stumble down a steep and rocky grade to find an agitated patient who begins assaulting you, your partner, and a security guard upon your arrival. To make matters worse, despite your best efforts, you cannot radio for backup because, as you learn later, one of the rented repeaters has gone down, and your signal cannot be picked up.

1. What could you have done to prevent this scenario from occurring?
2. What would your next action be if you were in a dangerous situation and your chain of communication has broken down?

The most commonly used of the VHF high-band frequencies for emergency medical purposes are in the 150 to 160 MHz range. The UHF band extends from 300 to 3,000 MHz, with most medical communications occurring around 450 to 470 MHz. At these frequencies, communications are entirely free of skip interference and have minimal **noise** (signal distortion). The UHF band has better penetration in dense metropolitan areas, and UHF reception is usually quite adequate inside buildings. The UHF band, however, has a shorter range than the VHF band, and energy at UHF is more readily absorbed by rain and environmental objects, such as trees and brush.

The 800 MHz frequency commonly used by EMS systems offers excellent penetration of buildings and has minimal interference and reduced channel noise. Because of this, it works quite well in metropolitan areas; 800 MHz also allows for **trunking**, in which multiple agencies or systems can share frequencies. An 800-MHz radio can also be linked to a computer system to transmit voiceless communications. The use of trunked systems has allowed the dispatcher to reprogram the radios so that agencies that do not routinely talk to each other can easily do so at the scene of a mass-casualty incident (MCI), a rescue, a hazardous materials incident, or other special operations.

The **Federal Communications Commission (FCC)**, the agency that controls frequency allocation in the United States, has set aside medical VHF band assignments for general emergency radio communications.

Cellular Telephones

Cellular telephones operate on 3 watts (W) of power or less. Mobile antennas are much closer to the ground than base station antennas, so communications from the unit are typically limited to 10 to 15 miles over average terrain. Base station antennas are usually located on high sites to increase the coverage area.

Cellular telephones are becoming more common in EMS communications systems. These telephones are simply low-power portable radios that communicate through a series of interconnected repeater stations called "cells" (hence the name "cellular"). Cellular telephones are also popular with other public safety agencies, particularly as more cell sites are constructed in rural areas. At some larger events, **cells on wheels (COWs)** are brought in to increase cellular site availability Figure 4-1. The Sprint Nextel Corporation and NASCAR are an excellent example of companies that have partnered together at a major sporting event to increase cellular capability at the event. SEMS providers can find out if any communications companies are coming to their event, and if so, they can use them to assist with communications.

Many cellular systems make equipment and airtime available to EMS services at little or no cost as a public service. The public may be able to call 9-1-1 or other emergency numbers on a cellular telephone free of charge. However, should an MCI or disaster situation occur at your special event, this easy access may result in overloading and jamming of cellular systems. SEMS providers should have a backup communications plan in their service to circumvent these overloads. For example, the radio system should have built-in redundancy when possible; this means if one frequency is down, the system will automatically switch to another. A mobile command post may be brought in as a backup communications method. Satellite phones are another alternative for a backup communications system. These can be brought to the event and then activated if needed. If satellite phones are going to be the backup communications system, usually two to ten satellite phones should be brought to the event (depending on the size of the event) and the SEMS team must have the information

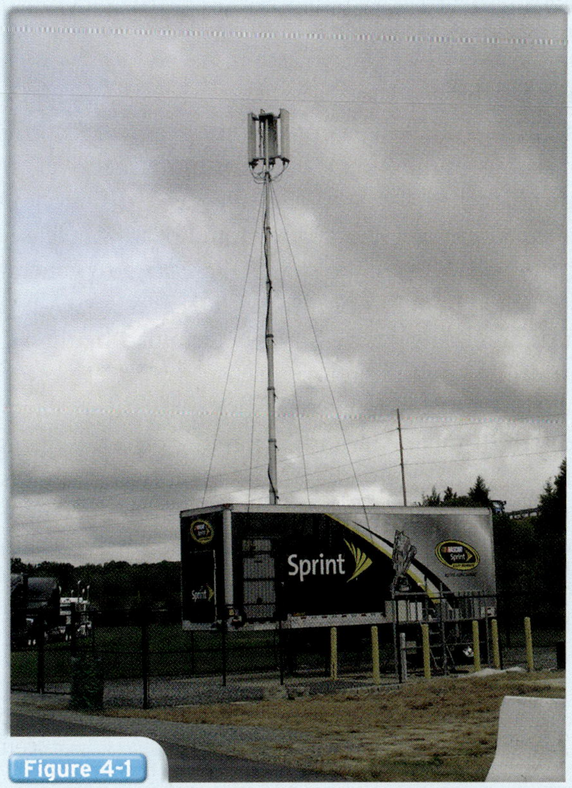

Figure 4-1

A cell on wheels (COW).

on how to activate the phones. A backup plan can even include the possibility of personnel to serve as runners to convey information should a system fail. Events of national significance sometimes have a communications trailer with special capabilities that allow different types of radios to communicate with each other in the event that different or additional radios must be added to the communications system. Finally, there should always be a list of contact details for the event.

Modes of Radio Operation

Assigned radio frequencies may be used in a variety of systems. In a **simplex** system, portable units can transmit only in one mode (voice or telemetry) or receive (voice) at any given time. A simplex system requires only a single radio frequency. A network that uses two different frequencies at the same time, to permit simultaneous transmission and reception (like a telephone), is referred to as **duplex**. Another alternative is to combine two or more signals for simultaneous transmission on one frequency, which is called a **multiplex**.

Building Blocks of a Communications System

Although EMS communications systems vary considerably from one to another, most systems serving moderate to large populations are constructed of the following components.

Base Stations

The **base station** is a collection of radio equipment consisting, at minimum, of a transmitter, receiver, and antenna. The base station serves as a dispatch and coordination area and ideally should be in contact with all other elements of the system. Base stations generally use relatively high power output (45 to 275 W); the maximum allowable power is determined by the FCC and printed on the station's license.

The base station must be equipped with an antenna located in suitable terrain, preferably on a hill or high building, close to the base. The antenna system has a vital part in transmission and reception efficiency. A good antenna system can compensate for FCC limits on power output and human-made signal distortion in the area.

Mobile Transmitter/Receivers (Transceivers)

A mobile transmitter/receiver, or mobile **transceiver**, is a two-way radio mounted in a vehicle. Mobile transmitter/receivers come in a variety of power ranges, and the power output largely determines the distance over which the signal can be effectively transmitted. A transmitter in the 7.5-W range, for example, will transmit for distances of 10 to 12 miles over slightly hilly terrain. Transmission distances are greater over water or flat terrain and reduced in mountainous areas or where there are many tall buildings. Mobile transmitters with higher outputs have proportionally greater transmission ranges. Today, the typical mobile transmitter operates at between 20 and 50 W.

Portable Transmitter/Receivers

In everyday EMS operations, portable, handheld radios are useful when providers must work at a distance from their vehicle but need to stay in communication with the base or with one another **Figure 4-2**. **Portable radios** can also be useful at a SEMS event, allowing providers to communicate with each other when they are at different locations within the event. Cellular telephones may also be used for that purpose, provided coverage is available **Figure 4-3**.

Portable units usually have power outputs of up to 5 W and, thus, have limited range by themselves, although the signal of a handheld transmitter can be boosted by retransmission through the vehicle.

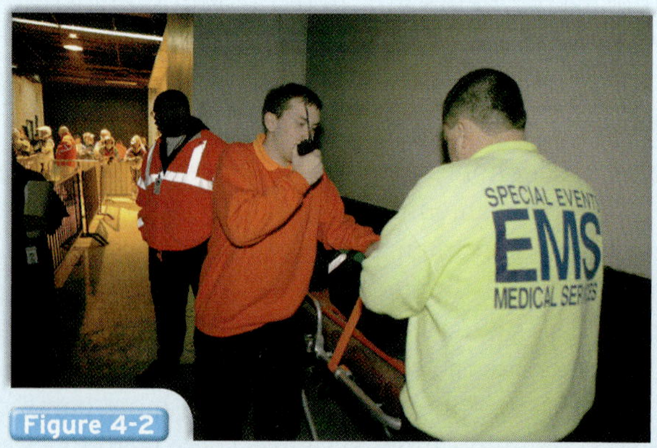

Figure 4-2

A portable radio is useful for communicating with other providers at different locations within the event.

Repeaters

A **repeater** is a miniature base station used to extend the transmitting and receiving range of a telemetry or voice communications system Figure 4-4. Repeaters may be stationary in one location (fixed repeaters) or carried in emergency vehicles (mobile repeaters). A repeater picks up a weak signal and retransmits it at a higher power on another frequency; thus, it extends the range of low-power portables and allows more members of the system to hear one another. At a SEMS event, engineers assess the topography of the event and set up repeaters in positions where they can best receive and send signals.

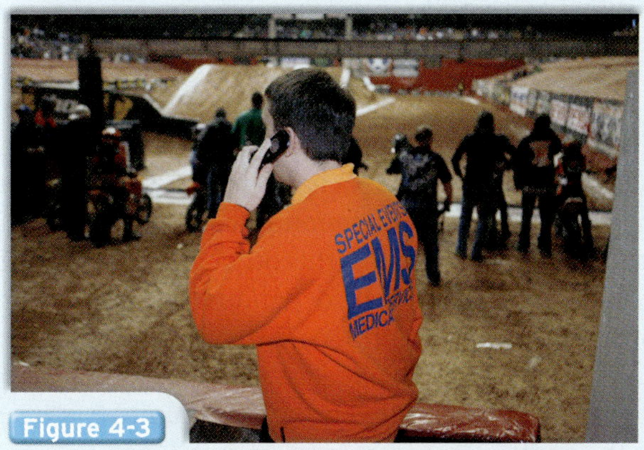

Figure 4-3

Cellular phones can be useful in SEMS operations.

TIP A good general guideline for event managers is: Do not skimp on security, medical services, or radio systems! These three areas are crucial to a successfully managed SEMS event.

Backup Communications Systems

In addition to radio communications, most systems use landline (telephone) backup to link various fixed components of the system, such as hospitals, public safety services, and poison control. Telephones may also be patched into radio transmissions through the base station, enabling, for example, communication between providers using radios in the field and a provider using a telephone. Cellular telephones are becoming an increasingly important part of EMS communications,

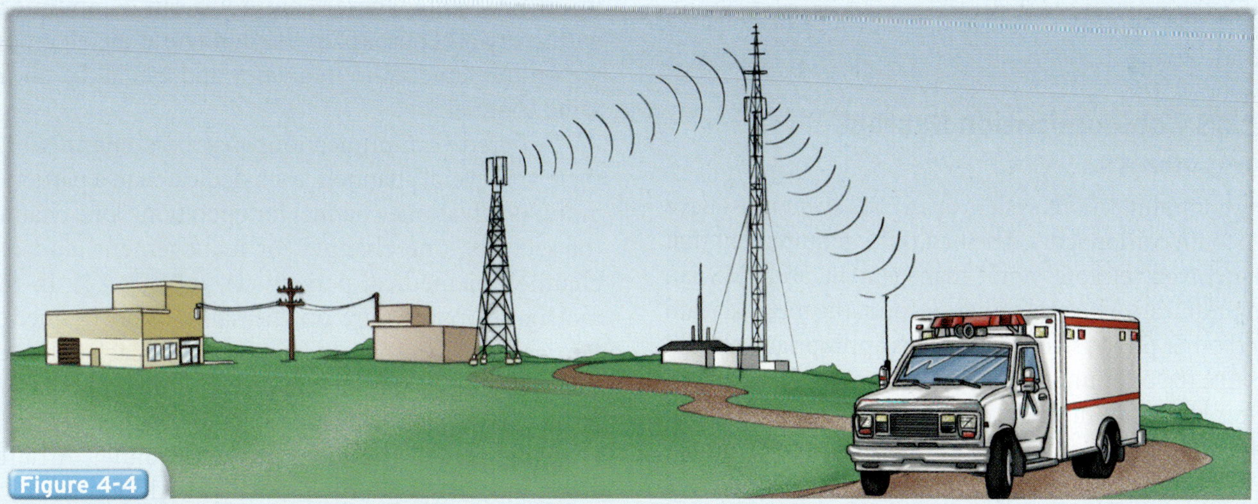

Figure 4-4

A message is sent from the control center by a landline to the transmitter. The radio carrier wave is picked up by the repeater for rebroadcast to outlying units. Return radio traffic is picked up by the repeater and rebroadcast to the control center.

overcoming many of the problems of overcrowded EMS radio frequencies. Cellular phones are cheaper than radios and generally give a much clearer signal. Furthermore, they enable a provider in the field to communicate with anyone who has a telephone.

TIP It is essential to be able to communicate with other providers and event personnel to ensure an efficient response.

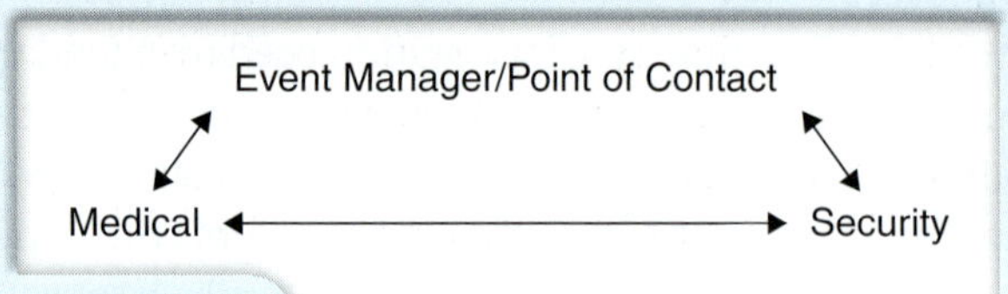

Figure 4-5 A simple communications matrix, used for a small event. Everyone in this matrix is on the same radio frequency and may communicate on one channel.

Communications at a SEMS Event

An important planning consideration for each venue is its communications capacity. Communications needs must take into account the size, terrain, and complexity of the event. Fortunately, many small, medium, and even some large special events have simple communications needs. Most events can operate on one channel.

In general, it is best to specify—in advance—what phone number will be used for internal emergencies, where that phone will ring and who will be responsible for answering it.

SEMS Communication System Components

Any communications system at a SEMS event must have two main components. The first is the requirement that all involved vendors, venue management, and EMS can communicate with each other. Second, the medical team (and other public safety agencies as appropriate) should be able to communicate internally (among themselves). Internal communication is especially important—and difficult—if the venue is geographically dispersed, such as at fairgrounds or athletic facilities with large areas designated for parking. Communication is best handled by installation of an on-site repeater for utilization by the EMS providers.

Communication Matrices

Depending on the size and type of an event, there are several different ways a communications matrix can be set up. A communications matrix is the configuration of a radio system. It can be simple, tiered, or complex. Each group is assigned a channel for communication. If needed, groups may communicate with other groups either directly by using the other group's channel, or through a dispatcher, depending on the size and complexity of the event. A communication matrix may be configured to accommodate one frequency or several frequencies, depending on the communication needs for the event.

A simple communications matrix is one in which the event manager (or point of contact), the medical personnel, and security communicate with each other by radio **Figure 4-5**. This configuration is usually used for small events where each group can communicate with every other group. In this configuration, all groups are on the same radio frequency and can all be on the same channel.

A tiered communications matrix is one in which there are several channels, each dedicated to a particular group (such as one channel for operations, one channel for security, one channel for management, and one channel for medical personnel) **Figure 4-6**. In this matrix, all parties are on the same radio frequency. Parties in each group may speak with each other on their respective channels. If needed, members of one group may speak with members of another group by crossing over to the other group's channel. A tiered communications matrix is usually used for a small- to medium-sized event.

A complex communications matrix accommodates for a central dispatcher who may communicate with a multitude of groups **Figure 4-7**. As in the tiered matrix, in a complex communications network, all parties are on the same radio frequency, and parties in each group speak with each other on their respective channels. If needed, members of one group may speak with members of another group by crossing over to the other group's channel. However, as mentioned, the difference in a complex communications matrix is that it includes a dispatcher who directs radio traffic. This model must include trained dispatch in order to be effective. A complex communications matrix is usually used for larger events such as college football games or pro-football games.

Finally, a communications matrix for multiple radio frequencies may be needed if outside agencies will be involved, such as a fire department Figure 4-8.

Unlike the other matrices discussed, in this matrix, parties may be on different radio frequencies. This model requires a trained dispatcher who not only directs radio traffic, but also relays the communication between parties. This type of communications matrix is used when the event involves multiple agencies or multiple jurisdictions, for example large, complex events such as NASCAR events or a presidential inauguration.

There are advantages and disadvantages to each type of communications matrix. The type of matrix should be designed to suit the specific event.

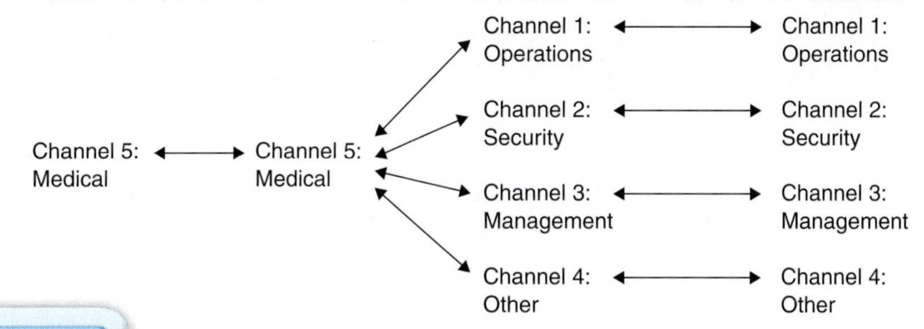

Figure 4-6

A tiered communications matrix, generally used for a small or medium-sized event. Everyone in this matrix is on the same radio frequency, but each group is assigned a different channel. For the purpose of simplicity, this diagram only shows the Medical channel communicating with the other channels.

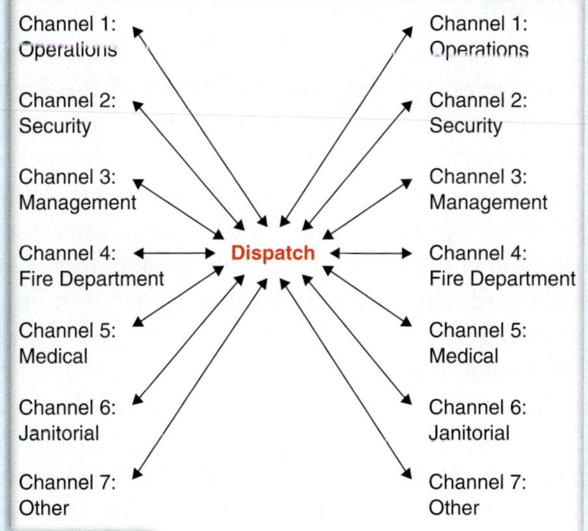

Figure 4-7

A complex communications matrix, used for a large event such as a football game. Everyone in this matrix is on the same radio frequency, but each group is assigned a different channel. Dispatch directs all communication.

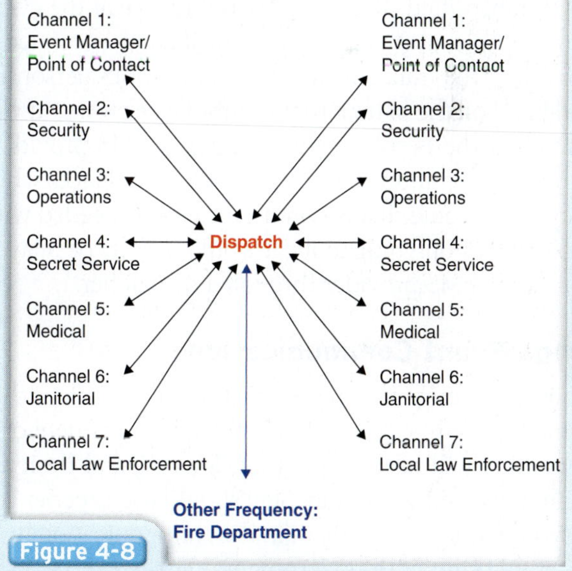

Figure 4-8

A communications matrix for when multiple radio frequencies are being used, for events involving multiple agencies and multiple jurisdictions (usually large events such as NASCAR events, inaugurations, etc). Each group is assigned a channel. Dispatch relays and communicates information between parties.

Communication With Off-site Public Safety Agencies

If working with off-site public safety agencies, there should also be protocols enabling the dispatch center or **public safety answering point (PSAP)** to route its incoming calls back to the venue. (This will not apply to all events.) By having fail-safe communications and established protocols, the PSAP and other public safety agencies are protected from liability that could occur as a result of believing that an incident is being handled when, in fact, the on-site emergency teams are not aware of the incident—a situation that could occur if proper communication backups are not in place. Reciprocally, these procedures provide backup to the on-site public safety agencies by allowing the off-site response to occur if the on-site agencies are taxed or unable to get to the location of the emergency.

Transport

Depending on how the event is managed, SEMS providers may or may not be the personnel who transport the patients to the hospital. If there is an ambulance at the event, SEMS providers will usually conduct the on-site patient care as well as the transport to the hospital, returning to the event once the patient has been transported. If there is no ambulance at the event (for example, at smaller events), or if another service is providing the transport for the event, SEMS personnel will hand off the patient to the ambulance crew and will remain at the event for the duration. SEMS providers will rarely communicate directly with ambulances while they are en route. If any communication is needed with incoming or outgoing units, it would usually be relayed from the SEMS provider through a dispatcher.

Mega-Event Communication

Communication at a mega-event should be viewed as running a temporary EMS communications network. Personnel will need to plan for, lay out, and design a mini-communication hub. Staff should use experienced dispatchers and place them in the communication hub, or, if working with governmental agencies, the Joint Operations Center (JOC). There may be channels within the matrix that do go through dispatch, but all channels should be monitored in the communication hub or JOC. The communication center can be located anywhere, but it must be permanent and receive clear two-way communication. Key personnel may need to know where the center is located, but in certain situations, the location of the communication center may need to be kept secret. Despite the size of an event, it is important to keep the communication structure and process as simple as possible.

Radios

What kind of radios are going to be used at the event? All radios must be FCC compliant. If event personnel rent radios, SEMS providers must talk to the vendor and explain exactly what is needed. Radio coordination is definitely a priority that needs to be worked out with the special event organizers; SEMS providers should not just trust that the event organizers will handle it.

Exclusive EMS channels should be avoided whenever possible. All communications should be on the main channel or security channel. Large events require multiple channels. The use of each channel must be specified before the event. An example of how channels could be allocated is as follows:

- Channel 1: stage operations
- Channel 2: transportation
- Channel 3: operations
- Channel 4: camp ground
- Channel 5: security
- Channel 6: first aid
- Channel 7: fire department/transport

Dispatch

Dispatch may or may not be used at a SEMS event, depending on the size and complexity of the event. An event may be small enough for event personnel to simply talk to each other on one radio channel, or could be complex enough to require official dispatching capabilities. If dispatch capabilities are not necessary during the entire event, one option is to increase your resources during peak flow times to accommodate increased needs.

If dispatch is used, it may be accomplished by telephone, pager, fax, or two-way radio that may include **push-to-talk** technology. Push-to-talk devices can include mobile phones or walkie-talkies, known as half-duplex devices. These devices allow the voice to be transmitted when a button is pushed and allow the listener to hear when the button is released. Most telecommunications equipment today uses digital technology rather than direct or analog transmission and radio tubes. Digital technology offers many advantages in terms of speed, privacy, programmability, and the global positioning system.

Because we know from experience that emergencies usually happen in clusters, the communication center must have the ability to monitor certain events and assign them to side channels, or channels other than the main channel. This assignment of communication will require monitoring of the event if the dispatcher is not actively involved in the incident to ensure that there is both continuity and safety in the communication between and within on-site work groups and/or allied organizations. It is important in active incidents to monitor radio traffic. This ensures an up-to-the-minute report of the status of the incident. Additional communications resources such as these may not be necessary for smaller events, but they are especially useful for larger events with significant communications infrastructure.

Emergency Transmissions

In the event that there is an emergency involving SEMS personnel, the SEMS provider will need to urgently communicate. An example of an urgent situation is when a SEMS provider is assaulted or requires immediate assistance for another reason.

In the preplanning stage, SEMS personnel must determine how urgent communication will be handled. The method for sending an emergency broadcast may already be predetermined by your local jurisdiction (for example, three loud tones may indicate that an emergency broadcast is about to be given), or one may need to be developed based on the unique characteristics of the special event. One option is for the SEMS provider to press the orange button on his or her radio, which sets off an alarm at the dispatch center (this feature is not available on all radios, so it is important to know the radios' features ahead of time, for example if they are being rented). Another option is for the SEMS provider to hold down the button on the radio and in a loud voice, say, "URGENT." When this occurs, everyone else on the channel is to remain quiet so that dispatch and the SEMS provider with the urgent situation may communicate. Regardless, once the method for urgent communication has been determined, all personnel working at the event must be informed of it.

Radio and Electronic Transmission Etiquette

The first and most important rule of communication etiquette is to first listen. Nothing is more annoying than someone who "keys up" in the middle of another conversation without first checking to make sure the repeater is free. If the repeater is in use, providers should wait for a pause in the conversation and simply announce their call sign; they should then wait for one of the other stations to acknowledge their call.

When using the repeater, leaving a couple of seconds between exchanges will allow other stations to join in or make a quick call. Most repeaters have a "courtesy tone" that will help in determining how long to pause. Repeaters have a time-out function that will shut down the transmitter if the repeater is held on for a preset length of time (normally 3 or 4 minutes). This ensures that if someone's transmitter is stuck on for any reason, it will not hold the repeater's transmitter on indefinitely.

The effectiveness of an EMS communications network depends less on the technical hardware than on the people who use it. Communicating effectively by radio under emergency conditions requires skill and experience. Effective radio communication in EMS requires knowledge of the rules that govern the communications and an understanding of conventions for transmitting medical information by radio. Communications should be kept simple, brief, and direct.

You Are the SEMS Provider

CASE 2

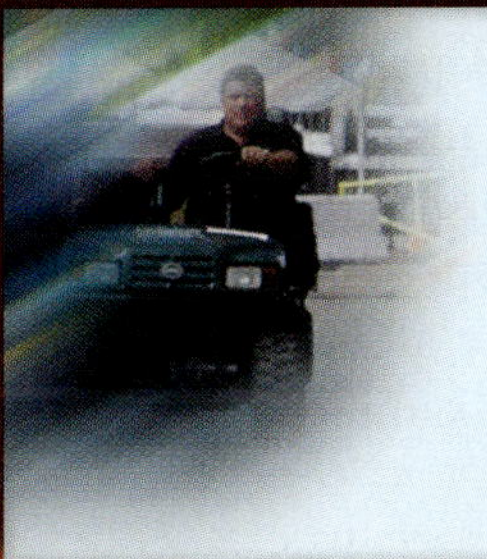

Your service is covering a charity walk on a sweltering day in the middle of summer. You and the other SEMS providers are stationed at the rest stops and around the lunch area. Currently, your staff members are casually moving among the crowd and appear to be engaging in light conversation with the event's participants. Suddenly, you spot a man stumbling around, looking confused.

1. How should you approach him to find out what is going on?
2. How should you communicate this to your fellow SEMS providers?

FCC Regulations

As mentioned earlier, the FCC is the agency of the US government assigned to regulate all radio and television communications in the United States. For radio, the FCC issues licenses, allocates frequencies, establishes technical standards, and establishes and enforces rules and regulations for the operation of radio equipment. FCC officials monitor transmissions on various frequencies and conduct spot checks of base stations to ensure that they are properly licensed. Fines can be imposed for failing to follow the FCC rules and regulations.

The FCC requires that communications over frequencies allocated for emergency medical use be confined to that use. According to the FCC, "Except for test transmissions, stations licensed to ambulance operators or rescue squads may be used only for the transmission of messages pertaining to the safety of life or property and urgent messages necessary for the rendition of an efficient ambulance or emergency rescue service." The use of obscenity and the transmission of messages unrelated to the provision of medical services are forbidden.

Clarity of Transmission

The basic model of communication, whether by radio, intercom, telephone, or face-to-face, involves a sender, a clear message, a receiver, and a feedback loop. The feedback loop is when the sender ensures that the exact message that was sent is received and interpreted properly by the receiver. The first principle of communicating by radio is clarity.

A number of guidelines can help improve the clarity of transmissions:

- Before you begin to transmit, listen to make sure the channel is clear. If another radio transmission is in progress, wait until the parties have finished transmitting before you try to get on the air. Cutting in on someone else's transmission will only ensure that neither of you is adequately heard.
- Once the channel is quiet, press the transmit key for at least 1 second before you start speaking to ensure that the beginning of your message is not lost.
- Start your transmission with the identifying information: give the number or the name of the unit being called first, then your own identification (for example, "First Aid, this is SEMS Mobile 1"). That way, the party being called is alerted immediately and will be listening when you give your own identification, so they can reply at once, "Go ahead, SEMS Mobile 1." If you say, for example, "SEMS Mobile 1 calling First Aid," the recipients might listen only when you have mentioned their identification and, therefore, will miss your identification. Their inevitable response will be, "This is First Aid. What unit is calling?" That extra transmission is a waste of time.
- Keep your mouth close to the microphone, but not too close. About 2 to 3 inches is usually ideal.
- Speak clearly and distinctly, pronouncing each word carefully.
- Do not shout! Shouting distorts the signal. Speak in a normal pitch; very high- and low-pitched sounds do not transmit well. Whispering is not effective for transmitting.
- Do not talk with your mouth full. It muffles transmission.
- Keep calm and keep your voice free from emotion. You do not have to imitate a talking computer, however; a normal conversational tone is fine. Just keep your voice and mind free of panic, anger, excitement, and other feelings that can distort your transmission and your judgment.
- Keep your transmissions brief. Airtime is precious, and emergency medical frequencies are not the place for long philosophic dialogues. Try having your radio reports taped at some point to critique your own transmissions and perfect your style.
- If you have a long message to transmit, break up the message into 30-second segments, checking at the end of each segment to determine whether it was received and understood.
- Do not waste airtime with unnecessary phrases, such as "be advised." Also bear in mind that courtesy is taken for granted; there is no need to use airtime for social graces such as "please," "thank you," and "how nice to hear your voice."
- When speaking a word or name that might be misunderstood, spell it out, using the international phonetic alphabet or a similar system. Suppose, for example, you are asking

the hospital to notify the patient's family doctor whose name might be mistaken for that of another doctor on the staff; you might say, "Notify Dr. Wilby. That's Dr. WHISKEY-INDIA-LIMA-BRAVO-YANKEE, Wilby."

- When presenting numbers that might be misunderstood, transmit the number as a whole, then digit by digit. For example, if the respirations are 16, you would say, "The respirations are sixteen—that is, one-six."

Terminology

Each phase of the communication process requires using terminology understood by the people with whom providers are communicating. Patients might need providers to explain medical conditions in terms that patients know and understand. When relaying information to the other medical personnel, providers can use the medical terminology they have learned to make radio reports clear. The old saying, "When in Rome, do as the Romans," applies here. Using medical terminology and avoiding slang terms demonstrates professionalism and respect for everyone with whom providers work.

Content of Transmissions

Radio transmissions for EMS should be brief, to the point, and professional in tone. Here are some guidelines about what should and should not be included in EMS radio communications:

- The first thing to remember when you get "on the air" is that anyone may be listening. It is essential to protect the privacy of the patient at all times. Do not use the patient's name on the air, and do not transmit personal information about the patient because this would violate the Health Insurance Portability and Accountability Act (HIPAA) guidelines on confidentiality.
- Do not assume that your cellular telephone offers you protected conversations. There are scanners on the market that can tune into the local cellular frequencies. Do not say anything on the radio or the cellular phone that you do not want everyone in town to hear.
- Use "we," not "I," to refer to yourself, and use proper names and titles to refer to others when necessary.
- Do not try to be a comedian or a critic. There is no place for unprofessional behavior, sarcasm, or other poor conduct on emergency medical radio frequencies.
- Do not use profane language on the air. Aside from the reflection on your professional character, the FCC might issue civil monetary penalties, revoke a license, or deny a renewal application. In addition, violators of the law, if convicted in a federal district court, are subject to criminal fines and/or imprisonment for up to 2 years.
- Use professional language, but do not show off. Once again, remember that the object of the exercise is to communicate information, not to stun your listener into awe and admiration. Using proper medical terminology is advisable when done correctly.
- Avoid using words that are difficult to hear. The word "yes," for example, is easily lost in transmission; use "affirmative" instead. Similarly, use "negative" instead of "no."
- Use standard formats agreed on by your EMS service for transmission of information. The patient's history, for example, should always be presented in the same order. When the listeners know what they are listening for, they are less likely to miss parts of the transmission.
- When you finish transmitting, obtain confirmation that the transmission was received. When you receive instructions by radio from the dispatcher or from medical control, echo the order back to make certain you have understood it correctly.
- Question any orders you did not hear clearly or did not understand.
- Use EMS frequencies only for emergency medical communications.

TIP

Communication plans at and during the event must be clear. Prior to the event, it is crucial to review the emergency response plan with everybody who will be involved on event day. A clear communication system is key in making sure incidents are handled smoothly, should they occur.

You Are the SEMS Provider SUMMARY

CASE 1

1. **What could you have done to prevent this scenario from occurring?**
   Without superior planning and a thorough understanding of radio systems, SEMS and event personnel could endanger both patrons and their own employees. Instead of piecing together an unknown system, event promoters should be encouraged by SEMS personnel to install radio systems from the ground up. Radio installation companies will enable promoters to address factors such as terrain, area, and volume of traffic. Some communities even have complex multi-tiered radio systems, such as the 800 MHz, that SEMS personnel can access for event purposes. However, most places and events will need to build a new system from the ground up. Testing any new system's abilities throughout the event location is also an essential part of ensuring communication safety.
2. **What would your next action be if you were in a dangerous situation and your chain of communication has broken down?**
   At this point in the scenario, it would be very beneficial to have a cell phone. In this case, see if any other providers or personnel in the area have a cell phone available. Always remember that bringing a cell phone or creating a backup method of communication is crucial when experimenting with new systems. It is also important to always know the phone numbers of points of contact for the event.

CASE 2

1. **How should you approach him to find out what is going on?**
   Politely engage him in conversation and gauge his response to your questions, such as, "Hello, sir, how are you doing today?" or "How are you enjoying the fair?" His response allows you to ascertain that the man has a mild case of heat exhaustion, which you quickly treat at the nearest station.
2. **How should you communicate this to your fellow SEMS providers?**
   An example of how you might communicate about this event would be, "First Aid, this is SEMS Mobile 1." After First Aid acknowledges your transmission, you may continue with, "We are transporting one patient back to First Aid," or, depending on the urgency of the patient's condition, "First Aid, this patient is going to bypass First Aid and go directly to transport." You may include details about the patient's condition as needed. In cases where the communications matrix involves dispatch, you may communicate with them, and your message will be relayed to the intended receiving party. For example dispatch may say, "SEMS Mobile 1, this is Dispatch. We have a call backstage." You would reply, "Dispatch, this is SEMS Mobile 1 responding." In all cases, ensure that your communication is clear and professional.

Ready for Review

- Communication at a SEMS event requires special consideration.
- Radio frequencies are designed by their cycles per second, or hertz (Hz). Radios that operate at 800 MHz are common in EMS systems because this frequency offers excellent penetration of buildings and has minimal interference and reduced channel noise.
- Cellular phones are becoming common in EMS communications. At some larger events, COWs are brought in to increase cellular site availability.
- Assigned radio frequencies may be used in a variety of systems, including simplex, duplex, and multiplex.
- The base station is a collection of radio equipment consisting, at minimum, of a transmitter, receiver, and antenna.
- A mobile transmitter/receiver, or mobile transceiver, is a two-way radio mounted in a vehicle.
- Portable, handheld radios are useful when paramedics must work at a distance from their vehicle but need to stay in communication with the base or with one another.
- A repeater is a miniature base station used to extend the transmitting and receiving range of a telemetry or voice communications system. At a SEMS event, engineers will assess the topography and set up repeaters where they can best receive and send signals.
- A backup communications system is an important feature of a SEMS communication network.
- Dispatch may or may not be used at a SEMS event, depending on the size and complexity of the event. An event may be complex enough to require official dispatching capabilities.
- The communications network for a SEMS event should be planned depending on the type and scope of the event. Plan details such as what phone number will be used for internal emergencies, where that phone will ring, and who will be responsible for answering it.
- There are various types of communication matrices that can be used at a SEMS event: simple, tiered, complex, and a matrix for multiple radio frequencies. Each type of communication matrix has advantages and disadvantages. The communication matrix should be tailored to the event.
- If the event includes working with off-site public safety agencies, the venue must have established communications to ensure that all relevant parties are aware of emergency incidents and that providers are responding to them.
- SEMS managers must work with event organizers to determine what kind of radios are going to be used at the event.
- Avoid exclusive EMS channels whenever possible. All communications should be on the main channel or security channel. Large events may require multiple channels.
- The FCC is the agency of the US government assigned to regulate all radio and television communications in the United States.
- All radios must be FCC compliant. If event personnel rent radios, SEMS providers must talk to the vendor and explain exactly what is needed.
- Certain larger events require a dispatcher. The communication center must also be able to monitor the event to ensure continuity of communication between and within groups.
- Mega-event communication should be similar to a temporary EMS communications network. The physical location of the communication center may need to be a secret in certain situations.
- In the preplanning stage, SEMS personnel must determine how urgent communication will be handled. Options include sending an alarm to the dispatch center (if one is being used), or holding down the button on the radio and in a loud voice, saying, "URGENT."
- The first and most important rule of radio communications is to first listen.
- The basic model of communication involves a *sender*, a clear *message*, a *receiver,* and a *feedback loop*. The feedback loop is when the sender ensures that the exact message that was sent is received and interpreted properly by the receiver.
- Radio transmissions for EMS should be brief, to the point, and professional in tone.

Vital Vocabulary

base station Assembly of radio equipment consisting of at least a transmitter, receiver, and antenna connection at a fixed location.

cells on wheels (COWs) Temporary cell phone towers that can be brought in to increase cellular site availability.

communications matrix The configuration of a radio system, which can be simple, tiered, or complex; which includes multiple channels for different groups to communicate with other members of their group, or other groups; and may be configured to accommodate one frequency or several frequencies depending on the communication needs for the event.

duplex Radio system using more than one frequency to permit simultaneous transmission and reception.

Federal Communications Commission (FCC) The federal agency that has jurisdiction over interstate and international telephone and telegraph services and satellite communications, all of which may involve EMS activity.

frequency In radio communications, the number of cycles per second of a signal, inversely related to the wavelength.

hertz (Hz) Unit of frequency equal to one cycle per second.

multiplex Method by which simultaneous transmission of voice and ECG signals can be achieved over a single radio frequency.

noise In radio communications, interference in a radio signal.

portable radio A handheld radio that can be carried on a person and is used for communications away from a vehicle.

public safety answering point (PSAP) An official term for a dispatch center; a designated location where incoming calls to public safety are routed during an event; helps ensure that all incidents are communicated to SEMS providers.

push-to-talk A method of communication that uses a half-duplex communications system. By pushing a button on the communication device, a person can send; by releasing the button, a person can receive.

repeater Miniature transmitter that picks up a radio signal and rebroadcasts it, extending the range of a radio communications system.

simplex Method of radio communication using a single frequency that enables transmission or reception of voice or an electrocardiogram signal but is incapable of simultaneous transmission and reception.

transceiver A radio transmitter and receiver housed in the same radio; a two-way radio.

trunking Sharing of radio frequencies by multiple agencies or systems.

ultrahigh frequency (UHF) band The portion of the radio frequency spectrum between 300 and 3,000 MHz.

very high frequency (VHF) band The portion of the radio frequency spectrum between 30 and 150 MHz.

CHAPTER

Safety Concerns 5

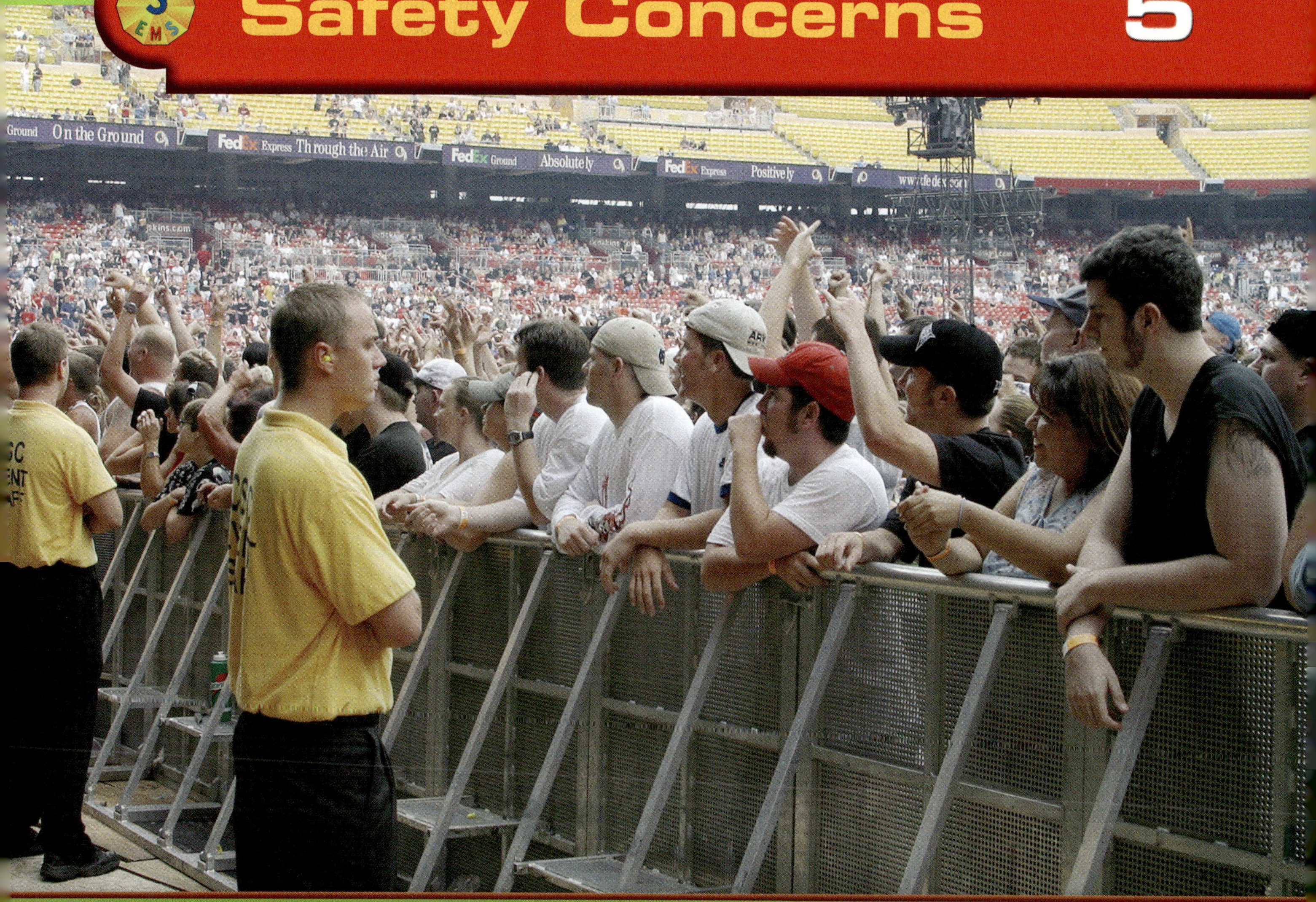

LEARNING OBJECTIVES

- Outline common security concerns surrounding a special event, including violence, alcohol and drug use, gangs, and terrorism.
- Understand how certain medical conditions pose a threat to safety.
- List the common precursors to violent incidents.
- Understand the role of demographics of an event and the importance of predicting the crowd mentality.
- Establish emergency planning techniques in order to effectively prevent and react to crowd behavior problems.
- Describe safe vehicle and helicopter operations in a crowd.
- Explain what preplanning considerations should be taken to ensure the safety and efficacy of emergency medical services (EMS) equipment in a special events setting.
- Know the precursors, signs, and actions to take when dealing with sexual assault.

Introduction

Special events medical services (SEMS) providers must prepare for a number of concerns relating to safety. Significant effort is required to account for the safety of all SEMS providers. The SEMS manager should consider a variety of security and medical concerns as well as vehicle and helicopter operations and the use of specific EMS equipment. In addition, there may be specific safety concerns unique to a particular event.

Security Concerns

It would be impossible to address every special situation that may arise during a SEMS-covered event. Instead, SEMS providers must know the particular nuisances that are inherent to a special event. As mentioned in previous chapters, preplanning is crucial. SEMS providers should do some research and, when possible, talk to other EMS providers who have serviced similar special events. They should do a walk-through and ensure that all personnel are notified of any possible security issues. They should also consider relevant threats to security; this can be as simple as an event that has a high incidence of alcohol consumption or as extreme as gang violence. If servicing a high-profile event or covering an event with a high-profile individual, SEMS managers must methodically review the various security concerns that could arise, such as terrorist incidents. They should use resources that are available in their area. Local police, security agencies, state police, and even federal agencies may have information to share about possible threats to the venue or other security concerns.

TIP

In the preplanning stage, SEMS personnel must determine how urgent communication will be handled. One option is for the SEMS provider to hold down the button on the radio and in a loud voice say, "Urgent!" When this occurs, everyone else on the channel is to remain quiet so that dispatch and the SEMS provider with the urgent situation may communicate.

Unfortunately, violence can occur at special events. Where crowds gather, violence is always a potential problem, no matter the reason for the event. Even an event with a good intention, such as a community fair, can produce unfortunate issues. News sources repeatedly report on special events that are the site of violent encounters. Certain types of special events such as music festivals, protest rallies, and sporting events with large crowds interacting in a small area; events that include alcohol consumption; and events that attract individuals who may be looking to incite a crowd disturbance are especially prone to violent incidents. If the energy level is high, such as at a rock concert or a high-stakes sporting event, attendees may become very worked up. These crowds have a higher risk for a violent

You Are the SEMS Provider

CASE 1

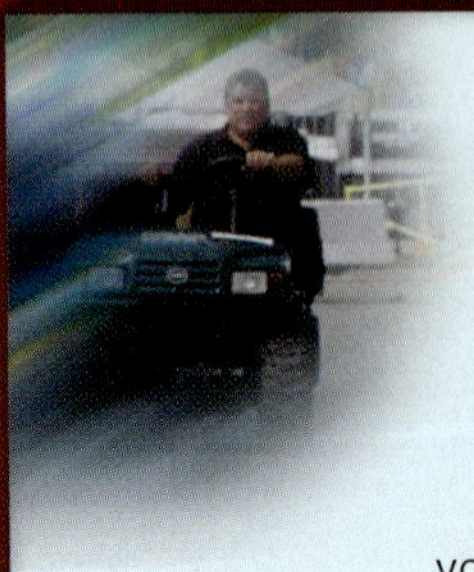

It is a warm fall day on a local college campus when two rival football teams meet on the field. This will be the 98th meeting between these fierce rivals. The two university teams are separated by only 20 miles, and both teams are nationally ranked. The entire state seems to have tickets for this game, and the stadium is crowded with over 100,000 people. Tailgating begins early in the morning and, because it is a night game, continues for several hours.

You are on a mobile medical team, stationed near the student section. Late in the fourth quarter, both teams are tied when you get a call about an unconscious person in the stands. As you approach, you see the patient is dressed in the opposing team's colors. Several of his friends are yelling at other spectators who are fans of the rival team. You kneel down next to your patient to begin your care when someone in the crowd throws a beer. A fight breaks out.

1. How do you respond? Do you continue your care?
2. How could you have anticipated this situation?

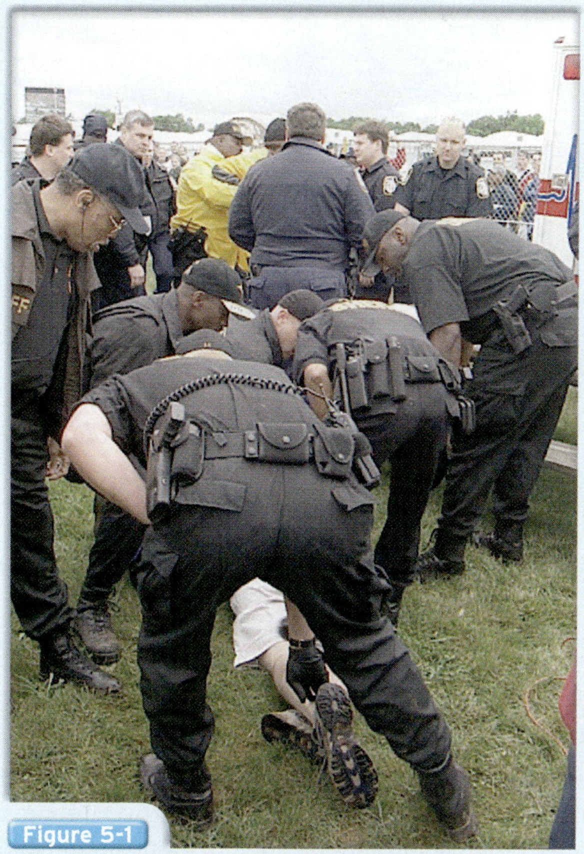

Figure 5-1

Violent encounters may occur at special events and could necessitate a security takedown. SEMS providers should not begin patient care until safety concerns are addressed.

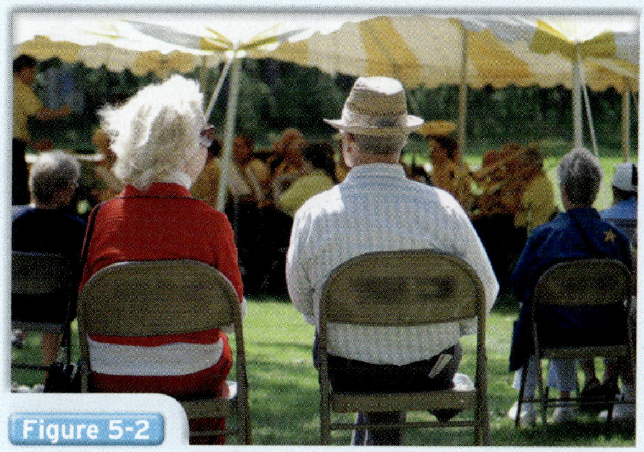

Figure 5-2

An older crowd may require chairs, warming or cooling stations, or wheelchairs.

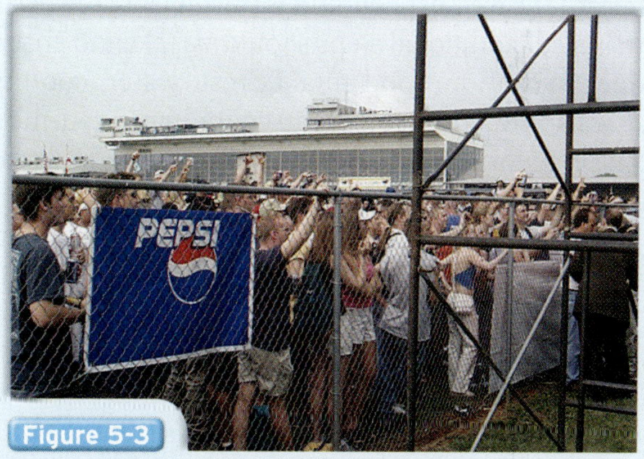

Figure 5-3

A younger crowd may have a higher incidence of trauma and emergencies related to substance abuse.

encounter Figure 5-1. Finally, incidents at which drug use is likely, such as some music festivals or concerts, may also pose a threat of violence, or at least will have emergencies related to this factor.

Crowd Dynamics

Crowd Demographics

Different types of events draw different types of spectators, and the issue of crowd demographics plays an important role in response planning. SEMS providers should try to anticipate the **crowd demographics**, especially age distribution, for a given special event to determine possible medical needs.

It is important to consider the age of the attendees. Will a large percentage of the crowd be a certain age (or will the crowd contain many different age groups)? Crowds consisting of middle-aged or older adults may require medical support such as chairs, water, cooling and warming stations, and wheelchairs Figure 5-2. Crowds consisting of adolescents or young adults may require more trauma and wound care and may have emergencies related to substance abuse Figure 5-3. Events with younger crowds tend to be more "high energy" or risk-oriented, which can lead to more incidents of violence or substance abuse. However, these are not hard and fast rules. An older crowd may require more trauma or wound care due to an increased incidence of falls and lacerations, and an older crowd can still engage in substance abuse. Be aware of the event's average age group, but consider other factors such as the type of event and the event's history.

Younger crowds tend to need additional assistance in hot or cold weather, because they are more likely to

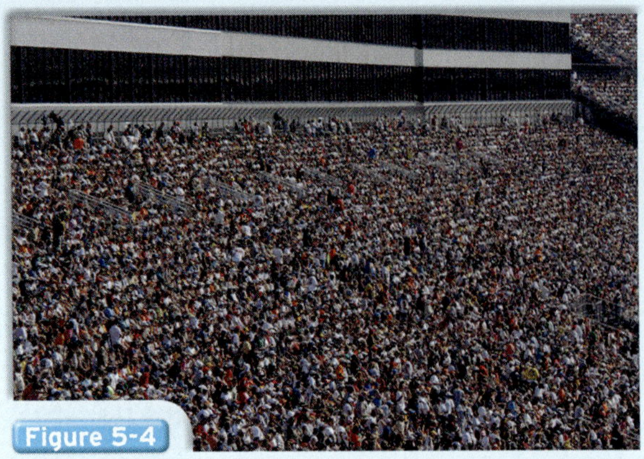

Figure 5-4

With very large crowds, expect a range of demographics and emergencies.

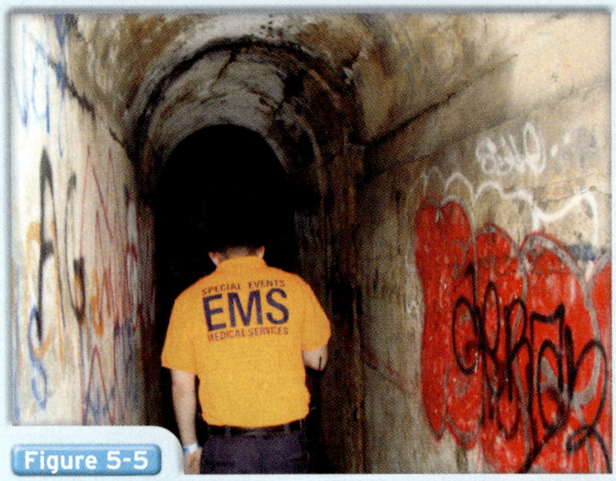

Figure 5-5

Events that are associated with drug culture will likely have higher rates of injury. This photo shows a location at a rave concert where a patient fell from above. Also note the access/egress issues this tunnel would present.

disregard the weather conditions. If younger crowds are anticipated, additional steps should be taken to ensure proper hydration, food intake, rest, water, cooling, and warming. Younger event-goers may need more monitoring for preventative and maintenance measures (eg, encouraging them to stay hydrated, seek shade). Some crowds may be so large that you may need to anticipate all ages and types of emergencies Figure 5-4.

The type of event can help SEMS providers anticipate the crowd demographics. For example, if an older folk musician is performing, SEMS providers should prepare for attendees to be consistent with the main fan base—an older, calmer population—and prepare for preexisting medical conditions like angina and chronic obstructive pulmonary disease. If a genre of music is affiliated with a drug culture, a concert within the same genre will likely attract attendees who participate in substance abuse. For example, if a younger rap group or metal group is performing, the crowd is likely to be younger and more aggressive, leading to a higher rate of injuries and drug use Figure 5-5.

TIP

When planning to cover an event, consider the possibility of renting wheelchairs. At any large event or at an event where attendees could sustain leg or foot injuries, it is prudent to have wheelchairs available. This should be a standard consideration when preplanning.

Crowd Energy

The behavior or energy level of a crowd may be affected by the event (eg, type of music, rivalry between sporting teams, or a religious revival). When preplanning SEMS coverage of an event, try to anticipate the crowd's energy level. Once at the event, observe the crowd to gauge the energy level and note whether it matches with the energy level you expected Figure 5-6. If it does not, take measures to adjust your plan (for example, request additional equipment or backup if you believe you will need it).

Crowd Activities

Certain events may include rough or violent crowd activities such as moshing, crowd surfing, and crowd surging, which are often precursors to violent encounters. These activities are discussed next.

Moshing

Moshing is a modern version of the punk tradition of slam dancing. It is popular among young men. Individuals enter into the "pit," an area located in front of the stage, and flail around, wildly smashing into each other Figure 5-7. With the teaming forces of the music, the adrenaline, and the physical contact, a mosh pit quickly becomes an active and hazardous place. Injuries from moshing are common.

At a recent concert, a young man was moshing, and, after being knocked to the ground, he was stomped

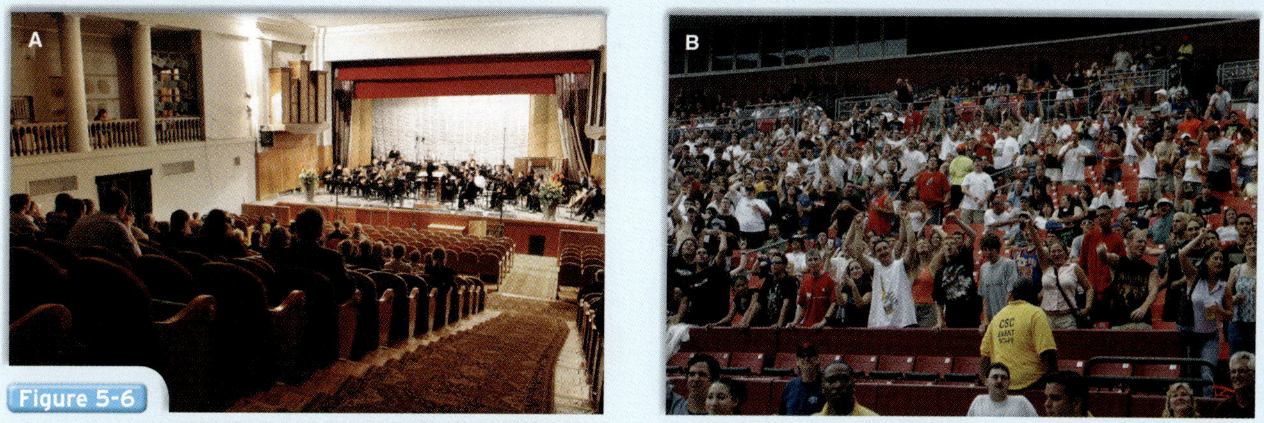

Figure 5-6

Try to gauge the energy level of the crowd. **A.** This is likely a low-energy crowd. **B.** This is likely a high-energy crowd.

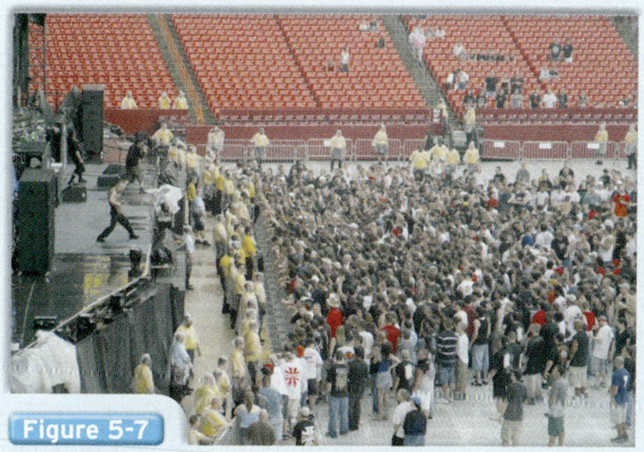

Figure 5-7

A mosh pit can be a very dangerous place and may be a precursor to violence, injury, or sexual assault.

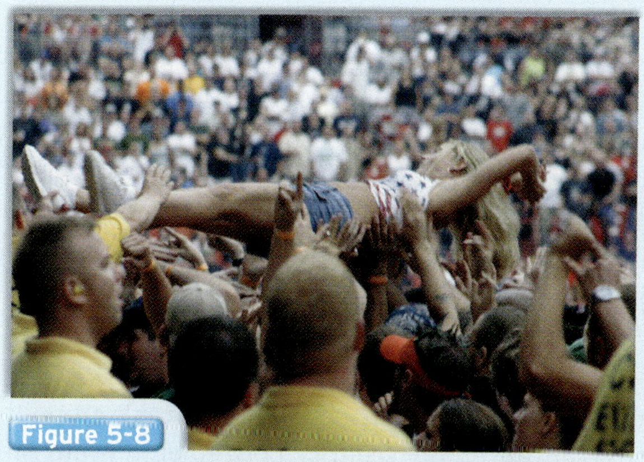

Figure 5-8

Crowd surfers may be injured from a fall or sexually assaulted.

by the crowd until he lost consciousness. After he had been fully examined, it was evident that the patient had sustained a subdural bleed. Broken bones, spinal cord injuries, sexual assaults, and rapes are the most frequent types of injuries and violent acts that occur in mosh pits. SEMS personnel should coordinate with security to plan for a safe extraction of a patient and should only enter a highly charged mosh pit alone in the direst of circumstances.

Bull in the ring (or "bull in the middle") is a modified form of moshing. It occurs when one person is surrounded by a crowd and must break through the crowd by smashing into people. Bull in the ring often occurs in mosh pits or when two rival groups meet. Once alcohol is added to the mix of violent bodily contact and high-energy music, the situation could spark violent encounters. With bull in the ring, SEMS providers can expect to see the same type of injuries as with moshing, including head and spinal injuries and broken bones.

Crowd Surfing

Crowd surfing usually begins with stage diving, which is when someone dives off the stage and into the crowd. The stage diver lays on top of the crowd and is passed around ("surfing" through the crowd) Figure 5-8. The two main safety hazards of crowd surfing are falls to the person surfing and sexual assault (primarily to women). When a crowd surfer is dropped by the crowd, he or she can sustain injury from the impact of hitting the ground and may be trampled by the crowd. SEMS personnel should work with security to move the patient to a safe location for treatment.

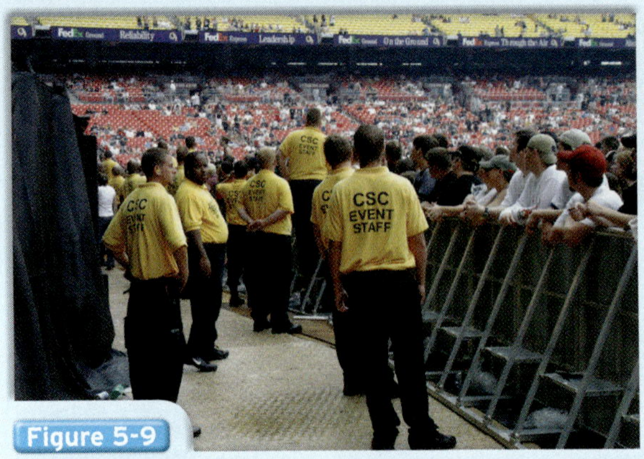

Figure 5-9

A barricade may be used to help prevent crowd surging.

For cases of sexual assault, it may be difficult for SEMS personnel to learn of the assault and treat the patient privately in such a public setting. The provider will usually not learn of the assault until he or she interviews the victim. Wrap the patient in a sheet or blanket and follow your service's sexual assault protocols. Such an incident is not only a SEMS issue but is also a law enforcement issue.

Crowd Surging

Crowd surging is when a crowd moves as a group, for example to overtake security personnel to jump onto the stage at a performance. To prevent crowd surges, many venues will place a security barricade in front of the stage Figure 5-9. **Barricade operations**, generally taught to security personnel, is a skill set on how to safely protect and remove people in distress who may become pinned against a barricade (eg, near a stage). If a SEMS provider is assigned to floor duty or in front of the stage, it is best if he or she is trained in barricade rescue operations, though this may not be possible in all cases. SEMS personnel should be aware of typical security procedures in the event of a crowd surge and should meet with the event security prior to the date to discuss protocol and expectations from SEMS staff in response to such an incident. In general, a SEMS provider should not try to assist in managing a crowd surge unless he or she is trained in barricade operations and security has agreed during preplanning to SEMS assisting in this role.

> **TIP**
> In a crowd surge, you may be tempted to try to help security deal with the surge, but unless you are trained in barricade operations, you should stay back and allow the trained professionals to rescue the patients from a violent crowd. Otherwise, you may become a victim.

Front-to-Back Crowd Issues

It is important for SEMS providers to recognize differences in front-to-back communication; patrons at the rear of the crowd often have access to less information than those at the front. As a consequence, people toward the back of a crowd may cause problems, such as moving forward to try to see what is happening in the front of the crowd. This pressing forward can crush people and cause injuries; in severe cases, it can cause death. Lighter crowd density at the rear allows for freer movement; more dense crowds at the front may be immobile and under great pressure. Security personnel often attempt local control of the crowd from the front, urging people not to push, but this type of control is relatively ineffective during a serious crowd incident.

Crowd Behavior

Crowd psychology is an important, yet unpredictable part of any event. The mood and behavior of a crowd are important considerations; people's behavior is affected when they are in a crowd. With experience, SEMS providers will learn to sense the mood of a crowd. There are some concepts of crowd behavior that SEMS-trained personnel should understand.

Pack mentality (also called mob mentality) occurs when individuals in a large crowd base their decisions on what they believe to be the collective standpoint, rather than basing decisions on their own beliefs and thought processes (essentially no longer thinking for themselves). Pack mentality can lead to members of a group performing unthinkable actions that they would never otherwise do, such as acts committed in riot situations. Similarly, SEMS providers must be aware of **herd mentality**, in which people react as a herd does when startled or enraged. This reaction can be initiated by an aggressive security or SEMS response; the crowd

TIP SEMS providers should be on the lookout for pack or herd mentality, which may lead to rioting.

reacts by initiating violence or generally becoming dangerous and unpredictable. SEMS providers should never take an aggressive tone and should refrain from making inflammatory statements. These are examples of overly aggressive responses that could incite a crowd.

Physiologic Effects of Being in a Crowd

Crowded places may give attendees a feeling of **crowd syndrome**, meaning that they may begin to feel sweaty, hot, faint, paranoid, and short of breath due to the density of the crowd, intense volume of performers (such as at a concert), or flashing lights. Usually, finding a quiet, private place away from the crowd can help treat these symptoms.

Psychological Effects of Being in a Crowd

A chaotic event in the crowd or epidemic hysteria can have an impact on the crowd's emotional state and can produce a wave of panic. For example, if a show is sold out or is late to start, the crowd may become irritated. If a fight occurs, the crowd may become angry or scared and react by rioting or panicking Figure 5-10. Humans are animals of instinct and often have the same inherent panic reactions as any other animal. Once people sense fear and panic, it may be difficult for them to calm down in a crowd setting.

Crowd panic is a problematic issue and can be extremely dangerous. A trigger such as a fight in the middle of a crowd or a loud startling noise (such as fireworks or gunfire) can create widespread panic. People may not think rationally when they are part of a crowd; they react with herd mentality. The stress levels caused by being in a chaotic crowd lead people to make decisions based solely on self-preservation. One effort that is vital in preventing and dealing with a crowd panic situation is ensuring that the entrances and exits provide a safe route into the facility as well as a safe route of egress.

Once a crowd becomes irritated, it is extremely difficult to control. Crowd incidents often occur at music-related events such as concerts and festivals, but can occur at any type of event. Consider the potential for violence at a sporting event where rival teams are

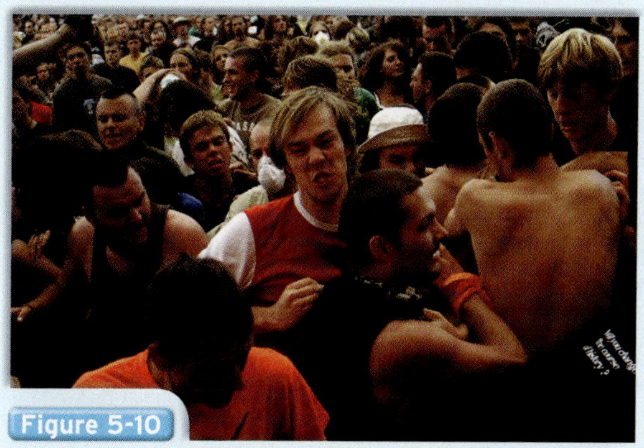

Figure 5-10

If a fight breaks out in a crowd, expect injuries related to the fight and other emergencies among attendees in the vicinity of the fight.

competing. Even seemingly benign events can experience crowd issues. For example, several people were killed due to crowd incidents during visits from Pope John Paul II in Zaire and Brazil.

When a crowd pushes, the pressure on people within the crowd can be extremely forceful. Consequently, most deaths from crowd incidents are not due to trampling, but rather asphyxia. People may become stacked on top of each other while being pressed and crushed. People also try to push off each other in an attempt to find more space, and this can cause additional injuries. As the crowd pushes, the shock wave from the push ripples through the crowd. It causes additional injury and may be strong enough to remove people's clothing and shoes. Incidents within a crowd cause additional psychological effects on people in the crowd as well. Anxiety levels increase, causing additional breathing problems and emergencies. The heat that is caused by many people being pressed together can cause additional emergencies, such as weakness and fainting, which are exacerbated by anxiety.

Preplanning for Crowds

Egress Choke Points

Choke points are locations where a pathway has less capacity, the normal direction of movement changes, or there is a confluence of traffic streams. These areas result in conflicts or accident exposure. Examples include directional changes where there are inadequately

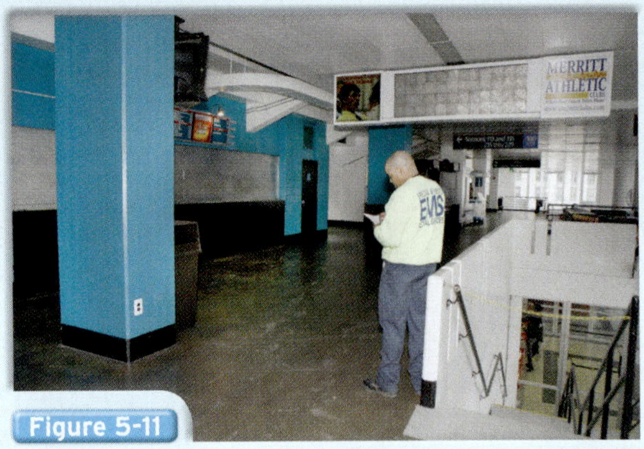

Figure 5-11

A choke point. In this example, during an event, lines will form in front of the vending area and block the stream of traffic.

guarded openings to lower levels, at stair approaches, and landings at the ends of escalators Figure 5-11. Crowd pressure at such locations has resulted in people being pushed over guardrails or down stairs, or in the structural failure of guardrails.

Note any entries or exits that could be problematic. National Fire Protection Association standards dictate that all doors must swing out and that all exits must be unobstructed and be clearly marked. This code came about as a result of the Coconut Grove Fire that occurred on November 28, 1942, in Boston, Massachusetts, where a fire killed 492 people and injured hundreds more. Exit doors at the site had not been clearly marked. The main door was a revolving door instead of a door that swung outward, and other exit doors had been welded shut to stop patrons from leaving without paying their bill. Fire codes were changed across the country due to the problems identified as a result of this fire.

During preplanning, it will be important to predetermine potential choke points and plan for emergencies in these areas, or even work with event management to change pathways to decrease the number of choke points, if possible.

Capacity Calculations

Many indoor events will have seating areas; therefore, capacity of the event is already predetermined, at least for those areas (the capacity will equal the number of seats). However, at events where a standing crowd gathers in a defined space to watch entertainment (such as at a street theater or a music event), the general guideline is for a clear, flat, open space with a reasonable view of the performance, with two people per 3 ft^2 (1 m^2). For example, an average concert crowd of 16,000 people would require a minimum of 24,000 ft^2 (8,000 m^2), which is approximately 2 acres. Even this is not a very large area, and the people will be very close together. Some experts feel that this formula is ineffective because it assumes that people will stand regimentally in the space allotted to them, and no consideration is given to how people will interpret space (eg, if they dance, thereby potentially moving outside their allotted space). Some experts say this area needs to be 2 to 3 times this amount to allow for people to have a comfortable amount of personal space.

Crowd Management

Within any SEMS situation, the keys to success are assessing factors that can affect crowd behavior and mood, preplanning for foreseeable challenges, and addressing any adverse factors. In most cases, problems with crowd behavior can be anticipated, such as overcrowding, drug or alcohol use, delays in the performance, or a trigger such as a fight or emergency.

Controlling crowd capacity is a key concern. If the maximum capacity is exceeded, discomfort and frustration could take over the crowd and lead to panic. By adhering to the venue's capacity (eg, not overselling the event), the venue can eliminate this risk.

SEMS providers must be professional and nonjudgmental at all times. For example, it would be inappropriate for a provider to display loyalty to a particular team at a sporting event because this may provoke an angry response from excited fans. SEMS providers must be realistic when it comes to security risks, recognize environments that have the potential for violence, and avoid any conduct that may provoke the crowd to respond in a violent manner.

When violence does occur, SEMS personnel should immediately and discreetly alert security of any potentially violent situations and remove themselves and patients from the situation as quickly and safely as possible. Often, SEMS personnel must venture into a crowd with a high level of activity to retrieve a victim. It is essential to understand that in their excited state crowd members can turn on the SEMS providers. As such, providers must have specific procedures in place for what to do in these situations.

Removing a victim from a violent crowd can be challenging. All efforts to remove a victim from a crowd should be preplanned with event security. The questions to ask are:

- How will the SEMS team enter?
- Who will set the perimeter?
- How will the SEMS providers' safety be ensured?
- Where is the exit route to private locations?

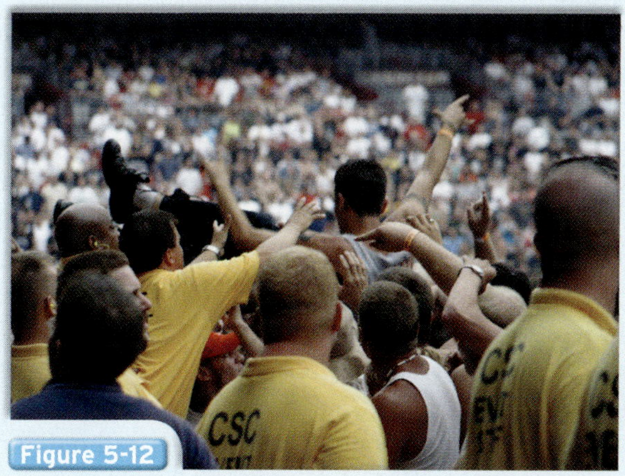

Figure 5-12

It may be necessary to lift a patient over a crowd to remove him or her from the crowd, but this is a last resort.

Remember to preplan for how to access individuals in the middle of a dense, uncontrolled crowd, and also how to handle an incident in a mosh pit and an incident involving a crowd surge. In some cases the only way to remove patients from these areas may be by lifting them up and moving them overhead to the exterior of the crowd, though this is a last resort Figure 5-12.

TIP During patient treatment, do not stay in crowds for long periods. Move the patient to a safe, secure location as soon as possible.

Supervision is a second key consideration in crowd management. Security officials are generally the most common form of supervision. During the preplanning process, SEMS providers should inquire about the security personnel who will be on site during the event. While venue security is certainly not a SEMS responsibility, failure to ensure adequate security personnel may create problems for SEMS providers. If they frequently cover events with security issues, it may be wise for SEMS providers to obtain training in security-related matters such as barricade operations, crowd control, and hazard mitigation.

If you work at many events in one area, or many events at the same venue, it is a good idea to create a working relationship with the companies in your area that provide security services because you may work with them frequently. Meeting with security personnel throughout the year will allow you to understand their capabilities and educate them about your needs. This open line of communication will go a long way in securing the safety of all concerned. Consistent and repetitive training will prepare security staff to prevent panic and react to problematic situations.

Finally, remember that at a special event it is important for people to feel safe and comfortable. A comfortable crowd is a happy crowd, and a happy crowd is often a safer crowd. When preplanning the event, carefully assess all possible risks, and work with the event and risk managers to mitigate the potential for injury. For example, if the event location borders a busy freeway, it might be wise for event personnel to erect a fence blocking access and also to post security personnel at that location to ensure that no one climbs the fence.

You Are the SEMS Provider

CASE 2

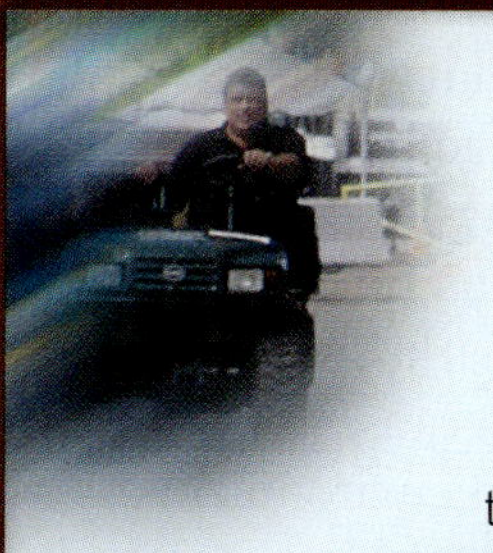

You are providing SEMS coverage at an indoor rock concert. There are about 8,000 attendees at the venue. Adrenaline rushes as the show proceeds with a growing level of excitement, and everything seems to be sound. Suddenly, there is a disturbance among the people. Before you can react, the crowd surges forward. In an instant there are more than a dozen people on the ground, lying face down. They are visibly distressed and are using all their strength in an attempt to stand up, but people in the crowd do not assist and seem not to notice. The people on the ground continue to struggle while the crowd continues to push and trample them. You realize that the area has succumbed to pandemonium.

1. What should SEMS providers' first response be?
2. How should providers access and treat these patients?

Alcohol and Drug Use

Alcohol and drugs are serious variables that can be difficult to predict and plan for. In general, SEMS providers should expect a greater incidence of alcohol-related and drug-related emergencies at events where spectators are adolescents or young adults. Alcohol and drugs may lead to more trauma, altercations, and car crashes. The concern for alcohol-related and drug-related events should be a primary one at rock concerts, hip-hop concerts, music festivals, and sporting events, so be sure to preplan for it at such events; however, remember that alcohol and drugs can be present at any type of event.

Alcohol Consumption

Because intoxicated people are often more aggressive than sober people, alcohol often contributes to violent behavior, accidents, and mishaps. Researchers at the National Institutes of Health have concluded that while alcohol does not trigger aggressive behavior, it can be a facilitator of violent events. In their bar violence study, researchers found that men who reported experiencing violence in a bar were also more likely to report having problems with alcohol in general; researchers found that women who experienced violence in a bar setting were more prone to demonstrating high levels of anger and consumed higher-than-average levels of alcohol.

TIP

Treatment of minors and treatment of intoxicated persons are two separate issues. When treating an intoxicated minor remember that a minor generally is not legally able to refuse treatment. To refrain from treating a minor can be a tricky matter for all persons involved. Review your state's laws and your organization's policy concerning treatment of minors, and proceed accordingly.

Drug Use

SEMS providers will deal with various kinds of drugs, both illegal and legal. The landscape of the drug world is ever-changing. SEMS providers should make an effort to stay up-to-date on new and emerging drug use trends by communicating with local hospitals and law enforcement as well as any local, state, or national databases. This section presents some of the most commonly occurring drugs at special events such as raves, club parties, rock concerts, and outdoor festivals.

Ecstasy

Ecstasy (also known as MDMA, X, E, the love drug, or the hug drug) is a methamphetamine derivative that is generally sold as a capsule or tablet but can also be found as a powder. It has gained popularity because it alters and intensifies a person's sensory perception, producing stimulant and hallucinogenic effects. It causes people to lower their inhibitions and has earned a reputation as a "soft" drug (implying that it is less dangerous), but nothing could be further from the truth. The long-term effects of ecstasy use are well documented. Ecstasy damages brain nerve endings involved in cognitive processes and memory. It also negatively affects the production and function of serotonin, a brain chemical that helps regulate mood, sleep, and appetite. Damage may be long term and permanent. Even short term, ecstasy can have seriously negative side effects, including:

- Increased heart rate
- Increased blood pressure
- Dehydration
- Overheating
- Teeth grinding
- Jaw clenching
- Confusion
- Depression
- Sleep problems
- Drug craving
- Severe anxiety
- Paranoia
- Muscle tension
- Nausea
- Blurred vision
- Rapid eye movement
- Faintness
- Chills
- Sweating
- Altered level of consciousness (LOC)

Additionally, because it causes poor judgment, ecstasy may lead to sexual assaults or increased accidents (for example, a motor vehicle collision in which the driver was under the influence of ecstasy).

One of the major concerns for SEMS providers is that ecstasy also causes a marked increase in body temperature (hyperthermia). Because ecstasy users are usually found in hot, crowded environments such as clubs or dance floors, this condition can become critical. When unchecked and untreated, hyperthermia can lead to heart, liver, or kidney failure; seizure; or coma. Factors that induce hyperthermia include dehydration, alcohol consumption, physical exertion, and heat, all of which are often present in environments associated with ecstasy use.

Ecstasy users are usually exerting themselves (eg, dancing) and also may believe the myth that water is an antidote to ecstasy overdose. For either or both of these reasons, they may drink copious amounts of water in very short time periods, potentially causing hyponatremia. Combined with the fact that ecstasy also affects kidney function (inappropriate antidiuretic hormone) by slowing or stopping the kidney's ability to process fluid in the body, this effect could be life-threatening. SEMS providers should follow local protocol to help avoid this situation, ensuring that the patient does not exceed a normal intake of water.

TIP

Ecstasy users often present with extreme thirst but have reduced renal function. Excessive water consumption can be damaging to the patient.

Methamphetamine

Methamphetamine (also called speed, ice, meth, or crank) is the second most abused drug in the United States (following marijuana). The drug can be smoked, inhaled, injected, or taken orally. It is a white, crystalline powder made out of common over-the-counter medications and household products such as cold medicine, ether, paint thinner, and table salt. Methamphetamine is a stimulant with dangerous neurotoxin properties and has a powerful effect on mood, energy, and appetite suppression. The effectiveness decreases with time and usage so that a user must use higher doses more often to achieve the same effect. Over time, users find they have difficulty functioning and experiencing pleasure without the drug.

Side effects of methamphetamine persist indefinitely due to neurotoxicity and can include:

- Agitation or restlessness
- Excited speech patterns
- Heightened physical activity
- Heightened aggression or violence
- Psychotic behavior and hallucinations
- Skin lesions (from compulsively picking at the skin)
- Suicidal thoughts
- Confusion
- Chest tightness
- Chest pain
- Heart palpitations
- Shortness of breath
- Uncontrolled movements of the head, neck, mouth, arms, or legs (known as tics)

Treatment considerations for patients who have taken a methamphetamine include the same treatment as for other stimulant drugs: maintain oxygen saturation levels, prevent seizures with adequate sedation if allowed per protocols, and monitor vital signs.

LSD

The hallucinogen **lysergic acid diethylamide (LSD)** (also known as acid, yellow sunshine, tab, or dose) alters a person's sensory perception and causes hallucinations. It is generally taken orally or can be transdermal and is generally odorless and tasteless.

LSD's effects take anywhere from 30 to 90 minutes to be felt, but once they are felt, they are intense. The episode is known as "tripping" and can be pleasurable or terrifying for the user. Side effects include:

- Pupil dilation
- Increased heart rate
- Increased blood pressure
- Increased body temperature
- Sweating
- Dry mouth
- Muscle tremors
- Numbness
- Weakness
- Nausea

Treatment for a patient using LSD is primarily supportive. Try to limit sensory stimulation as much as possible. SEMS providers should watch for users who are having an adverse reaction (commonly called a "bad trip"). In this case, SEMS providers may consider sedating the patient for transport.

Date Rape Drugs

Date rape drugs are drugs used to sedate a victim, allowing the perpetrator to commit acts of sexual assault or rape. Gamma-hydroxybutyric acid and Rohypnol are the most common examples of these types of drugs and may be found at festivals and dance parties.

Gamma-hydroxybutyric acid (GHB) is a central nervous system depressant that has sedating and intoxicating effects. GHB was readily available as an over-the-counter fat reducer and muscle-building product before the Food and Drug Administration pulled the drug from the shelves due to reports of seizures and comas. The drug may still be purchased in Mexico and over the Internet. GHB is available as a clear liquid, tablet, or white powder and is clear, tasteless, and odorless. This date rape drug may be slipped into a victim's drink, intensifying the drug's sedation effect and rendering the victim comatose.

Symptoms of GHB intoxication range from sleepiness, loss of muscle tone, and forgetfulness to seizure-like activity. Respirations and heartbeat are depressed, progressing to a coma-like state that generally lasts about 2 hours. At lower doses, GHB may make the victim violently ill. If the drug renders the victim unconscious and causes vomiting, the victim's airway may be compromised. The drug alone is powerful enough in higher doses to completely depress respiratory efforts and cause the patient to slip into a deep coma, possibly resulting in death.

Treatment for a patient who has ingested GHB is supportive, making sure there is adequate ventilatory support for patients in respiratory depression. There is no antidote for GHB ingestion.

Rohypnol (flunitrazepam; commonly called rophie or roofies) is a benzodiazepine (the same drug family as Valium). It is illegal in the United States but may be prescribed as a sedative or treatment for insomnia in other countries and is readily available in Mexico, Canada, and over the Internet. Rohypnol has gained popularity as a chemical-assisted rape drug because it is colorless, odorless, and tasteless and has amnesia-causing properties. Alone, the drug produces incapacitating effects that last up to 12 hours; when mixed with alcohol or other depressants, the drug's sedative effect can be lethal. Victims of this drug often report **anterograde amnesia**, which means they do not have a clear memory of events that occurred during the drug's effects.

Effects of Rohypnol begin within 30 minutes after it is consumed and last for 8 hours, with peak effects occurring about 2 hours after ingestion. Symptoms include decreased blood pressure, drowsiness, dizziness, confusion, and as mentioned, memory loss. Overdose can lead to death due to central nervous system depression.

Treatment for a patient who has ingested Rohypnol requires advanced life support, with possible administration of flumazenil (Romazicon). Naloxone hydrochloride (Narcan) has no effect on Rohypnol, but its administration may be considered because Rohypnol is sometimes used in conjunction with other drugs. Naloxone hydrochloride reverses respiratory depression caused by depressant drugs.

> **TIP**
> People may mix substances for an intensified or different effect. One such example is the "hillbilly cocktail," a mixture of GHB, grain alcohol, and marijuana.

Ketamine Hydrochloride

Ketamine hydrochloride is a veterinary anesthetic in the form of a dry white powder that can be snorted, smoked, or (rarely) injected. Street names include special K, K, vitamin K, cat Valium, and Fort Dodge. The effects of ketamine begin after a few minutes and last less than an hour. Ketamine causes a dreamlike dissociative state and hallucinations. Users of ketamine will often be seen with an unsteady gait (known as high-stepping), which is caused by blocked neurotransmitters.

SEMS providers should be aware that a person on ketamine may have a bad reaction, causing violent paranoia, agitation, and confusion. Users could sustain severe injuries due to trauma and still function because they have no pain inhibitions. Users are also capable of great physical feats of strength.

Users may also experience an inability to move or communicate, feeling very far away from their bodies (a phenomenon known as "the k-hole"). This experience may cause the user to exhibit repetitive motion or speech, which may happen more often and with greater intensity with increased dosages; as the drug wears off, the cycle of the behavior becomes less frequent and less intense.

Extreme caution should be exercised when dealing with suspected ketamine overdoses. SEMS providers should never directly touch a patient who may be experiencing a ketamine overdose—the drug is transdermal and can pass into the provider's skin. Always ensure the safety of your crew because ketamine users may exhibit erratic or violent behavior; involve law enforcement when warranted and always wear appropriate personal protective equipment such as gloves, eye protection, and a mask. Keep the patient warm and treat for shock.

> **TIP**
> Ketamine, like many club drugs, causes dissociation between the body and the brain. Therefore, a patient may not be physically able to control his or her movement, potentially causing serious safety issues. SEMS providers should always keep safety in mind when treating a patient suspected of using such a drug.

General Management Concerns

Remember that you may have difficulty getting an accurate patient history from a patient who is on drugs, either because he or she has an altered LOC or because the patient does not want to admit to taking drugs. A patient may even purposely try to mislead you, complicating treatment of these patients.

When dealing with people who are intoxicated or who have used drugs, SEMS providers should always be professional. They should not be judgmental, provoke the person, or escalate the situation in any way. Providers should try to isolate the situation from the crowd as quickly and safely as possible. When dealing with an intoxicated minor, providers should review the laws in their state, always erring on the side of caution and summoning law enforcement if there is any doubt or discrepancy.

> **TIP** Professionalism is not just a catch phrase—it is a matter of personal safety. There is no place for your personal political feeling or views while you are working. You must work without prejudice or malice. If you find a particular special event so personally objectionable that you feel unable to act in a professional manner, you should not work that special event.

Gangs

Like other public safety personnel, SEMS providers may encounter members of gangs. Once again, providers must do their homework. Knowing the type of special event they will be protecting (eg, concert, cultural festival, or motorcycle rally) will enable them to work with venue security and local law enforcement to identify the probability of gangs. SEMS providers should monitor the crowd and identify any possible signs of gangs. Gang signs can be numerous, and providers should work with law enforcement to identify known gangs, affiliates, and the signs that they are present. Gangs quite often communicate using nonverbal signals (sometimes referred to as "throwing signs" or "stacking"), and providers should be able to identify these hand signals Figure 5-13. Gang presence may be indicated by a group of young people all wearing the same color either on their hats, shirts, shoes, or shoelaces. If the special event is taking place in a known gang area, learn whose territory the special event is being held on because that gang tends to be dominant and may try to protect its territory from rival gangs.

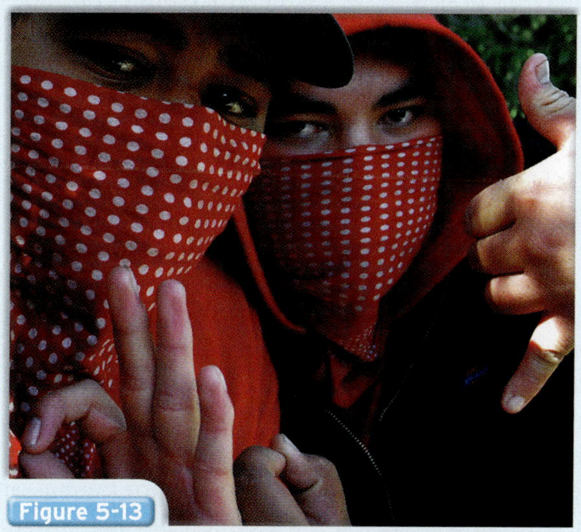

Figure 5-13

Gang members often communicate by special gang hand symbols.

When treating gang members, providers should be professional. Respect is critical in this world. If gang members feel like a provider somehow disrespected them or caused them embarassment, tensions could escalate and the provider could even be marked for revenge by the gang. The gang world is difficult to work in. Providers must never treat two rival gang members in the same room or area and must, therefore, have a second, separate treatment area available at special events where gangs may be present.

Sexual Assault

SEMS providers increasingly encounter victims of sexual assault at special events. The precursor to most of these events is a heightened crowd agitation. People may do things they would not do in everyday circumstances, such as commit a sexual assault. Others may be too afraid to stand up to the mob and refuse to help the victims as they endure assault and humiliation.

As medical providers and public health advocates, SEMS providers must do everything in their power to prevent sexual assaults from happening. Working with security personnel and special event organizers to ensure the area is safe for all attendees is the responsibility of everyone involved in planning and running the event. SEMS personnel should know that while event security is not their primary job, being vigilant to potential problems is crucial. For example, are all of the lighting fixtures in the area working? If not, SEMS providers need to report this to ensure property lighting for security purposes. Are there suspicious people in the area? Every person working an event should be on the lookout for anything or anyone suspicious. Remember, SEMS providers are there to work, not to enjoy the event. Paying attention to the surroundings can prevent safety problems.

When treating a victim of sexual assault, keep in mind to never judge the victim or the validity of his or her statement; nor should you imply in any way that the assault could be his or her fault. Remember to treat sexual assault cases as crimes, documenting and preserving all evidence. A SEMS organization should have a protocol in place to deal with sexual assaults. A sample is provided in Figure 5-14.

Behavioral Concerns

After working with special event security and law enforcement to ensure the safety of SEMS staff, special event staff, and people attending the event, the next order of business is to identify and treat potentially life-threatening medical conditions. Often providers are required to care for a patient who has an intense emotional or psychiatric disturbance, which could be caused by a physical problem such as hypoxia or a low blood glucose level, or which could relate to a preexisting psychiatric problem. For example, providers may be servicing a special event for war veterans and need to care for a patient with post-traumatic stress disorder. These types of incidents can be difficult and require patience and professionalism. Providers must remain calm and avoid sudden movements as well as any nonessential treatment that may further upset the patient. They should avoid providing treatment or advice for ailments other than the original complaint.

Vehicle Operations in a Crowd

Vehicle safety was discussed in Chapter 3 but deserves additional mention here. Driving a vehicle through a crowd creates a startled-herd effect described earlier in this chapter. As a policy, providers should never attempt to drive an ambulance or any full-size vehicle through a crowd because of the danger it creates. This policy also includes carts, bikes, trucks, support vehicles, and scooters. However, there will be times when, because of the situation or distance that must be covered, the use of a cart is unavoidable Figure 5-15. To preplan for vehicle operations in a crowd, providers should speak to the venue staff and together answer the following questions:

- Are vehicles expected to be used at the event? If so, what type of vehicle?
- Who will provide the vehicles?
- Who will drive the vehicles?
- Where will the vehicles be kept?
- Do vehicles need to be secured? If so, how should they be secured?
- Are vehicles protected from the elements?
- Are vehicles accessible to the general public?
- What routes will be used?
- How close to the main body of the crowd are the primary and secondary egress routes?

> **TIP**
> Be careful when considering using bicycles as a vehicle at a special event. There are many drawbacks, including danger of injury to the crowd and rider, a potentially slower response, and the inability to carry much equipment. Also, bicycles are quiet; therefore, people in the crowd will not move out of the way until they see the bicycle.

Remember the drawbacks to using bicycles as a response vehicle at a special event. When SEMS providers ride bicycles to a response, there is an increased danger of injury to the crowd and rider. The response time is often slower than on a cart, and not much equipment can be carried on the bicycle. Finally, bicycles are quiet; therefore, people in the crowd will not move out of the way until they see the bicycle (or may not move out of the way at all).

Ambulances should not move from their designated positions. At special events with high audience densities, it may be best to have medical personnel on foot or using carts. Never use large vehicles or bicycles in dense crowds to remove patients. The use of any type of vehicle should be curtailed in a crowd.

It should go without saying that providers should never land a helicopter in a crowd. The best landing zone is outside the venue, a minimum of a quarter mile away. The maximum distance is close enough that it is still advantageous and beneficial to the patient to be flown. There is no hard and fast rule for maximum distance, but providers should refer to their jurisdiction's rules and regulations governing helicopter evacuation. Occasionally, SEMS providers will encounter patients who require air transportation to a hospital or specialty medical facility. Neurologic injuries, burn trauma, and chest trauma are just a few examples of the potential injuries providers may see that could require this type of transportation. Providers should use local protocols to decide when to use aviation to transport a patient.

I. Introduction

A. The terms sexual assault and sexual abuse refer to any act of sexual contact or conduct performed upon one person by another without mutual consent, or with an inability of the victim to give consent due to age, or mental or physical incapacity. This protocol should also be used for other forms of sexual assault (sex crimes perpetrated against adults) and sexual abuse (sex crimes perpetrated against children and adolescents).

B. By state law, rape is defined as any sexual penetration, however slight, using force or coercion against the person's will. Although the majority of victims are women, children and men are also victims.

C. Rape is an act of physical violence and not an act perpetrated for sexual gratification.

II. Objectives

A. It is of the utmost importance that the rape survivor feels acceptance and support, regardless of his or her emotional response.

B. Do not evaluate or pass judgment on the credibility of the circumstances of the assault, recognizing that any response from a rape victim is within the appropriate range.

C. Providing help to victims of sexual assault requires special sensitivity. Social, cultural, and religious practices may cause victims additional stress if they are concerned about discriminatory treatment as they are seeking support.

III. Recognition

A. History: Procedures include the following:

1. Document time, date, and place of the attack.
2. If the patient volunteers the information, ascertain all body areas violated in the attack.
3. Confirm whether the patient bathed since the attack.
4. If the victim is still wearing the clothing worn during the assault, suggest he or she take other clothing to be worn home.
5. If the patient changed clothes after the attack, the clothing must be brought along to the hospital in a *paper* bag. Plastic bags trap moisture and promote mildew, which destroys vital evidence.
6. Document all marks or evidence of trauma.
7. Document other significant physical findings.
8. Obtain medical history, including possibility of pregnancy.
9. Document all treatment given.

B. Physical exam: *Unless a life-threatening condition occurs*, the following protocol should be followed:

1. Explain all procedures to be performed prior to undertaking them.
2. Obtain consent if possible. Do not assume that your presence automatically implies consent to treatment in part of the patient.
3. Limit the physical exam to any evidence you can visually obtain without causing any further emotional distress to the patient.

IV. Treatment

A. Basic life support (BLS)

1. If time permits, obtain consent for all treatment given.
2. Specific protocols may need to be followed after assessing the ABCs (eg, respiratory or cardiac problems).
3. Obtain vital signs.
4. Stabilize injuries necessitating immediate attention (eg, fractures, bleeding).

B. Advanced life support

1. Perform all BLS procedures as outlined above.
2. Follow the specific protocol after assessing the ABCs dependent on the patient's condition.

V. Caution

A. All sexual assault patients should be transported to an appropriate medical facility where rape evidence exams are performed, unless a medical condition dictates otherwise.

B. If the victim changed clothes after the attack, the clothing must be brought along to the hospital in a paper bag.

C. Attempt to notify the receiving facility of your impending arrival.

Figure 5-14

A sample emergency medical services protocol for sexual assault.
Modified from J. M. Behar, "Emergency Medical Services Protocol for Sexual Assault," Ohio Department of Health, August 2004.

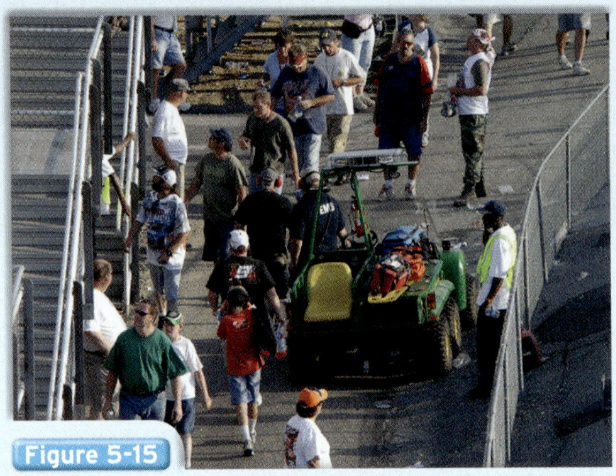

Figure 5-15

Always preplan for vehicle operations, including determining which vehicles will be used and their routes of travel to various areas of the venue.

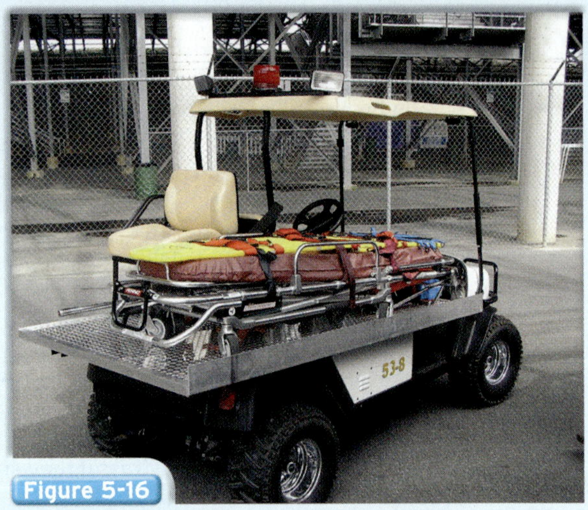

Figure 5-16

A cart with a medical transport module.

If air transportation is necessary, special steps must be taken to handle landing a helicopter in a crowded area. By their very nature, helicopters draw a crowd. However, having sufficient landing space is important to prevent injury. According to the US Coast Guard, a typical landing zone is 200 square feet; the average hospital helicopter landing zone is 500 square feet. Crowds should be kept even farther back to protect bystanders. SEMS providers should discuss helicopter transport with the venue staff to answer the following questions:

- What is the available terrain?
- Is there a secured area that can be used?
- Is there an area nearby (ie, within a mile radius) that can be secured for the landing zone?
- How should providers get to the landing zone?
- Are there enough security personnel to make the landing area safe for the helicopter and the crowd?

The goal of SEMS providers is always quality patient care, but the safety must be a priority.

Equipment Considerations

The equipment that EMS providers use every day in the field is not designed specifically for the special events setting. Providers should never use any of the new equipment on the market, such as a gator or cart with a medical transport module Figure 5-16, until they have been trained in their usage. Most departments have developed in-house programs to train staff to use these tools. Some manufacturers also have safety programs on their vehicles' operations.

Before the special event, SEMS providers should rehearse using all available equipment such as stair chairs, Reeves Sleeves, stretchers, and any other equipment their service may use. They should rehearse their response in bleachers or in a venue's seating, where lifting and moving a patient safely can be challenging due to limited spaces. Providers should rehearse patient movement in all areas of the special event venue to learn what will and will not work. For example, if they are planning to use a stretcher as a primary patient moving device, they need to ensure that such movement is possible, especially if working on varied terrain such as grass, gravel, asphalt, stairs, ramps, and naturally occurring obstacles. They should also rehearse removing patients from chairs and determine the minimum number of SEMS providers needed to safely achieve the desired outcome.

Terrorism

Since September 11, 2001, Americans are more aware of the threat of terrorism, which has heavily impacted the field of SEMS. Events such as NASCAR races, dignitary events, and political rallies are considered Events of National Significance and have high potential for terrorist activity. In planning for any event, the subject of safety and terrorism will likely come up with the venue manager. Venues may be particularly vulnerable to security risks if they do not have direct control over the selection of vendors. A selection process is usually completed by the special event organizers, but thereafter, vendors are granted broad access to the venue. The job of a SEMS provider is to be an extra set of eyes and ears; all SEMS professionals should note suspicious objects, people, activities, or anything that is out of place at the event. This includes reporting people without IDs in restricted areas, people acting suspiciously, and packages or bags that have been left unattended.

SEMS providers must have access to all areas of the venue and must ensure that all possible precautions are taken to account for all SEMS vehicles and SEMS personnel. SEMS vehicles must be secured to prevent unauthorized persons from accessing vehicles and equipment. The identities of all SEMS personnel should be provided to the event organizers at least 3 days prior to the start of the special event. At the security gate entrance, there should be pictures of these individuals and their identification for a positive ID check. The most common identification credential is a photo identification badge worn by the provider that displays a clear photo, the name of the provider, the service he or she is with, and the level of access. If the SEMS service is small or only a small number of personnel are needed, photo identification is not as important, but for high-profile special events where a number of services are present, an ID check is essential. At such high-profile events, the coming and going of SEMS services could inadvertently create a gap in security. In these large and complex special events, a security photo array at the entrance is essential in addition to strict adherence to uniforms. With these special events, no personnel substitutions may be made 3 days before the event, and credentials must be required to avoid unauthorized access.

You Are the SEMS Provider

SUMMARY

CASE 1

1. **How do you respond? Do you continue your care?**
   It is important to avoid taking sides or participating in the altercation. Obtain assistance from security, and attempt to move the patient away from the scene as quickly and safely as possible. You can then care for the patient in a safe environment.
2. **How could you have anticipated this situation?**
   Considering the fierce historic rivalry between the teams and the fact that tailgating (and, therefore, alcohol consumption) occurs all day long, this event obviously has the potential for violence. In the preplanning stages for such an event, you must determine how to respond to violent events, and you must have a plan for contacting security for additional assistance. Always be sure to meet with security before such an event to preplan your response.

CASE 2

1. **What should SEMS providers' first response be?**
   As always, a clear approach for this type of scenario should have been thoroughly preplanned. The approach should indicate that SEMS providers not enter the scene until security personnel have ensured that it is safe and have given SEMS providers the verbal go-ahead on the radio to enter. Always remember provider safety.
2. **How should providers access and treat these patients?**
   Once scene safety has been ensured, SEMS providers should follow their preplanned method for accessing this area of the concert. Considering that at least 12 attendees are potentially injured, 4 to 6 SEMS providers should approach the scene (2 or 3 SEMS providers to triage patients, backboard if needed, and bring them outside the incident area; and an additional 2 or 3 SEMS providers staged outside the incident area to provide treatment to the patients). The first task is to triage the injured patients. This should be immediately followed by transferring injured patients to a separate area where they can be assessed and treated. This area should be far enough away from the incident site to ensure that it will remain safe, even if the incident worsens. Preplanning should have also addressed how patients would be moved in such an incident—with carts or on foot. During all of this, SEMS providers will need to stay alert to the potential for crowd violence and escalation of the incident, and may even need to leave the scene should it again become unsafe.

Ready for Review

- Ensuring the safety of SEMS providers should be a primary consideration before responding to any situation.
- There are a wide variety of safety considerations for special events, so providers must strive to be knowledgeable and aware of the specific threats posed by a particular event or venue.
- It is important to preplan for safety concerns by talking with other services that have worked similar special events, doing a walkthrough at the venue, and training personnel about relevant security issues.
- In high-energy situations, crowds may become overexcited and more easily incited to violence. Providers must recognize environments with the potential for violent encounters and work to avoid provocation.
- When violence does occur, providers should immediately and discreetly alert security of any potentially violent situation and remove themselves and the patient from the situation as quickly and safely as possible.
- Because SEMS providers will often be working at events with large crowds, it is helpful to be familiar with crowd dynamics.
- Consider the crowd demographics when preplanning for the event, especially age distribution, to anticipate medical needs.
- Older crowds (those consisting of middle-aged and older adults) may require medical support such as chairs, water, cooling and warming stations, and wheelchairs.
- Younger crowds (those consisting of adolescents or young adults) may require more trauma and wound care; they may have emergencies related to substance abuse.
- Consider the crowd's energy level. Will they be dancing? Sitting? Knowing the energy level can help providers predict the types of emergencies likely to occur.
- Violent crowd activities such as moshing, crowd surfing, and crowd surging, are often precursors to violence. Special care should be taken in these instances to ensure the safety of the crowd, venue staff, and SEMS providers.
- Moshing may lead to injuries such as broken bones and spinal cord injuries or violent acts such as sexual assault or rape.
- Crowd surfing may lead to injuries from falls from a height or sexual assault.
- The risk of crowd surging requires that SEMS providers assigned to floor duty or stationed in front of the stage be specially trained in barricade rescue operations. Without proper training, SEMS providers should not try to rescue patients from a violent crowd.
- Remember the concept of front-to-back crowd issues. Patrons at the rear of the crowd often have access to less information than those at the front and may push forward in an effort to find out what is happening at the front of the crowd.
- SEMS providers should understand the concepts of pack mentality and herd mentality. Pack mentality is when individuals in a large crowd base their decisions on what they believe to be the collective standpoint. This can lead to people performing unthinkable actions. Herd mentality is when people react as a herd does when startled or enraged, possibly becoming dangerous and unpredictable.
- Crowded places may give attendees a feeling of crowd syndrome, meaning that they may begin to feel sweaty, hot, faint, paranoid, and short of breath. Relocating attendees to a quiet, private place away from the crowd can help treat these symptoms.
- Crowd panic can be triggered by something specific such as a fight in the crowd or a loud noise. It is vital in preplanning to ensure that entrances and exits provide safe routes into and out of the facility.
- Most deaths from crowd incidents are due to asphyxia. Crowd pushing can be extremely forceful, stacking and crushing people in the crowd. The shock wave from the pushing may be strong enough to cause additional injury. Anxiety may lead to additional emergencies, such as breathing problems.
- Preplanning considerations for crowds include analyzing the venue for choke points (areas where a pathway has less capacity, the normal direction of movement changes, or there is a confluence of traffic streams). Expect emergencies in these areas, and work with event personnel to improve event layout if possible.
- Events with standing crowds may not allot enough space to attendees. Discomfort increases the likelihood of emergencies related to panic and violence, so consider this when preplanning for events with standing crowds.

- Always remain professional and nonjudgmental. Do not take sides in any incident.
- When violence occurs, SEMS personnel should immediately and discreetly alert security of any potentially violent situations and remove themselves and patients from the situation as quickly and safely as possible. Specific procedures for such situations must be determined during preplanning and understood by all SEMS providers working at the event.
- Removing a victim from a violent crowd can be challenging. All efforts to remove a victim from a crowd should be preplanned with event security.
- SEMS providers should expect a greater incidence of alcohol-related and drug-related emergencies at events where spectators are adolescents or young adults.
- Alcohol and drug use can facilitate acts of violence.
- When dealing with intoxicated people, SEMS providers should always remain professional. They should try to isolate the patient from the crowd as quickly and safely as possible.
- SEMS providers will encounter event attendees on drugs, especially at raves, rock and hip-hop concerts, and outdoor festivals. SEMS providers should make an effort to stay up-to-date on new and emerging drug use trends.
- Remember that it may be difficult to get an accurate patient history from a patient who is on drugs.
- Gangs pose a unique security threat. Providers should always work with venue security and local law enforcement to identify the probability of gangs. Gang members should be treated in a respectful and professional manner.
- SEMS providers may encounter victims of sexual assault at special events. The precursor to most of these events is crowd agitation. SEMS providers must work with security personnel and special event organizers to ensure safe areas and remain vigilant to potential problems during the event.
- All SEMS professionals should be on the lookout for potential acts of terrorism or suspicious behavior or articles.
- A photo identification badge and ID checkpoint are essential at large, complex special events to prevent unauthorized entry into secure areas.
- After ensuring safety, providers must identify and treat potentially life-threatening medical conditions. They may be required to care for a patient who has an intense emotional or psychiatric disturbance. They should remain calm, avoid sudden movements, and avoid any nonessential treatment.
- While in general, providers should never attempt to drive an ambulance or any vehicle through a crowd, there may be instances when this is necessary, so this must be addressed in the preplanning stage.
- When necessary, SEMS providers should preplan for safe helicopter landings for air medical transport of patients.
- Preplanning efforts should include rehearsal using all available equipment and response in a variety of settings (eg, bleachers or venue seating) to ensure that the equipment will allow adequate patient movement and treatment during the event.

Vital Vocabulary

anterograde amnesia Loss of memory relating to events that occurred after an injury or episode of drug use.

barricade operations Generally taught to security personnel, a skill set on how to safely protect and remove distressed individuals who may be pinned against a barricade, such as near a stage.

bull in the ring A modified form of moshing that occurs when one person is surrounded by a crowd and must break through the crowd by smashing into people.

choke point Any area that prohibits the crowd from moving freely and can cause a pedestrian backup, such as doorways, riot gates, or places where people naturally stop to talk, blocking the pathway of others.

crowd demographics Statistical characteristics of a crowd, such as age, race, and sex distribution.

crowd panic The occurrence of widespread alarm in a group of people; responses of people in the group may vary or be amplified because of the fact that they are in a group.

crowd surfing Laying on top of a crowd of people and being passed around; this often begins with stage diving (diving off a stage into a crowd).

crowd surging Crowd movement as a group, for example to overtake security personnel to jump onto the stage at a performance.

crowd syndrome A collection of physical symptoms that may occur when a person feels anxious in a crowd; symptoms include sweating, shortness of breath, and feeling hot, faint, or paranoid.

ecstasy (MDMA) A drug officially named methylenedioxymethamphetamine and generally sold as a capsule or tablet; it alters and intensifies a person's sensory perception, producing stimulant and hallucinogenic effects and lowering individuals' inhibitions; may lead to hyperthermia or hyponatremia.

gamma-hydroxybutyric acid (GHB) A central nervous system depressant that is colorless and has a salty taste; it has sedating and intoxicating effects and is used to perpetrate date rape.

herd mentality A situation in which people in a crowd react as a herd does when startled or enraged, initiating violence or generally becoming dangerous and unpredictable.

ketamine hydrochloride A veterinary anesthetic and a phencyclidine hydrochloride (PCP) derivative; street names include special K, vitamin K, cat Valium, and Fort Dodge; can be absorbed through another person's skin.

lysergic acid diethylamide (LSD) Also called acid, a hallucinogen that alters a person's perception and can cause intense hallucinations; it can transfer through another person's skin.

methamphetamine A highly addictive stimulant drug that affects mood, energy, and appetite; it comes as a white, crystalline powder and is made out of common over-the-counter medications and common household products.

moshing A modern version of the punk tradition of slam dancing wherein dancers start flailing around wildly and smashing into each other.

pack mentality A situation that occurs when individuals in a crowd base their decisions on what they believe to be the collective standpoint, rather than basing decisions on their own beliefs and thought processes; can lead to members of a group performing unthinkable actions.

Rohypnol A benzodiazepine sometimes used to perpetrate date rape because it can cause memory loss; commonly called rophie or roofies; produces incapacitatory effects that last up to 12 hours.

CHAPTER 6

Mass-Casualty Incidents and Terrorism

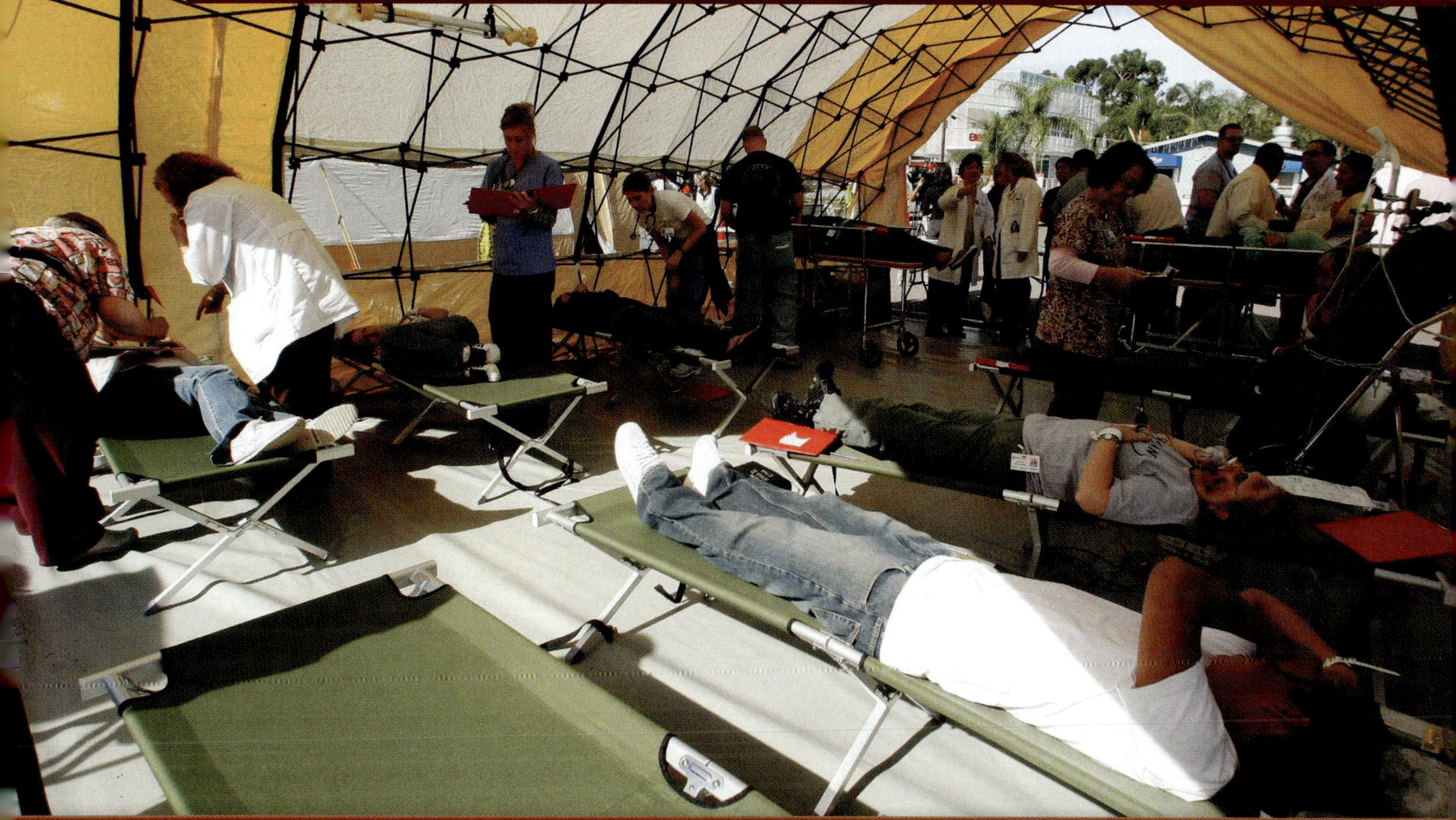

LEARNING OBJECTIVES

- Explain the difference between a temporary overwhelming patient load (TOPL) and a mass-casualty incident (MCI).
- Discuss the role of triage and list common triage systems.
- Briefly describe the National Incident Management System (NIMS) and how it may apply to a special events medical services (SEMS) event.
- List the positions for emergency medical services (EMS) providers per NIMS at an MCI.
- Discuss the roles and tasks for each MCI position.
- List considerations when preplanning a treatment area.
- Describe special considerations for handling a potential terrorist incident at a special event.

Introduction

Mass gatherings and special event medical personnel must remember number 5 of the SEMS 10 discussed in Chapter 1: a mass gathering is not the same as a **mass-casualty incident (MCI)**. There is always the potential for an MCI to occur, but these events are very rare. When providing SEMS coverage, providers must adjust their mentality. In normal everyday EMS functions, providers receive dispatches to emergency calls; they arrive, assess, and treat each patient; and they transport them to the appropriate hospital. However, at a mass gathering, providers do not transport every person who seeks care. It is not medically necessary to transport every patient at a special event because many injuries and illnesses that occur can be handled and resolved on site. The issue then becomes, who should be treated and released and who should be transported? Having established treatment protocols will help guide this decision process; MCI protocols will be determined by your state or your medical director. When working at a special event, providers must adjust their mindset and refrain from transporting every patient they are called to treat.

Regular emergencies at a special event can be handled adequately by SEMS providers. The NIMS will come into play if an MCI occurs. This chapter will discuss NIMS in more detail later. First, we will review the difference between a TOPL and an MCI.

TOPL Versus MCI

As discussed in Chapter 1, a **temporary overwhelming patient load (TOPL)** is not the same as an MCI. A TOPL is a brief period during which there is a larger number of patients than the available resources can handle, but this does not prevent the event from continuing and subsides without external resources being required. An MCI is an event that overwhelms the internal and external resources that are required to resolve the situation, resulting in an inability to resume the special event after the incident. The important factor to keep in mind is that a TOPL is simply a busy period or an unexpected spike in the patient load. After these patients are cared for, the special event can resume with no adverse consequences. With an MCI, the special event cannot return to normal.

Though the previously stated definition for an MCI is the most standard, some EMS systems have set numbers and rules that define an MCI and how to respond to it. For example, some systems define an MCI as any incident that has 10 to 25 injured or ill patients,

You Are the SEMS Provider

CASE 1

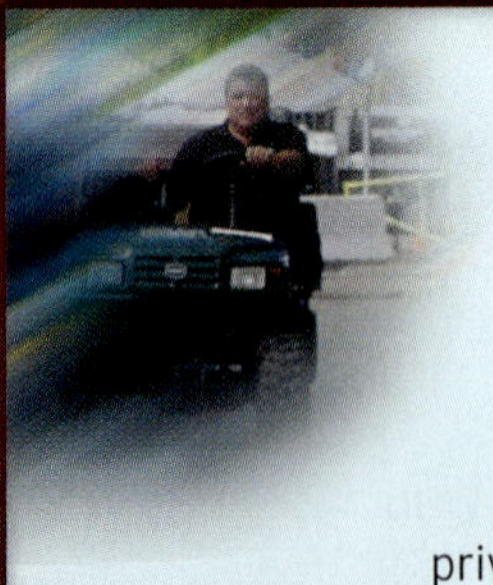

Your agency is selected to provide emergency care services for a local radio station's annual concert. The concert is a 1-day event at the end of the summer at the local football stadium. The radio station will have 11 bands and expects 40,000 people to attend.

The 5-year average temperature for the day is 87°F, and the relative humidity is above 60%. You are expecting an afternoon thunder shower because that date has historically experienced one in the late afternoon, according to your research.

You have four ambulances assigned to the special event, with a contract with the local private EMS service for another two ambulances and crews. You have two first aid stations—one on the inside and one on the outside. In total, you have roughly 21 personnel.

On the actual day of the special event, it is hot (90°F by 10:30 am) with 70% relative humidity. Your patient hourly cycle rate is six patients per hour, which is double the rate you had originally estimated during the preplanning stage. Between 12:30 and 2:00 in the afternoon, there are 26 patients in the first aid station. Then three emergency calls come in. Suddenly you realize that all of your resources are now in use.

1. How will you handle this situation?

or an incident that may escalate to 10 to 25 patients. In such systems, this criterion activates the prehospital MCI response. Other jurisdictions may define an MCI as any incident that generates 26 or more injured patients, or a minor emergency that will likely escalate into 26 or more injured patients. Some systems define an MCI as a single incident that overwhelms normal responding resources. Finally, some agencies define an MCI as six patients in one place at one time.

In the mass gathering special event arena, SEMS does not have one definition for an MCI. Remember, one's viewpoint when working as a SEMS provider must be different than one's viewpoint when working as an everyday EMS provider. At a special event, providers only triage, treat, and transport when necessary. Several times during an event they may feel overwhelmed by the sheer number of patients who have requested assistance at the same time, but they must remember that this is a TOPL, not an MCI. For example, if at a 30,000-person event, in half an hour 30 people come to the first aid tent needing water (temporarily overwhelming resources), this situation is not an MCI; it is a TOPL.

To decide whether an event is a TOPL or an MCI, providers must consider other factors. Is the sudden influx of patients due to a temporary situation that will improve with time? In the previously mentioned case, yes, the day will likely become cooler in the afternoon and evening, and the patient load will decrease. Or is the patient load due to an incident, such as a structural collapse, which can prevent the event from continuing? Providers must also consider whether, after the incident resolves, the event can continue without significant change or variation. They must assess the incident by stepping back and considering a larger frame of reference, including:

- The source of the event
- The scale of the event
- The ability to return to normal after the event
- Whether it was a structural event
- The number of priority patients

By systematically looking at an event and answering the questions laid out in this chapter, as well as employing SEMS skills and experience, a SEMS provider should be able to distinguish between an MCI and a TOPL.

TOPL events are temporary and can be systematically worked through with existing resources or a small increase in resources. The period will pass, but this does not mean that it will not repeat during the special event. This phenomenon can be **dispersed**, meaning it can take place in more than one place at an event, or **local**, occurring in one location at the event. Consider this scenario: 125,000 people are at a NASCAR event on a warm, humid day in June. Early in the day, the vendor runs out of water to sell. By early afternoon, SEMS is receiving calls all around the facility for people who are dizzy and dehydrated. Several units have to be dispatched to handle the calls due to the large size of the venue. In this case, the calls were dispersed. On the other hand, consider a cart running over several attendees in a crowd. In this case, the incident is confined to one location and is therefore local. The same number of patients may result from these scenarios, and it may take the same number of units to assess and treat these patients, but by no means would the event have to stop as a result of either incident. A busy period that passes does not require MCI protocols to be enacted. At the conclusion of the TOPL, the special event may proceed uninterrupted. Providers who mistake a TOPL for an MCI risk inadvertently disrupting an event to draining a system of vital resources, leaving an area vulnerable if those resources are needed.

The most common TOPL event occurs when multiple patients approach the aid station at the same time. This requires a modified or informal triage system. Multiple calls for unrelated patients could quickly outnumber providers. Providers may temporarily need more resources to handle individual calls. The problem posed here is where to obtain these resources. Is the event in a large city where providers can call for aid from neighboring EMS agencies, or is it miles from the nearest assistance? The need for additional resources must be considered during the preplanning phase. Preplanning, as discussed in Chapter 2, is the key to making sure providers know from where they can get aid if needed, and how long it will take for that aid to arrive. Again, this is only a temporary situation; there is no need to implement the MCI system.

A TOPL may escalate to an MCI if multiple patients overwhelm current resources for the foreseeable future and create an overwhelming patient load. An MCI occurs when there is an influx of patients that exceeds current resources as well as the resources that can be called in. MCIs are often dramatic and sudden, and the special event will not be able to continue. Examples are bleacher collapse, violent weather events, or an unforeseen violent event. A specific example occurred in 1998 at the Tibetan Freedom Concert in Washington, DC Figure 6-1. Lightning struck the crowd while the

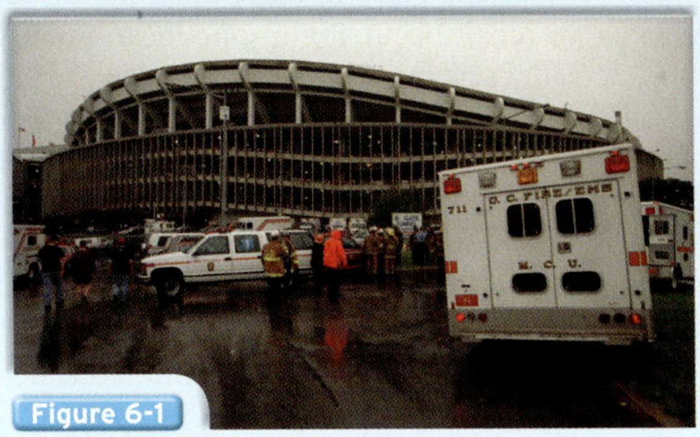

Figure 6-1

The Tibetan Freedom Concert in 1998 had to be canceled due to a lightning strike, which caused an MCI.

music was playing and produced a large number of priority patients, causing both an MCI with structural damage to the venue. Due to this incident, the concert had to be canceled.

It is important to differentiate between a TOPL and an MCI because in an MCI different protocols need to be enacted. A TOPL is the most common situation SEMS will see in a mass gathering.

Triage

Whether the incident is a TOPL or an MCI, SEMS providers will likely need to perform triage. There are many different triage systems in use and there may be a preference for one or another in the area where you work. Two of the more common triage systems are START triage and SALT triage, which will be briefly discussed here.

START triage stands for Simple Triage And Rapid Treatment. It uses a limited assessment of the patient's ability to walk, respiratory status, hemodynamic status, and neurologic status. START triage begins with providers asking people to move to a specific area if they can walk. The remaining patients are then assessed and triaged accordingly. Providers quickly open the airway of any patient who is not breathing, and patients who begin to breathe are placed into the recovery position until further treatment is possible. Patients' hemodynamic status and neurologic status are rapidly assessed so that the patient can be assigned a triage category. Pediatric patients can be triaged with JumpSTART, a pediatric version of START triage.

SALT triage stands for Sort, Assess, Lifesaving interventions, and Treatment and/or Transport. The initial step in this system is to identify which patients can understand verbal instructions; these patients are then moved to a collection point. The SALT method differs from others in its lifesaving intervention steps, which include bleeding control, opening the airway, two rescue breaths for children, needle decompression for tension pneumothorax, and auto-injector antidotes. Patients are then sorted into one of five categories.

National Incident Management System

Since the September 11, 2001, attacks on the United States, all EMS providers have been required by presidential directive to take courses in, and function under, the **National Incident Management System**, also known as NIMS.

With the introduction of the federal government's NIMS standards, all EMS providers and agencies know that there are now many considerations in appropriately planning for and successfully resolving an MCI, including:

- Scene size-up
- Triage
- Movement of patients to the casualty collection points
- Treatment
- Transportation of patients for definitive care

A well-designed incident management system provides both for responder safety and the efficient triage, treatment, and transportation of patients. SEMS providers must be well-versed in NIMS procedures because they may be the ones to immediately respond to the scene when the MCI happens. If an MCI is not managed correctly from the beginning, it becomes very difficult, if not impossible, to regain control and manage the incident correctly later on. In the chaos of an MCI, providers must control the scene immediately. Someone must be assigned the role of scene commander, someone must triage patients, and

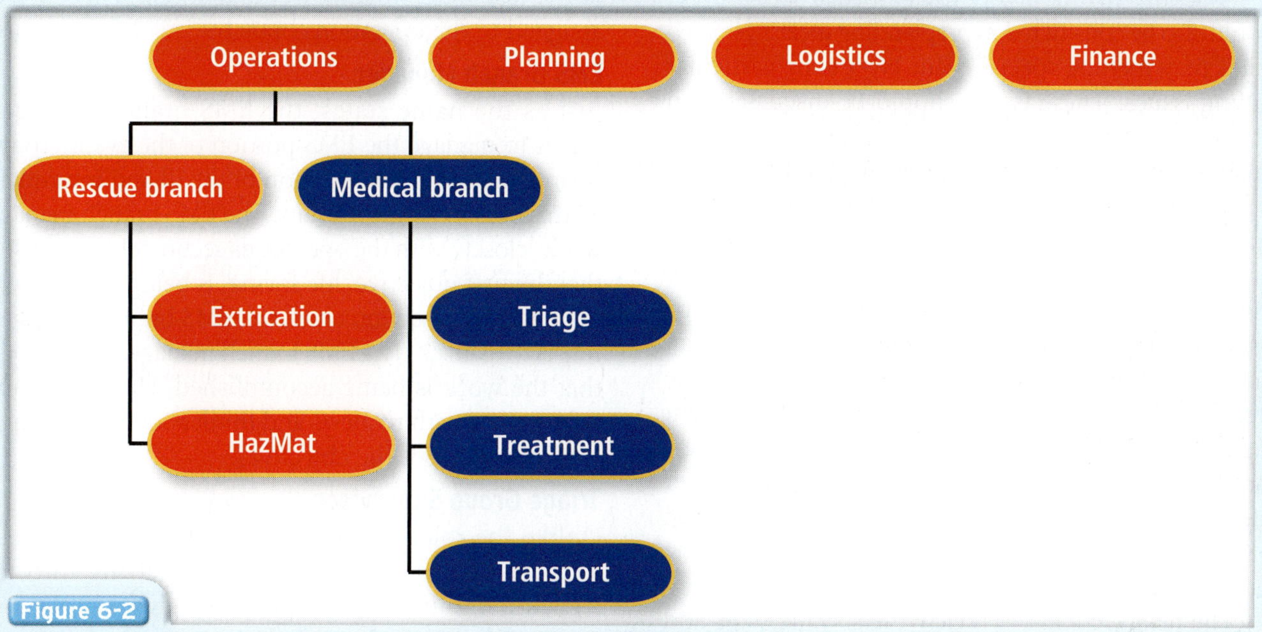

Figure 6-2

Incident command structure. Not all positions will be filled in every incident; however, the incident commander is ultimately responsible for all activity. Subordinates may be appointed to assist in managing the incident.

someone must gather and manage the information. SEMS providers and agencies should be familiar with and rehearse the mass-casualty procedures for their jurisdictions. In most cases, these procedures and plans are written by the local EMS agencies, either on a city, county, or state level. Note that some event medical companies may not have access to these plans; this is something that must be considered and addressed during the preplanning stage. Also, some states have EMS protocols that allow for different levels of care at an MCI. Reimbursement may be an issue if you do not follow these guidelines. Know your local laws.

Staffing for an MCI is not easy and depends on the resources and capabilities of SEMS and surrounding services. The number one priority in an MCI is the effective treatment and stabilization of the affected patient population. Providers will find this impossible if the initial steps are not taken to deal with the incident correctly. These initial steps include:

1. Establish incident command.
2. Size up the incident.
3. Assign an operations section chief, if needed and if manpower allows.
4. Assign an EMS branch manager.
5. Assign the triage, treatment, and transportation group supervisors.
6. Begin working, solving problems with the tools available.
7. Manage resources.
8. Manage the event.
9. Manage information disseminated to the public.

Figure 6-2 shows incident command structure.

TIP

SEMS providers begin MCI preparation during preplanning. Preplanning of the SEMS response to an MCI must take into consideration the same variables that are considered during preplanning for the event itself. These include geographic variables, ingress and egress routes, parking lots that could be used as staging areas, road access and egress to major thoroughfare, the terrain of the event, and the size and scope of the incident.

Issues that may be unique to a particular special event should also be considered in preplanning meetings. Such issues may include special event layouts or particular staffing issues. These issues should be discussed and rehearsed to ensure that medical incident operations function efficiently. For example, at an equestrian event, as a horse crosses the finish line at top speed, it has a heart attack, runs into the crowd, and hits a parked car. This is an MCI because it produced an exceptional number of priority patients, and caused the event to be disrupted. The on-site medical crew had to establish an incident commander, move the bystanders, shield the sites from the crowd, perform triage, coordinate patient packaging and movement to incoming ambulances, coordinate with incoming units and medevac, gather information about patients and the incident, and finally, manage the information that was disseminated to the general public.

The next section will review the specific steps and roles for managing an MCI. At a special event, consider that there may be other personnel on site who can fill some roles. Rapid evaluation and improvisation should be emphasized.

Establishing Command

As discussed earlier, the first step in any MCI is for someone to establish incident command. In a SEMS event, this would be the role of the on-site supervisor. The incident commander's job is to oversee the incident and establish incident objectives based on three NIMS criteria:

- Life saving
- Incident stabilization
- Property preservation

Once these goals are established, the role of the incident commander is to ensure that the people doing the work are meeting the objectives.

Assigning Roles

Operations Section Chief

If manpower allows, the first position filled should be that of an operations section chief. It is the operations section chief's job to take the incident objectives and turn them into action. This person needs to formulate tactics to get the work done. Operations will utilize the resources given to them to manage the incident; operations is the backbone of the entire operation. Most of the resources—manpower and equipment—will be assigned to the operations branch.

EMS Branch Manager

Just as the name states, the EMS branch manager's role is to manage the EMS portion of the event. Triage, treatment, and transportation of the ill and injured are all this person's responsibility. The EMS branch manager works closely with the operations section chief to ensure that the first objective, life saving, is being met. As with the operations section chief, the EMS branch manager's role is to oversee. The EMS branch manager must ensure that the work is being accomplished. He or she must aid workers with requests and think about ways to help providers achieve the objectives.

Triage Group Supervisor

Unlike the roles discussed thus far, the triage group supervisor is a role that involves getting into the trenches of the incident. The triage group supervisor oversees all people performing triage, usually in teams of three to five people per team. He or she also oversees the crews moving patients, called litter teams, to the treatment area. Triage is performed where the patients are, if safe to do so, and the patients are then moved by the litter teams. If safety is a concern, such as in events involving hazardous materials or a weapon of mass destruction, triage may have to be delayed until the patients can be moved to a safer location or until specialty teams with the needed equipment, such as decontaminated equipment or special medications, arrive. These teams can then perform triage in the unsafe area, or "hot zone." The criteria used for triaging patients depends on the local area's triage plan. Patients are classified as red (priority 1; immediate), yellow (priority 2; delayed), green (priority 3; minor), and black (unsalvageable), depending on the injuries found Figure 6-3. The triage group supervisor must keep an accurate count of the total number of victims, including the number of patients in each category, and pass this information to both the EMS branch manager and the treatment and transportation group supervisors, who will be discussed next. Lastly, the triage group supervisor must ensure that all patients have been triaged and moved to the treatment area.

Treatment Group Supervisor

As the name suggests, the treatment group supervisor establishes the treatment area and ensures that all patients receive medical attention.

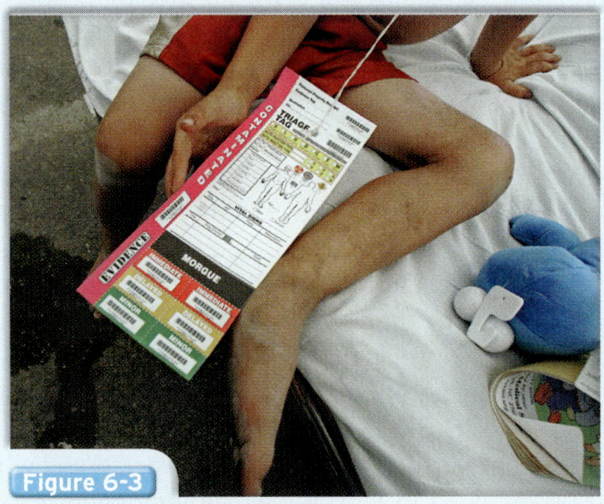

Figure 6-3

Triage at a special event.

Transportation Group Supervisor

One of the busiest people at an MCI is the transportation group supervisor. The transportation group supervisor's job is to move all patients to an appropriate venue for treatment. On a busy day in most cities across the country, a hospital emergency department is already overcrowded. Adding 50 to 75 patients will overload the emergency department. And no matter how prepared a hospital or EMS system believes itself to be, it is not ready for an influx of 20,000 patients, such as occurred in Bhopal, India in 1984. A gas leak killed over 3,000 people and sickened over 20,000 according to some estimates. To help avoid overloading an emergency department, the transportation group supervisor must consider the following questions:

- How will patients be moved (eg, ambulances, buses, helicopters, other options)?
- How will the transportation units get into and leave the loading areas?
- Where will patients be taken (eg, hospitals, clinics, urgent care centers)?
- How many patients can each facility take, and of what triage category?
- How will the patients be tracked? The Transportation Group Supervisor is responsible for tracking each patient's destination facility.

As with roles already covered, preplanning is crucial. Knowing the area's resources, hospital capabilities for receiving patients, transport options in the region, and the plans and forms an organization has in place will be vital to the transportation group supervisor's success.

The Treatment Area

The establishment of treatment areas follows the same guidelines as that of triage. There will need to be a red, yellow, and green treatment area for the patients to be placed into so they can receive appropriate care, as well as a black area for unsalvageable patients. Treatment areas need to be near the site of the MCI but must be

You Are the SEMS Provider

CASE 2

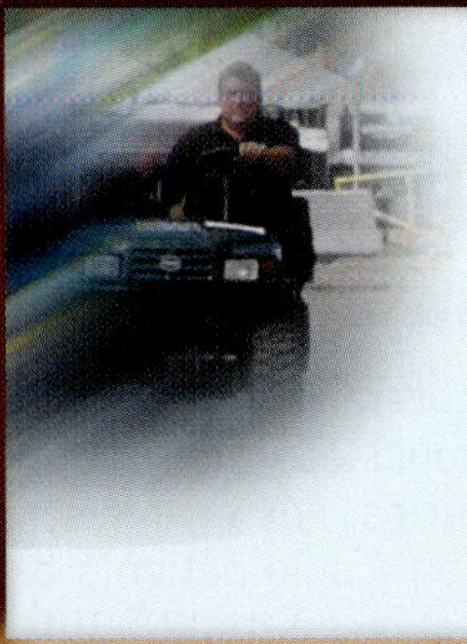

You are providing SEMS coverage at an open-air stadium concert in late spring with 15,000 attendees. There is a chance of rain, which looks likely because you see dark clouds forming. Suddenly, lightning strikes an area in the bleachers.

You and other SEMS providers respond to the scene and note that there are many injured people. During triage, you and your colleagues identify two critically injured patients, six patients with serious injuries, and at least a dozen walking wounded.

You have one basic life support ambulance on-scene, and you determine that you need significant additional resources because there are 20 people who need to be transported.

1. At this point, should you designate this as an MCI or a TOPL?

in a controlled area. This will allow for proper patient flow into and out of the treatment area. The area needs to be identified by a flag or other easily seen object. The existing first aid areas may be used if appropriate. The advantage to using the existing first aid area as the treatment area is that it is already established and functioning. Because the first aid station may quickly become overwhelmed at smaller special events, it is necessary to establish a separate treatment area in the event of an MCI. One option is to use the first aid station as a "green" treatment area for the walking wounded, separate from other treatment areas.

During preplanning, providers should remember that the treatment area must be able to accommodate the maximum number of potential patients should an MCI occur. If SEMS is planning to use the first aid area as the treatment area should an MCI occur, the first aid area must be flexible enough to accommodate more patients. This could mean setting up the first aid tent on a plot of grass that can accommodate an expanded first aid station. If the first aid station cannot be expanded to become a treatment area, providers must plan to have a separate treatment area at another location that can be set up should an MCI occur.

In preplanning, the following questions must be asked regarding the treatment area:

- Where will it be?
- Does the location allow for easy access by litter bearers bringing in field-triage patients?
- How large should the treatment area be, and can it be expanded if needed?
- Does the setup allow for access to needed medical caches?
- Is the treatment area adjacent to, and does it provide for, unimpeded access to the transportation area?
- Is there need for an on-site morgue, and how will it be secured?
- Is weather a consideration?
- How should the treatment area be secured?
- How should supplies be secured?

Should the incident involve hazardous materials, the SEMS provider will have to consider geographic concerns and may need to establish a remote treatment area outside the hot zone. If terrorist activities are suspected, close proximity to the actual incident site may not be prudent.

Another advantage to using a readily established aid station is the proximity and established plan for transporting patients. Due to preplanning and presite survey, the aid station will allow for direct and speedy access to the transportation area. This will prevent incoming patients in the triage area from crossing into and through the transportation area, which would lead to chaos and confusion on the scene.

As mentioned in Chapter 3, first aid stations should be clearly marked. An MCI treatment area must also be clearly marked. Each area should also appear on the event map (if the MCI treatment area will be different than the first aid station location, the incident commander should designate someone to prepare a separate map noting the MCI; this map will be used by SEMS providers, fire personnel, law enforcement personnel, and any other personnel who will be involved in working at the incident). If it is possible to give public service announcements at the venue, SEMS should request that an announcement be made explaining what patrons should do in an emergency and where help is located. In the event of an MCI, the announcement can be modified to communicate new information as needed. These announcements should be preplanned so that there is minimal confusion about what to communicate, should an MCI occur.

Every special event should have an MCI kit that contains cones, flags, patient triage tags, reflective vests, and a bullhorn Table 6-1. Providers should ensure that this kit is readily available and should know where it is stored. The entrance to the treatment area should be marked with cones or flags Figure 6-4.

Special shelters should be considered in the treatment area to shield patients and SEMS providers from the elements. These shelters will depend on the resources available. Possibilities to consider range from a pop-tent to tent to specially designed vehicles. The availability of these resources must be determined during the preplanning phase. In addition to offering protection from rain or other inclement weather events, shelters can provide shade during hot and sunny weather. Because providers will be working outside at most events, having a tent can help providers

TIP

When providing SEMS coverage during an MCI, consider factors that could lead to escalation of the number of injuries. For example, is weather a consideration (could patients become hypothermic? Overheated?) SEMS providers will need to anticipate an escalating scene and act to address it.

TABLE 6-1 Supplies in an MCI Kit

Triage tags - Red (Immediate) - Yellow (Delayed) - Green (Minor) - Black (Unsalvageable)
Clipboard
Pens
Four rolls of barricade tape - Red (Immediate) - Yellow (Delayed) - Green (Minor) - Black (Unsalvageable)
Triage flags
Road cones
Incident command vests (minimum of four) - Command - Triage - Treatment - Transport
Bullhorn
Incident command tracking capability (may be as simple as a dry erase board or as complex as a computer program)
Either a dry-erase board or MCI management software

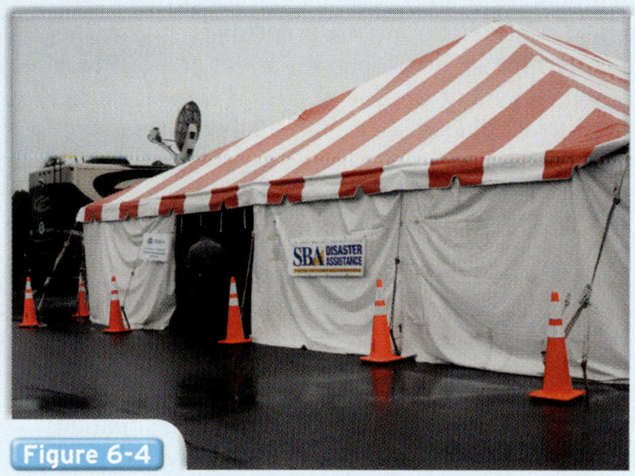

Figure 6-4

The treatment area, like the first aid station, should be marked with cones or flags.

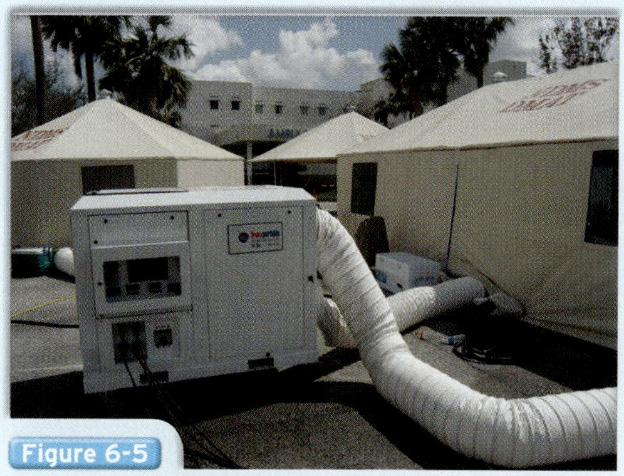

Figure 6-5

A climate-controlled tent.

effectively treat patients with heat-related emergencies in a hot environment or warm a hypothermic patient in a cold environment. Providers should also consider climate-controlled alternatives such as trailers and climate-controlled tents Figure 6-5. More complex shelters will be needed for extended operations, or depending on the nature of the event.

Special MCI Considerations

Security

The number one concern for all venues in the new millennium is security. EMS crews must always be alert to potential security threats. All EMS personnel must have service-issued photo IDs. Photos and names of all personnel, including SEMS personnel, should be submitted to the event manager prior to the special event. The special event security staff should be given proof of a valid ID from each SEMS provider.

Primary Versus Secondary Causes

At special events, the patients may be spread over large areas Figure 6-6. Patients may be injured during the primary MCI or during secondary events, such as trampling and crowd crush injuries. Consider the example of a festival where someone sets off firecrackers. The crowd may mistake the noises for gunshots. Attendees may panic and run. The SEMS providers would find patients hurt at the site of the incident and secondary patients at riot gates if there were a choke point where people were trampled.

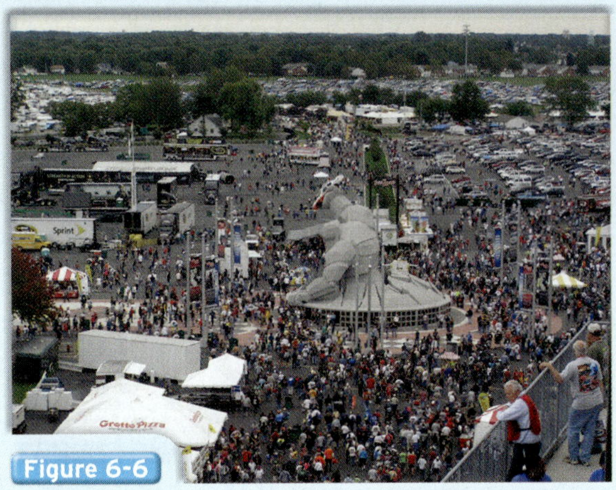

Figure 6-6

A special event may cover a large area, meaning that patients could also be spread over large areas should an MCI occur.

Suspected Terrorist Event

The majority of terrorist attacks against Americans involve conventional weapons—for example, bombs, rockets, and missiles. Like any event, at an MCI measures should be taken to ensure the safety and security of the responders and patients being brought to any treatment area for stabilization. A rule of thumb is, if the incident is known or reasonably suspected to be a terrorist event, locate triage, treatment, and transport operations no less than 1,000 feet from the event location and secure the area so that persons are monitored both entering and exiting.

Terrorist and hazardous materials events present logistic problems to the treatment areas. Patients are transferred from the incident location and will take longer to arrive, possibly with worsening conditions or with contaminants still on them, even after initial decontamination procedures. Additionally, due to the possibility of chemical exposure, these patients could present with conditions requiring special treatment medications and protocols; plan for these and stock in advance if possible. It might be necessary to incorporate trained hazardous materials personnel into the treatment area in these circumstances to provide stabilization efforts until transportation is available.

You Are the SEMS Provider

SUMMARY

CASE 1

1. **How will you handle this situation?**
During the preplanning phase, it is crucial to address how you will handle TOPLs such as this one. Preplanning in this example could include arrangements with EMS systems in surrounding towns to provide backup if needed. Contact information for these resources must be on-hand for easy and quick access. If an event has the potential to occur on a hot day, SEMS providers should consider, during the preplanning phase, the possibility of arranging for a climate-controlled tent or trailer that could be used in the event of a TOPL or MCI. Finally, be sure to bring extra supplies to provide for potential patient overloads such as this. Measures that could be taken to handle this incident include contacting surrounding agencies for additional personnel and supplies such as water, ice, and additional IV fluids, and if possible, identifying a nearby facility that has air conditioning and water available. For example, there may be a local hotel that would agree to allow SEMS providers to use their facility. However, note that handling incidents without having preplanned for them is a worst-case scenario.

CASE 2

1. **At this point, should you designate this as an MCI or a TOPL?**
Distinguishing between an MCI and a TOPL is important because instituting an MCI response for a situation that does not warrant such an alert can unnecessarily end the event. In this case, this incident is so extreme that it is in fact an MCI. The 20 transports will interrupt the event for a significant amount of time. Many additional ambulances will be required to deliver these patients to surrounding hospitals, and resources will be overloaded to the point that the event cannot continue.

Ready for Review

- Providers must remember number 5 of the SEMS 10: a mass gathering is not the same as an MCI.
- The approach at a SEMS event must be different than when providing everyday EMS care. At a mass gathering, it is not medically necessary to transport every patient. Many injuries and illnesses that occur at a special event can be handled and resolved on site.
- A TOPL is not the same as an MCI. A TOPL is a brief period during which there is a larger number of patients than the available resources can handle, but this does not prevent the event from continuing and subsides without external resources being required.
- An MCI is an event that overwhelms the internal and external resources that are required to resolve the situation, resulting in an inability to resume the special event after the incident.
- It is important to differentiate between a TOPL and an MCI; in an MCI, different protocols need to be enacted.
- To decide whether an event is a TOPL or an MCI, providers must consider the source of the event, the scale of the event, the ability of the venue to return to normal after the event, whether the event sustained structural damage, and the number of priority patients.
- When multiple patients approach the aid station at the same time in a TOPL, additional resources may temporarily be required. The need for additional resources must be considered during the preplanning phase.
- A TOPL may escalate to an MCI if multiple patients overwhelm current resources for the foreseeable future and create an overwhelming patient load. An MCI occurs when there is an influx of patients that exceeds current resources as well as the resources that can be called in.
- Whether the incident is a TOPL or an MCI, SEMS providers will likely need to perform triage. Two triage systems are START triage and SALT triage.
- START triage stands for Simple Triage And Rapid Treatment, and uses a limited assessment of the patient's ability to walk, respiratory status, hemodynamic status, and neurologic status.
- SALT triage stands for Sort, Assess, Lifesaving interventions, and Treatment and/or Transport. The initial step in this system is to identify which patients can understand verbal instructions; these patients are then moved to a collection point. The SALT method differs from others in its lifesaving intervention steps.
- The NIMS comes into play if and when an MCI occurs.
- There are many considerations in appropriately planning for and successfully resolving an MCI. These include scene size-up, triage, movement of patients to the casualty collection points, treatment, and transportation of patients for definitive care.
- The number one priority in an MCI is the effective treatment and stabilization of the affected patient population.
- The first step in managing an MCI is establishing incident command. The incident commander's job is to establish incident objectives based on three NIMS criteria: life saving, incident stabilization, and property preservation.
- The role of the operations section chief is to take the incident objectives and turn them into action. This person needs to formulate tactics to get the work done.
- The EMS branch manager is responsible for managing triage, treatment, and transportation of the ill and injured.
- The triage group supervisor oversees all people performing triage and oversees the crews moving patients to the treatment area. The triage group supervisor must keep an accurate count of the total number of victims, including the number of patients in each category, and pass this information to both the EMS branch manager and the treatment and transportation group supervisors.
- The treatment group supervisor is responsible for establishing the treatment area and ensuring that all patients receive medical attention.
- The transportation group supervisor is responsible for moving all patients to an appropriate facility for treatment. This person must plan the logistics of moving patients from the event to the facility that will provide definitive treatment.

- The treatment area must include separate areas for each triage category (red, yellow, green, and black). The treatment area should include enough personnel and resources to adequately handle treatment without wasting resources.
- Treatment areas need to be near the site of the MCI; however, they must be in a controlled area and must be identified by a flag or other easily seen object.
- The existing first aid areas may be used as the treatment area if appropriate.
- Every special event should have an MCI kit that is readily available and that contains cones, flags, patient triage tags, reflective vests, and a bullhorn.
- Special shelters should be considered in the treatment area to shield patients and SEMS providers from the elements.
- The number one concern for all venues is security. All EMS personnel must have service-issued photo IDs.
- Providers should remember that patients may be injured during the primary event or during secondary events.
- Terrorist and hazardous materials events present logistic problems to the treatment areas. Patients may require special treatment or may need to be decontaminated. It might be necessary to incorporate trained hazardous materials personnel into the treatment area in these circumstances.

Vital Vocabulary

dispersed Injuries or illnesses that occur in more than one place.

local Injuries or illnesses that occur in one location only.

mass-casualty incident (MCI) An event in which a large number of casualties are produced in a relatively short period, exceeding local logistic support capabilities. MCIs are usually the result of a single incident such as a military aircraft accident, hurricane, flood, earthquake, or armed attack.

National Incident Management System (NIMS) A Department of Homeland Security system designed to enable federal, state, and local governments and private-sector and nongovernmental organizations to effectively and efficiently prepare for, prevent, respond to, and recover from domestic incidents, regardless of cause, size, or complexity, including acts of catastrophic terrorism.

SALT triage A triage method that first identifies which patients can understand verbal instructions, then involves performing several lifesaving interventions.

START triage A triage method that uses a limited assessment of the patient's ability to walk, respiratory status, hemodynamic status, and neurologic status.

temporary overwhelming patient load (TOPL) A brief period during which there is a larger number of victims than the available resources can handle (though additional resources may need to be brought in), but this does not prevent the event from continuing and subsides without external resources being required.

CHAPTER

Weather and Outdoor Events

7

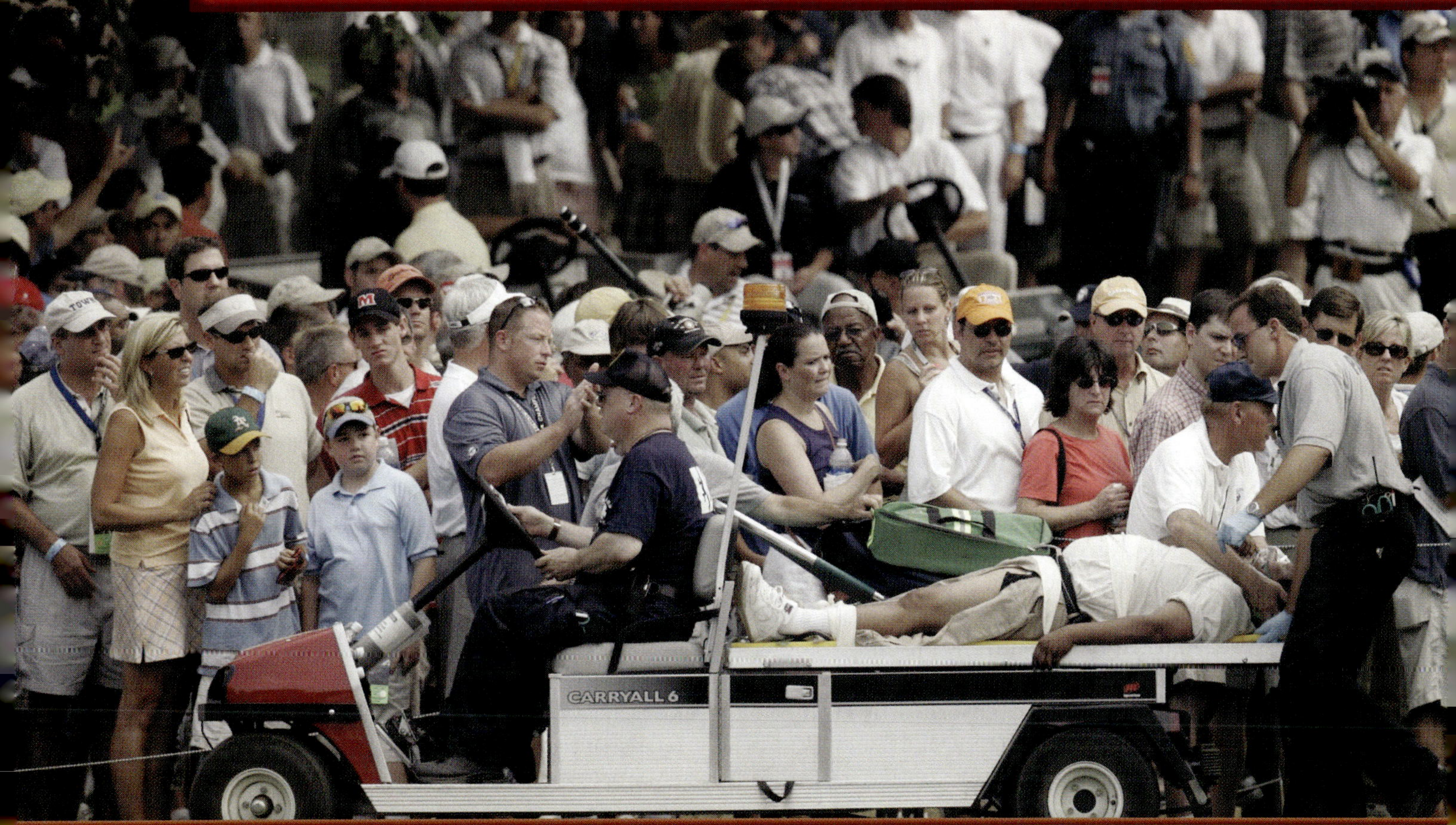

LEARNING OBJECTIVES

- Discuss considerations for events that will occur in hot weather.
- Explain the significance of dehydration and the rule of thumb for proper hydration.
- Discuss considerations for events that will occur in cold or wet weather.
- Discuss special considerations at road races and marathons.
- Discuss events that involve water, including river sports, open water sports, and multi-venue sports, and considerations for preplanning and working at these events.
- Understand the preplanning considerations that are unique to outdoor events.
- Explain the factors to consider when reviewing the weather history prior to an event.
- Describe situations that may have extremes of temperature, and how to effectively preplan for them.
- List items that should be taken into consideration regarding the venue's terrain.
- Discuss methods for responding to inclement weather should it occur.
- Describe types of lightning injuries and when they may occur.

Introduction

Outdoor events pose unique challenges for EMS providers. Weather and environmental factors constitute a major influence on the patient load. To review, the patient load is the total number of patients per hour a service can expect to treat at special events.

Weather Considerations

Hot Weather

In hot weather, SEMS providers can expect dehydration and heat-related illnesses (eg, heat exhaustion and, less commonly, heat stroke). Several conditions can worsen the morbidity and mortality from heat-related illness, including dehydration, fever, infection, lack of recent heat exposure, alcohol consumption, sunburn, lack of sleep, excessive clothing, diarrhea, or vomiting. Many medications, including amphetamines, antihistamines, anticholinergics, beta blockers, diuretics, psychiatric medications, sympathomimetics, neuroleptics, and certain illicit drugs can contribute to heat illness. Heat-related illness is one of the most preventable diseases. SEMS considerations should include efforts to prevent heat-related illnesses from occurring, including cooling stations, comfort stations, adequate water, cool or chilled water (which is more rapidly absorbed by the body and will assist with both rehydration and cooling), and adequate areas of shade and comfort Figure 7-1.

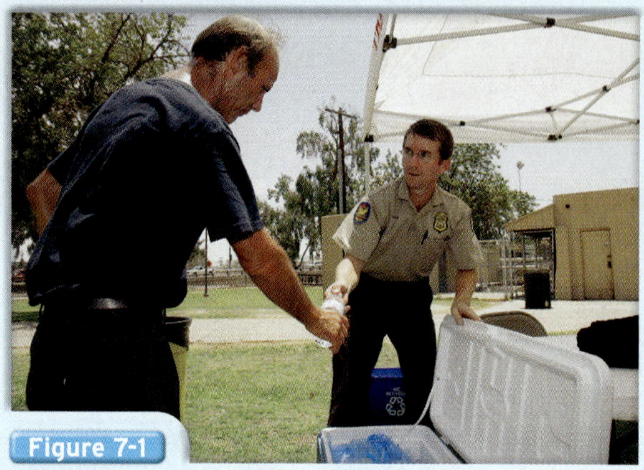

Figure 7-1

Initiatives such as cooling stations, adequate water, and areas of shade and comfort can help prevent heat-related illnesses.

Prior to the event, it is a good idea to discuss with event organizers how water will be made available to attendees and participants. As a SEMS provider, you may wish to recommend that there be access to free drinking water or allow coolers with non-alcoholic beverages to be brought in by patrons. It may be worthwhile to point out to event promoters during preplanning that it is okay to sell water, but this should not be the only option; if free drinking water is not available and patrons are not allowed to bring their own non-alcoholic beverages, this can lead to more heat-related and dehydration-related emergencies.

Also remember that during warm and hot weather, SEMS providers should expect wasp and beestings, as

You Are the SEMS Provider

CASE 1

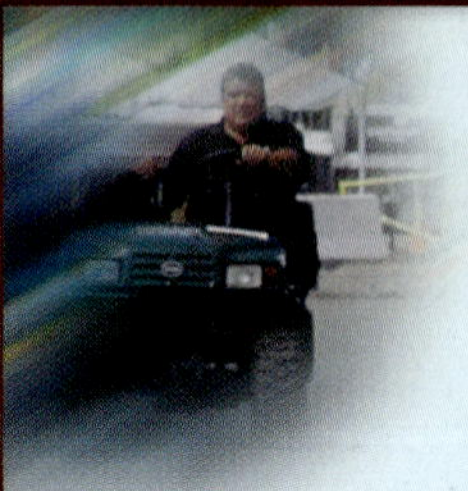

Your private service has been asked to provide EMS coverage at a 2-day music festival in mid-August. The festival will take place at a local race track. The special event organizers will primarily be using the infield and grandstand (which has an air-conditioned first floor). Parking is both on-site and off-site. For those days, the average temperature is 87°F (30.6°C) with high humidity. The special event organizers estimate a target attendance of 60,000 per day, but ticket sales are way down from last year's event. Your agency is providing EMS services for the special event. Also, the local jurisdiction insists on having their EMS resources present, the local hospital also has volunteered its services, and 400 security personnel in addition to an unknown number of uniformed police will be present. In previous years, the event had two first aid tents, but this year venue management would like to have only one. In addition, venue management is asking your service to provide three misting tents.

While reading reports from previous years, you note quite a few alcohol-related incidents.

1. In your initial size-up of the special event, what are your major safety and security concerns?
2. How many first aid stations and staff should be planned for this event?

TIP The combination of excessive heat without adequate hydration can be lethal.

wasps and bees are likely to congregate around garbage cans and areas with food.

Dehydration

A patient's condition can deteriorate rapidly by dehydration from extreme heat; the patient can degenerate into heat exhaustion and in the worst case scenario, heat stroke. Dehydration is not as common in the cooler months; however, remember that as people add layers and move around, they sweat and lose fluid, so dehydration in cooler temperatures is still possible.

The rule of thumb for proper hydration in hot weather is that a person should consume enough fluid to urinate every 45 minutes to an hour. This is a good rule of thumb even in cooler weather. During preplanning, event managers will need to ensure that they do not overlook the need to supply proper amounts of water for participants.

During the summer months, there is a heightened awareness of the importance of proper hydration. Unfortunately as the weather gets cooler, people are not as cognizant of its importance. Event organizers need to be aware that it is still important to make sure the participants are properly hydrated even during the cooler months.

Finally, remember that dehydration can occur more quickly in people with diabetes, older adults, and children, and it can exacerbate existing medical conditions. These populations need much earlier intervention. Also, medications for diabetes, such as hypoglycemic drugs and insulin, have side effects related to thermoregulation. These drugs contribute to rewarming problems.

Hyponatremia

Hyponatremia (an abnormally low level of sodium in the blood) may be seen in any event when an athlete takes in more water than the body can handle. This condition is more common in endurance events such as marathons and triathlons, though it could occur in athletes in other sporting events. When an athlete consumes more water than the body can process, the electrolyte balance in the bloodstream is diluted. To compensate, water seeps into the cells, which swell, and the body limits blood flow to the kidneys. This leads to a reduction in urine production. The sodium/potassium balance necessary for proper cardiac function and nervous function may also be affected.

Patients with this condition generally present almost identically to someone suffering from dehydration, with nausea, vomiting, lightheadedness, confusion, or dizziness. In more severe cases, patients may present with a headache from increased pressure on the brain due to the buildup of fluid. As the condition worsens, confusion, seizures, coma, and death can result from the pressure on the brain. It may be difficult for a SEMS provider to tell the difference between hyponatremia and dehydration. A detailed patient interview, including the history of present illness, is a useful tool. Questions to ask the patient include the amount of water he or she consumed, and the most recent time of and estimated amount of urination.

If in doubt, and the case is severe, transport the patient to a definitive care facility. Fluid replacement is essential in dehydration, but giving a patient with hyponatremia water can worsen the patient's condition by further diluting the patient's already low sodium levels.

The treatment of hyponatremia varies; some experts advocate giving the patient sports drinks that contain electrolytes while others argue that these drinks contain such low doses that the water in the solution will worsen the patient's condition. Be sure you know your local protocol. In most cases, the condition is minor and normal body functions will return after the event. Ensure that the patient is observed until he or she starts urinating out the extra fluid. In more severe cases, a normal saline IV solution may need to be administered (according to protocol). If this is necessary, the patient should be transported to a hospital for further care and observation.

Cold or Wet Weather

On cold and rainy days, SEMS providers should plan for cold-related illnesses such as hypothermia and frostbite as well as falls from slippery surfaces. Hypothermia should be considered at any event occurring in cool or cold weather, any event involving water, and any outdoor cool-weather or cold-weather event where alcohol is served (Figure 7-2).

Cold-weather events generally produce lower casualty rates. There are considerable variables that could affect these lower rates, including that winter events tend to have a smaller attendance. Additionally, participants are generally better prepared for cold weather, wearing coats, hats, and gloves. Finally, it is easier to get someone from a cold location to a warmer location than vice versa.

Also, note the time of year when the event is occurring, as this relates to when it will become dark outside. Once it becomes dark, it will become colder, and you will need to plan for this.

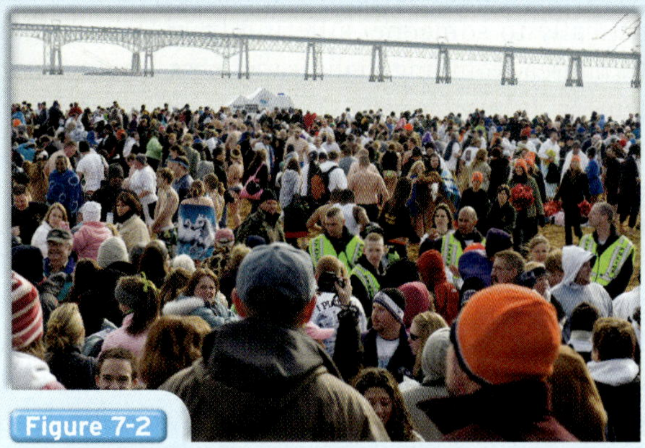

Figure 7-2

The chance for hypothermia will be increased at special events involving water in cold weather, such as this polar bear plunge.

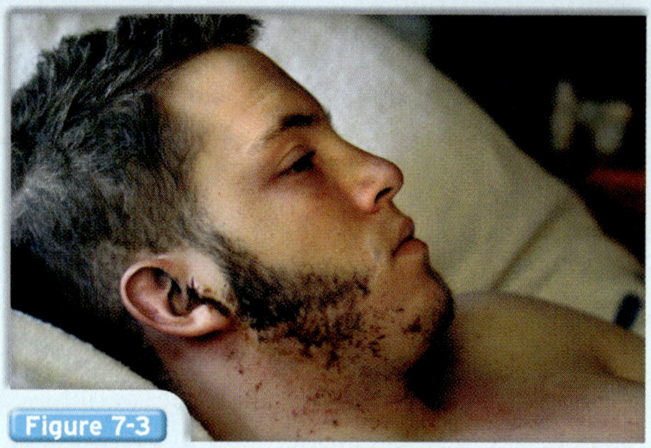

Figure 7-3

A burn from a lightning injury.

Lightning

SEMS may cover high-risk events such as outdoor fairs, festivals, and golf tournaments. At these types of special events, it is possible for people to be caught in the open by freak, fast-moving, violent weather phenomena. In such scenarios, people may seek shelter under a lone tree or lone metal structure, or engage in behavior that may increase their chances of being struck by lightning.

Lightning strike is one of the most common causes of death from isolated environmental or natural phenomena. Lightning injuries are sometimes mistakenly classified as electrical injuries, but there are some significant differences. First, lightning injuries usually do not cause significant tissue destruction along the path of the current to its ground point. Second, lightning strikes more commonly cause blunt force trauma, while electrical injuries do not.

Lightning injuries are grouped into three categories:

- *Mild*. These injuries result in little damage and include superficial burns, loss of consciousness, and confusion.
- *Moderate*. These injuries are more dangerous. They include burns, seizures, respiratory arrest, or cardiac arrest that resolves Figure 7-3.
- *Severe*. These injuries are often fatal and include respiratory and cardiac arrest, or traumatic injuries.

Serious injuries that can occur as a result of a lightning strike include:

- Cardiac arrhythmias
- Burns
- Internal injuries
- Rupture of internal organs
- Spinal cord injuries
- Paralysis
- Prolonged paresis

TIP One of the goals of SEMS is to increase patient survivability in lightning strikes by having in place a system, plan, and the resources to rapidly assess and treat patients.

A burn caused by lightning may have a feathery or zigzag appearance. Despite its unique appearance, the immediate life threats caused by lightning strike are airway obstruction, respiratory arrest, cardiac arrest, and trauma.

Any patient who you suspect to have a lightning-related injury must receive a complete trauma assessment, and the cervical spine should be stabilized. Triage may need to be performed, and patients with life-threatening injuries should be cared for first. As always, follow local protocols regarding these injuries.

Specific Outdoor Events

Outdoor sporting events and events involving water may require specific considerations during preplanning and while working at the event. These considerations are covered in the next sections.

Road Races and Marathons

Road races are popular for many reasons. They are often associated with fund-raising efforts, or may occur purely for competition. Marathons may be mega-events, requiring multiple first aid stations as well as hydration and cooling measures. Bike marathons are popular as well. They may be multiple day events. As a SEMS provider, it is important to remember that these events might draw participants who are not well conditioned. Also, it is estimated that any endurance athlete competing for more than 3 continuous hours experiences a 1 in 50,000 chance of death due to heart failure within the following 24-hour period, regardless of health status.

When these events involve large distances, it will be especially important to preplan how SEMS providers will reach patients at any location on the course Figure 7-4. At a bike race, for example, the patient could be 40 miles from a start line or finish line. When preplanning SEMS coverage for any long-distance race, it is important to give special consideration to the best locations for rest stops (which provide water and a place for participants to rest) and first aid stations. Such events will require multiple rest stops and access to plenty of drinking water. When preplanning, the SEMS provider should consider the terrain and course. It is usually a good idea to place rest stops or first aid stations around inclines, declines, or near long stretches on the course. If you expect the weather to be hot or humid, plan to have more stations.

It is a good idea to have a mobile SEMS unit centrally located (for example, at the middle of the course) so that it can get to any part of the race; do not place the mobile SEMS unit at the start line or finish line.

Road races and bicycle races are two situations in which it might make sense to have a mobile SEMS unit following the race. However, remember that if a mobile SEMS unit follows the race, it will be following the slowest component of the race, and this is not usually the group that needs the majority of care. There should be other SEMS providers stationed at various points along the race so that race participants are not solely dependent on the mobile SEMS unit.

Finally, in bicycle racing, the windchill effect from riding, even in warm or hot weather, can cause the cyclist to experience mild hypothermia. Keep this in mind when providing medical care at these events.

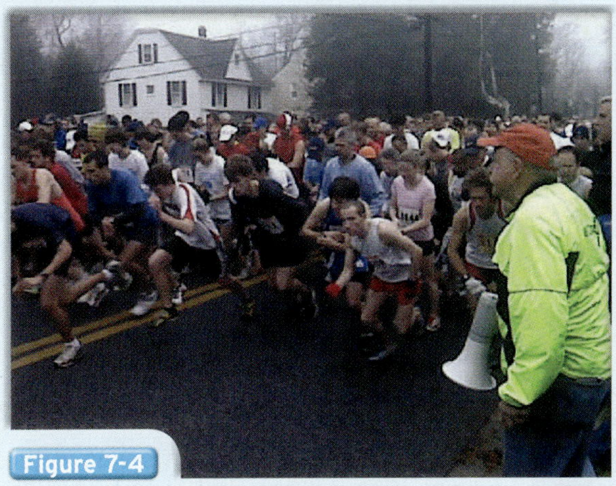

Figure 7-4

At road races, it is important for SEMS providers to preplan how to reach patients at any location on the course.

Events Involving Water

SEMS providers may work at events that involve water. These can be events where the entire event involves water, such as boat races, open swims, or polar bear plunges, or they can be events where only a portion of the event involves water, such as a triathlon.

These events may have constructed water platforms designed for a specific sport. Remember that not all arenas are created equal. We will discuss various water sports, including some extreme water sports and sports that occur in man-made venues.

River Sports

White water rafting and river kayaking are two main river sports Figure 7-5. A river's rapids are graded on a scale of one to six, with one being the easiest and six the most advanced, and involve a high probability of injury or even death. An example of grade 6 rapids is those leading to Niagara Falls. Participants are required to wear helmets, knee and elbow pads, and a personal flotation device. Training is required before descending the most difficult rivers.

Riverboarding is an extreme water sport in which an athlete lies prone on a boogie board with his or her face 6 inches from the water's surface Figure 7-6. The rider wears a wet suit for protection from the cold water and is equipped with small fins for navigation. Flotation devices and helmets are worn. Riverboards are also used to rescue victims in water rapids. The board allows the rider to rapidly access a victim who may have

TIP SEMS providers must always expect hypothermia at an event that involves water.

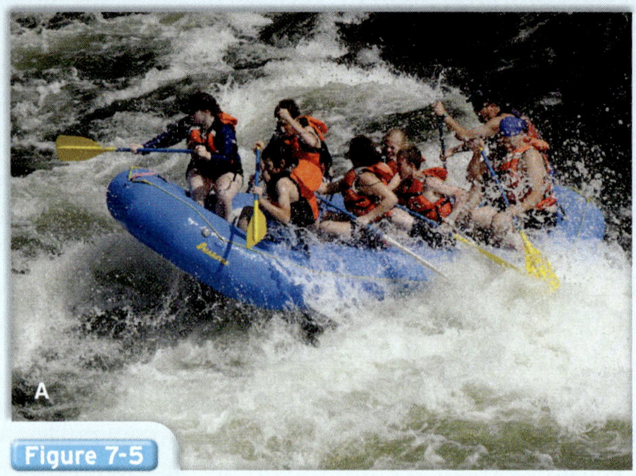

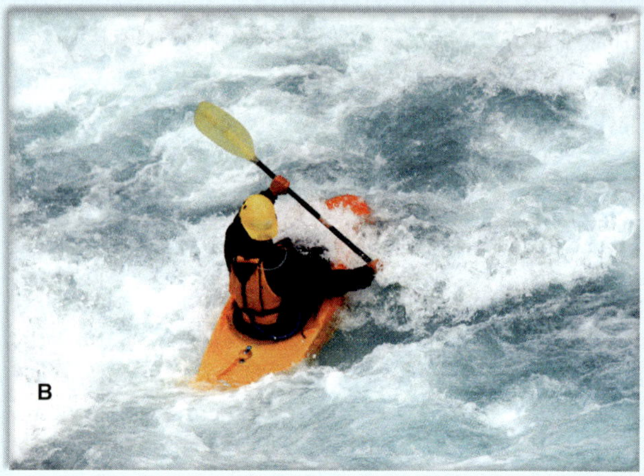

Figure 7-5

A. A white water raft. **B.** A river kayak.

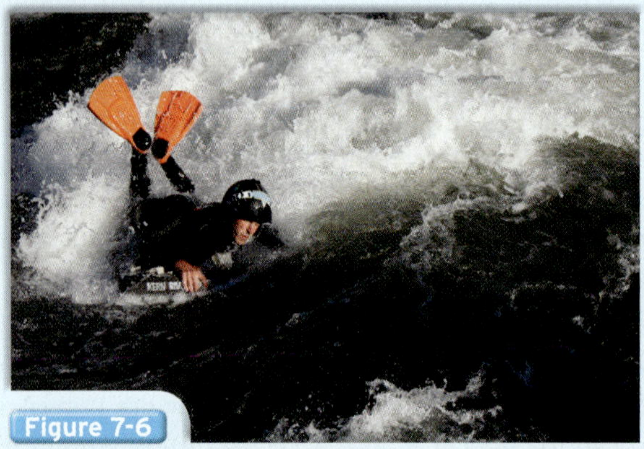

Figure 7-6

Riverboarders use a boogie board to travel down river rapids.

been swept downstream in either this sport or while performing other river sports.

Open Water Sports

SEMS providers may find themselves assisting with medical coverage at **open water sports** events, though many of these events will have specialty diving crews or water rescue crews. Open water sports are water sports held on the seas. Some are for everyone, while others require training and certification to participate.

Open swim is one of the oldest documented water competition sports. Because no equipment except a swimsuit is required and competitors range from novice to expert, a SEMS provider can expect to witness a wide range of possible issues at these events. Potential injuries range from simple muscle strains to cardiac arrest from either drowning or physical exertion. The most obvious SEMS concern is how to reach a swimmer who is in trouble. Some open swim races cover a distance of over 80 kilometers (over 50 miles) of water that can have hundreds of swimmers and potential patients. Specialty equipment for an event like this is a must, and these events may require higher ratios of equipment to participants.

Additionally, when an open swim is held in a natural outdoor body of water, riptides and marine animals are a danger to both participants and SEMS providers. A **riptide** is a current that runs perpendicular to the beach. It can pull a person out to sea very quickly and is an unseen danger. Both experienced and novice swimmers can be killed by this force. As a SEMS provider, knowledge of these concerns will be your best guard against you or a member of your team becoming a victim.

Open swim may be a component of a triathlon. **Triathlons** consist of three portions: a road race of 3.2 miles, a bike race of 24.8 miles, and an open water swim of 0.98 mile. These are the lengths for the events during the Olympics; lengths may vary at other triathlons. For example, iron man triathlons use different distances, but the components are the same (road race, bike race, and open swim). At triathlons, the SEMS provider must remember the special considerations for

> **TIP** Before working at an event involving water, find out if the event participants will be novices. If so, you can expect more injuries than if the participants have special training or certifications.

open swim events, but the added issue of fatigue must now be considered, along with considerations for bike races and road races.

Polar bear plunges, events at which participants jump into frigid water, are some of the most anticipated and attended fund-raising events in the United States. These events are sponsored by local civic and community organizations as a method to raise moeny for a specific charity. Plungers get sponsorship for their participation in the event. As the name suggests, participants earn pledged money by jumping into frigid water, usually a large lake or ocean. These events are typically held in January and February, when the ambient temperature can be around 20°F and water temperatures not much above freezing. Since hypothermia is a possibility, the dip is very short in duration. Spirits are very high at these events; however, these events present a real danger to the swimmers and the SEMS providers. In such frigid waters, hypothermia can set in within minutes and can be fatal in as little as 15 minutes.

An example of a dangerous polar bear plunge occurred at the Maryland event "Plungapalooza," one of the largest polar bear plunges in the United States. This event has an average of over 10,000 attendees and raises over 2 million dollars. However, on January 31, 2010, a severe cold spell caused ambient air temperatures to be in the lower 20s (°F) with windchills in the teens to single digits. The water temperature was estimated at 36°F. An estimated 15,000 people were set to participate in two groups of plungers. After the first group's plunge, several plungers had to be treated for hypothermia; three were transported to a nearby hospital for further evaluation Figure 7-7. While no permanent injuries or deaths occurred, the second group plunge was canceled. This event highlights how quickly an event can cause major patient care issues.

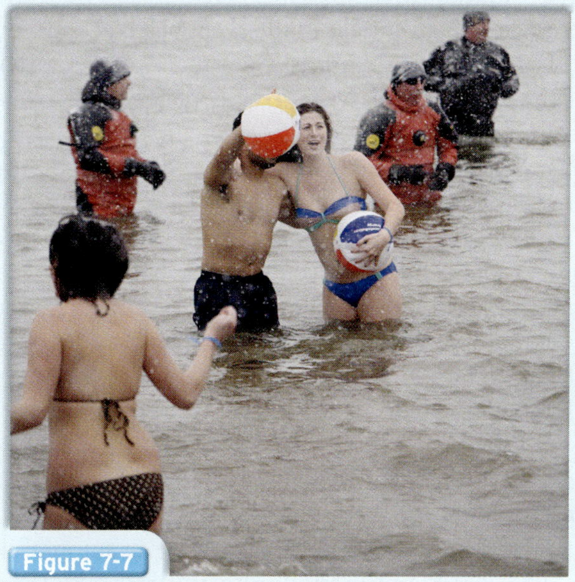

Figure 7-7

A polar bear plunge.

SEMS providers working at surfing events should note that surfers, like other extreme sports participants, may engage in reckless behavior that can produce dangerous rescue conditions if a need arises. Drowning is a common injury among surfers. Surfers do not, as a rule, have any safety equipment. Recently a "leash" was added to surfboards to connect the surfer to the board to prevent the surfer from losing the board, but this does not keep the surfer afloat and can even be dangerous.

Collisions are a significant threat to surfers. The majority of collisions occur with other surfboards. These incidents produce deep lacerations or severe puncture wounds. While most are minor, infection is always a danger. Finally, as mentioned, riptides are another danger.

Free diving is an extreme sport in which a person dives as deep as possible into water while holding his or her breath, not using any device to assist breathing. This extreme sport takes advantage of some unique physiological properties within the human body that allow the diver to endure a lack of oxygen that would otherwise cause death.

Before diving, professional freedivers may hyperventilate to postpone the stimulation of the breathing center in the brain. Since the oxygen level of the red blood cells is not increased by hyperventilation, a dangerous and potentially fatal situation can develop, known as shallow water blackout or deep water blackout. Shallow water blackout is more common and occurs at an average depth of only 15 feet. **Shallow water blackout** is a loss of consciousness that occurs while underwater in depths of about 15 feet or less, caused by hypoxia from holding one's breath. **Deep water blackout** is a loss of consciousness that occurs while ascending to the surface after a dive of at least 32 feet, and which is the result of a rapid drop in the partial pressure of oxygen on ascent. Shallow water blackout is more common and can be deadly; the diver becomes unconscious, is unable to

TIP Be aware of local laws and promoter requirements regarding which specific agencies must be notified about an event involving water. Some areas may require that the local fire department dive team or other dive team be notified when such an event is scheduled.

surface, and drowns. Most free divers wear a buoyancy belt to help them surface in the event of a blackout.

Lastly, scuba diving is a popular water sport in which the scuba diver wears a self-contained underwater breathing apparatus (hence the acronym "scuba"). While no professional competition exists for scuba diving, there are scuba diving events where large groups will participate in dives. SEMS providers may work at these events or at other events where scuba divers may comprise some of the rescue personnel. Therefore, event participants or rescue personnel may become your patients. The numbers for incidents involving divers will tell you why SEMS providers may be required at a large event where divers will be involved. A Japanese study performed in 2000 showed that a scuba diver, hour for hour, was between 36% and 62% more likely to suffer an injury than someone driving an automobile.

The most common diving injuries are those involving **barotraumas**, injuries resulting from pressure disequilibrium across body surfaces. Ruptured ear drums and damaged sinuses result from pressure changes that are not dealt with while diving. This is just one of the reasons why a certification is required to dive beyond certain depths.

Other diving injuries include **decompression sickness**, in which gas bubbles form in the body when a diver ascends too quickly. Decompression sickness must be treated promptly, usually in a decompression chamber. Administering oxygen to a diver with decompression sickness is all that can initially be done until transport to a facility with one of these chambers. Even with rapid field treatment and transport to an appropriate facility, fatality or permanent disability may still occur. Make sure the diver's watch or dive chart are transported with the patient to the hospital. These will contain important data on the depth of his or her dive and the air mixture that was being used for this dive.

Another danger from using compressed gases is **nitrogen narcosis**. It is a reversible change in consciousness that results from using nitrogen in the mixture of air. This narcosis produces a state similar to that of alcohol intoxication and is found in divers who breathe high pressure gas at depth. This can impair judgment and make diving very dangerous. Narcosis effects can begin for some divers at 66 feet (20 meters), at which point it presents as a slight giddiness. Most divers notice the effects by 132 feet (40 meters). At these depths, divers may feel euphoria, anxiety, loss of coordination, and lack of concentration. At extreme depths, hallucinogenic reaction and tunnel vision can occur. Nitrogen narcosis occurs quickly, and the symptoms usually disappear rapidly during the ascent.

Finally, **oxygen toxicity** can occur. Oxygen toxicity occurs when oxygen in the body exceeds a safe "partial pressure," described as PPO_2. In extreme cases of this type of toxicity, the central nervous system becomes affected, causing a seizure. This seizure can result in the diver spitting out his or her regulator, and with no one there to assist, the diver will drown. Fortunately, as deadly as this can be, it is also easily avoided by using special blends of air when diving below 180 feet (55 meters).

Multi-Venue Water Sports

Multi-venue water sports are sports that can be held either on rivers, lakes, or open oceans. In this category, the events that present the most concern are boat racing events, where boats travel as fast as 160 mph. Obviously, the faster the boat speeds, the greater the danger to the participant and crowds viewing the event.

Boat racing events present specific concerns for SEMS providers. Quite often these events are held near waterways that may have very limited access for EMS units. Dirt roads, single lane roadways, or parks with no roadways at all may be obstacles that the SEMS planner must address during preplanning. It is important to discuss these issues with the event promoter, and the SEMS planner should do an on-site inspection well before the event is scheduled. Also a site visit should be completed once obstacles such as spectator fences are placed by the venue.

Hydroplane racing is a type of racing in which specially designed watercrafts are raced. These boats have a cockpit similar to that of a jet fighter to protect the driver, and use a jet-powered turbine engine similar to that of a helicopter to propel them around a course. Scientific developments that have helped to address boat racing safety issues include Kevlar cockpits and seat belt systems designed to prevent the driver from being ejected from the cockpit of the boat. Safety precautions for the sport have developed to the point that there are now event age groups as young as age 9 years.

SEMS providers must expect injuries among boat race participants and among fans. Examples of the problems faced by a SEMS provider are highlighted by an incident that occurred in Pittsburgh, Pennsylvania, on August 7, 1988. The annual regatta was being held over the Fourth of July holiday and drew over 400,000 people. On this day, a Formula One boat traveling at over 160 mph crashed into the shore, injuring 24 spectators, half of whom were children Figure 7-8. Fortunately, preplanning had been thorough, and all patients were triaged and transported in less than an hour. Of the victims, 33% suffered injuries that required transport to a Level 1 trauma center. Clearly, providers

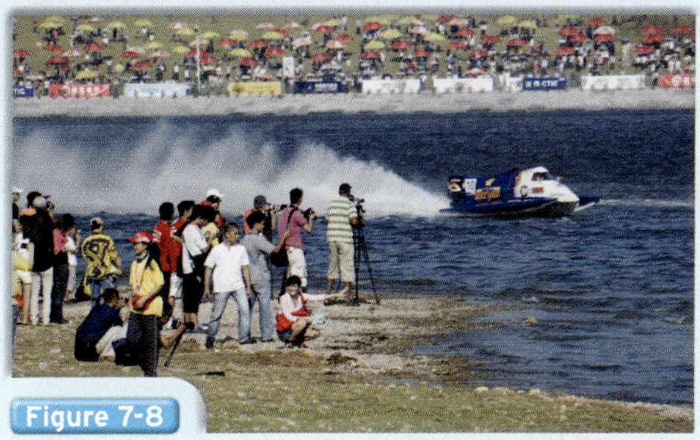

Figure 7-8

A boat racing event can lead to crashes within the crowd.

must be prepared for not only the routine calls, but also a mass-casualty incident that can develop within seconds.

Water skiing may be performed on almost any waterway deep enough for the use of a speedboat, such as a large river or pond, or in some instances, man-made lakes designed specifically for water skiing. This sport has developed to include slalom racing, ski jumping, and trick skiing. A personal flotation device is commonly worn, and at some water skiing events, helmets are also worn to protect the individual from head trauma. Speeds reached in the events can range from 18 to 35 miles per hour (mph). **Barefoot water skiing** is water skiing without skis. Speeds between 40 and 50 mph are required to perform this sport, so there is a greater chance for injury. Water surfaces feel like concrete when struck while traveling at these speeds. For this reason, barefoot water skiers must wear a wet suit with a built-in flotation device. Also, most barefoot water skiers will wear special padded shorts to protect the soft tissues of the upper legs and buttocks.

SEMS Considerations

General issues for a SEMS provider at a water-based event include remaining safe around water and ensuring that very thorough preplanning has been conducted, including preplanning how to reach patients and how transport units will access the venue.

Millions of people enjoy water sports safely. However, all water sports can be dangerous. Drowning is the fifth most common cause of accidental death in the United States, more common than death from fires and lightning strikes. In certain age groups, drowning is the most common cause of death after motor vehicle crashes. Additionally, for every death by drowning, four people are seen in emergency departments for problems caused while in the water. Most of these deaths and injuries are simply caused by a lack of proper safety gear. Nine out of ten people who die in boating accidents are drowning victims who did not wear a personal flotation device.

As mentioned, for the SEMS provider, the most important question is how to reach patients in the water. Any SEMS provider working at an event involving water must be a capable swimmer. A personal flotation device for each provider is a must. In some cases, special training exists, and only those who have received this training should work at the event. Swift water rescue courses, certified lifeguard courses, and scuba certifications are just a few of the special requirements that SEMS providers may need.

SEMS providers will also need to consider the equipment required to rescue a victim from one of these venues. Boats, scuba equipment, and special flotation devices designed to carry patients is just a partial list of the specialty gear that will be required. As usual, preplanning will be a key to success. Who will be providing this equipment? If it is your organization, where will you acquire the needed supplies? Do you need greater numbers of resources on the water, or will most SEMS providers be stationed on land? Most EMS services do not have speedboats readily available. You must also plan to care for spectators, especially at boat races. Because special equipment is required, preplanning cannot be

You Are the SEMS Provider

CASE 2

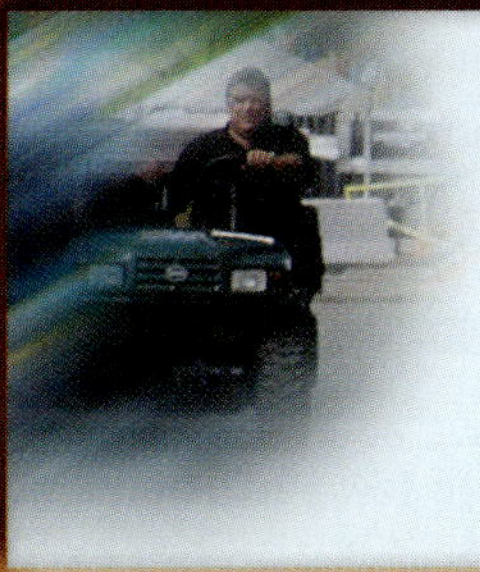

You are providing SEMS coverage at a speedboat racing event taking place in the fall. It is late afternoon and becoming cool. As you are watching one of the races, you see a speedboat start to lose control. Suddenly the boat hits another boat, becomes airborne, and flies out of the water and into the crowd of spectators.

1. What is the first thing you should do in this situation?
2. During preplanning, how can you plan for a major incident such as this?

stressed enough. With a successful preplanning phase, even if a tragedy strikes, you will be prepared to provide services to participants, spectators, or both.

Preplanning Measures

First Aid Tents

At an outdoor event, the first aid tents provide shelter from the elements. Also, if a suitable permanent structure is not available to serve as an on-site medical facility, it will be necessary to provide suitably equipped mobile first aid units. First aid tents and on-site medical facilities were discussed in detail in Chapter 3. At events that occur in hot weather, it will be important to provide an air-conditioned environment and plenty of water.

On-site Medical Facilities

At a large outdoor event, more than one medical facility may be necessary, depending on the size of the event, potential number of attendees, and number of expected emergencies. When multiple medical facilities are needed, it may be prudent to designate one as the main medical facility and have the others serve as satellite first aid stations. Satellite first aid stations should be equipped to handle minor patient care complaints with provisions such as bandages and ice packs. Patients who need greater attention (eg, IV fluid rehydration) need to be transported to the main care facility, which will be better equipped with the appropriate supplies and staff.

Outdoor Terrain

As mentioned in Chapter 2, it is important to consider the venue's terrain, especially at outdoor events Figure 7-9.

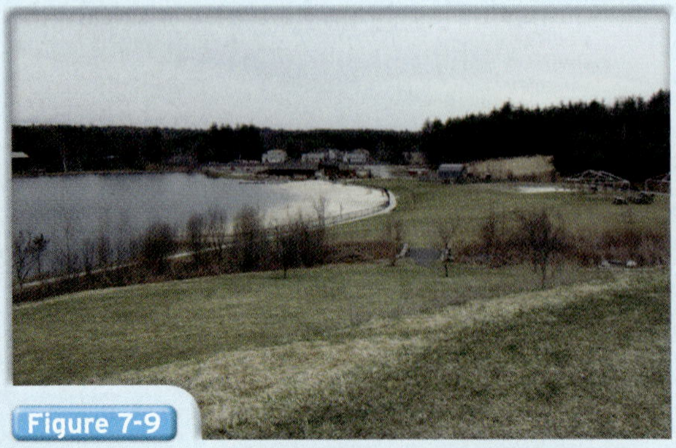

Figure 7-9

Terrains of outdoor events may vary, and every feature should be taken into consideration when preplanning the event.

TIP If dispatch is being used at the event, it may be a good idea for the dispatch center to be located off-site in case of power problems.

Review the following points about terrain, and consider them during preplanning:

- What is the type of surface:
  - Grass
  - Loose gravel
  - Asphalt
  - Concrete
  - Temporary flooring
  - Other
- What is the condition of the surface?
- Is the surface even or uneven?
- Are there areas that cannot be easily viewed?
- Where is the best vantage point?
- Where are the spectators located?
- How are the spectators contained?

Note that at larger events, the terrain can vary. For example, a community festival may take place partly on concrete streets and partly on grassy areas. A cart or gator may be handy for accessing patients across larger areas of terrain. If your service does not have carts or gators readily available, they may be available on loan from event organizers.

Weather History

SEMS providers must always consider the weather, geography, and type of special event, all of which are essential to an appropriate response. Weather impacts an emergency response in profound ways. Rain, snow, sleet, cold, and even hot, sunny weather are serious impediments to both patient care and responder safety. For example, during the 2009 presidential inauguration ceremony, rehearsals were held at night, and temperatures dropped to single digits. Such temperatures limit the time a provider can safely work outside and increase the patient load when people are ill prepared for the extreme temperatures. The same holds true in extreme heat. When preplanning for specific weather, remember that conditions will affect event attendees and also SEMS providers.

TIP It may be helpful to have additional vehicles such as a pickup truck to tow equipment and resupply outdoor events.

TIP Remember that in wet weather, dirt and grass surfaces can quickly become muddy and slippery.

It is essential to review the weather history for the past 5 years and find out the average temperature for each day of the special event. Find out the rainfall amounts, any extreme weather events, and the humidity levels. All of these factors need to be considered. Consider, for example, if it is traditionally the hottest week of the year or the coldest week of the year, you will need additional supplies to address the expected emergencies, and additional staff.

The **heat index** is the apparent temperature of bare skin when exposed to air with high moisture content. Dry air allows evaporative cooling of the skin's surface. The higher the humidity, the less the skin can cool itself with evaporative cooling. SEMS providers should consider the heat index when planning for an event.

Relative humidity is another factor to consider. It is the amount of water vapor in the air, compared to the amount of water vapor the air could hold. In addition to health issues related to respiration, humidity affects our ability to cool down. Humidity is important because evaporation rates depend on the humidity of the surrounding air. The more humid the air, the slower sweat will evaporate. This means that fewer water molecules are leaving the body, carrying away the heat. Therefore, consider humidity when planning for an event and plan for more heat-related emergencies if humidity could be high.

Also check if there is a **heat advisory**, a notice issued within 12 hours of the onset of extreme heat conditions, including the following: a heat index of at least 105°F (40.6°C) but less than 115°F (46.1°C) for less than 3 hours per day, and nighttime lows remaining above 80°F (26.7°C) for 2 consecutive days. If a heat advisory is issued, the likelihood of a heat emergency will increase.

Another factor to consider is windchill. **Windchill** is the apparent temperature of the air on exposed skin. The higher the wind speed, the higher the heat loss from the skin's surface and the greater the windchill will be. Thus, due to high wind speeds, it may feel colder than the thermometer actually indicates.

As in any endeavor, knowledge is power. Collecting information on temperature extremes, sudden changes in weather patterns, the heat index, relative humidity, and windchill is vitally important to the success of an operation. There are a number of reliable sources that can provide clues in predicting the weather, including verified news sites on the Internet, other EMS services, and the hosting service's files.

For all seasons, providers should plan for extremes in temperature and weather. Extremes occur most commonly in winter and summer, but they can occur any time and on any day. The types of extremes will vary from one environment to another, so it is vital to research the regional climate. Providers should visit national weather services website and examine the weather on the day of the event for the past 5 years, including the average temperature and rainfall. Granted, this will not illustrate exactly what the weather will be that day, but if for the past 5 years the temperature has been over 100°F (37.8°C), providers can plan for a hot weather response.

In most climates, summer has hotter, longer days and shorter, cooler nights (Figure 7-10). When planning for summer events, providers should keep these parameters

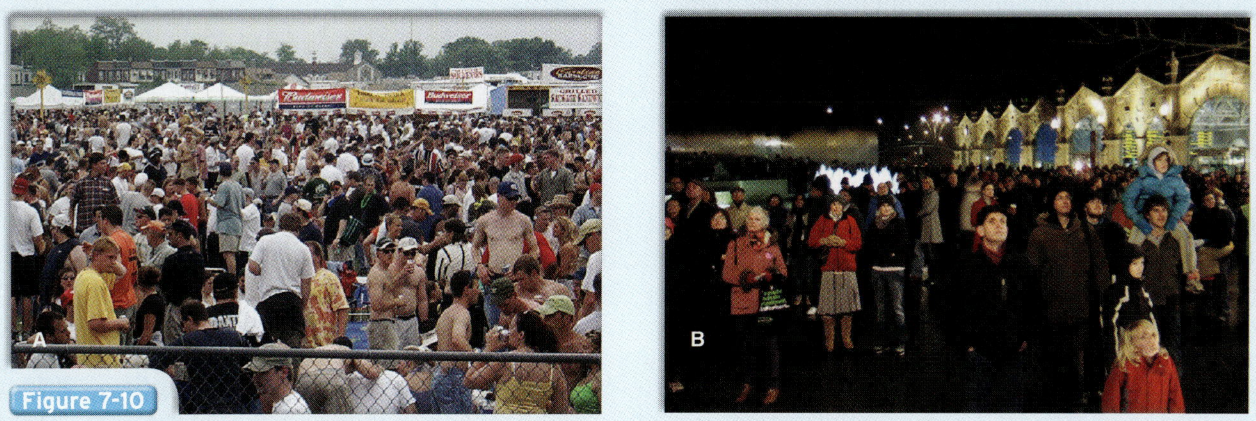

Figure 7-10 Because some events may have relative extremes of weather, SEMS providers must plan for and bring special equipment to cover all potential weather and temperatures. It may be hot during the day (**A**) and cool at night (**B**).

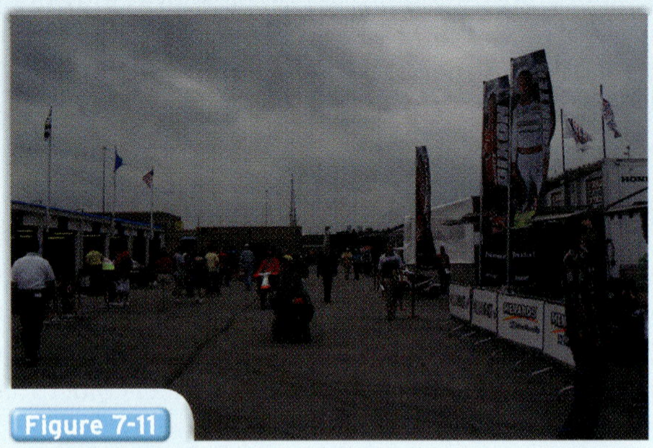

Figure 7-11

Sudden changes in weather can affect the event. For example, this storm delayed qualifying races at the Kansas Speedway on April 25, 2009.

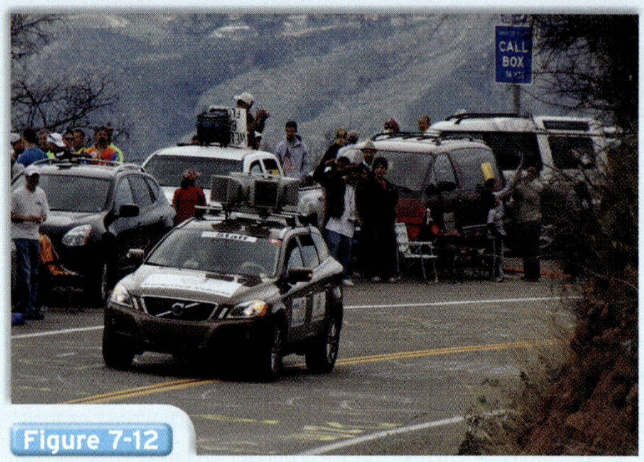

Figure 7-12

In certain situations, information may be communicated to event attendees via a roving PA system.

TIP For multiday events, it may be useful to provide a real-time weather update link on the event web site.

in mind for extended operations. For example, at the All Good Music Festival, a mid-July 3-day festival held each year in the mountains of West Virginia, SEMS personnel annually provide much-needed misting and cooling tents during the day as well as blankets and warming stations at night.

Before the event, track real-time weather changes. If you are covering a small event, keeping up with local weather reports on the television or Internet may suffice. For a multiday event such as a festival, SEMS providers should have a real-time link with a web site in order to continuously track the weather and plan for changes that could occur throughout the duration of the event.

Inclement Weather

SEMS providers must consider the possibility of sudden changes in weather Figure 7-11. Regardless of the time of year, sudden changes in weather patterns can occur and should be anticipated and planned for accordingly. Tornados, for example, can be produced in minutes and can cause great devastation to an area. In June of 2008, a Boy Scout camping event at Little Sioux Scout Ranch in Little Sioux, Iowa, was struck by an F3 tornado, killing 4 and injuring 48. Likewise, there have been several documented cases of spectators being killed by lightning strikes during a thunderstorm, such as in the early 1990s when three fans wearing radio headphones were hit by lightning and killed at a NASCAR race while walking from the grandstands. In 1998, another lightning strike occurred during the Free Tibet concert held in Robert F. Kennedy Memorial Stadium in Washington, DC, injuring 12 attendees, 4 of them critically.

During the event, SEMS providers should track any changes in the weather through the Internet or local weather report and should have a plan in case of sudden inclement weather. For example, it should be determined how this information will be communicated to the crowd and when decisions will be made to suspend or evacuate the special event.

A loudspeaker or bullhorn may be sufficient to communicate with small- or medium-sized crowds; larger crowds may require a public address (PA) system that may already be in place on the event stage. PA systems may also be mounted to vehicles so someone can drive around the event to distribute inclement weather instructions Figure 7-12. If the special event is held in a geographic area that is prone to sudden and violent weather events (eg, tornado or late afternoon thunderstorms), then your service should have a prepared announcement and method in place to communicate the emergency inclement weather plans to the crowd.

When inclement weather does occur, the decision will need to be made whether attendees should evacuate the site or be sheltered on site. For example, if a rapid summer storm with lightning occurred at a large outdoor event, it may not be safe for people to evacuate. In some situations such as this, it may be necessary to shelter the attendees in place—for example, under a grandstand.

If you will be working at an outdoor event where lightning is a possibility, you may wish to discuss having a lightning detector device on the ground that is monitored by staff. If a lightning detector is used, preplanning will also need to address at what point the event will be suspended and whether you will evacuate attendees or shelter them on site.

You Are the SEMS Provider SUMMARY

CASE 1

1. **In your initial size-up of the special event, what are your major safety and security concerns?**
Your major safety concerns should comprise the large number of attendees, the length of the event, the type of event and crowd demographic (eg, potential drug and alcohol use), the high temperature, heat provisions (especially water), and venue management's request to only have one first aid station. Your security concerns should involve how to effectively communicate and preplan with the various agencies involved, including the local jurisdiction, the local hospital, police, and security personnel. It will be important to have a clear chain of command, clear procedures for communication, preplanned ingress and egress routes, and a plan for how alcohol-related emergencies will be addressed. Be sure to discuss the event's alcohol sales policy; this will give SEMS providers an idea of whether the event is relatively strict or not (which may correlate to the number of alcohol-related emergencies that result). Finally, establish procedures for handling conflict and violence.

2. **How many first aid stations and staff should be planned for this event?**
Chapter 2 discusses staffing levels for special events. According to Table 2-2, an event with more than 25,000 attendees should have more than four SEMS providers and more than two first aid stations. The music festival presented in this case has an expected maximum of 60,000 attendees, which is more than double the 25,000 noted in Table 2-2. Assuming the same ratios presented in Table 2-2, the event would require anywhere from six to eight SEMS providers and three or four first aid stations, depending on other event factors such as likelihood of alcohol use, potential violence, venue terrain, and weather.
Considering this, the venue management's request to have only one first aid station raises concerns, as this would be very inadequate. Discuss causes for concern with venue management well in advance of the event, outlining the various types of emergencies you expect (heat-related emergencies, crowd-related emergencies, and alcohol-related emergencies) to help convince them of the necessity for more first aid stations.
Also, while misting tents are a good idea for this event, it will also be crucial that enough water be available to supply the misting tents. Additionally, adequate drinking water must be available for event participants and staff, and there must be a plan regarding how to bring in more water should the supply run out.

CASE 2

1. **What is the first thing you should do in this situation?**
SEMS providers should already know their procedures for a major incident such as this; there should be a preplan in place for an event that could overload resources. This incident will require specialized water rescue personnel, who should be requested immediately by the person designated to request additional personnel (which should be determined during preplanning). SEMS providers will need to move to the incident scene, bringing sufficient supplies to treat the expected injuries. Triage will likely need to be performed once SEMS providers are at the incident scene. This incident will likely have numerous injuries, including trauma to spectators and trauma to personnel in both boats. The patients could also become hypothermic as the day becomes cooler. Even if this incident had not occurred, SEMS providers should have planned for potential extremes of temperature, since during the fall it is often warm during the day and cool at night.

2. **During preplanning, how can you plan for a major incident such as this?**
It is impossible to preplan for every type of major incident that could potentially occur, but you do want to preplan for incidents that are quite possible. For a speedboating event, a crash into the crowd is a definite possibility and should always be planned for. SEMS providers should know how they will get resources to any potential crash site at the event and should always have plans and procedures in place for obtaining additional resources (personnel and supplies).

Ready for Review

- Weather and environmental factors constitute a major influence on the patient load, so these are important considerations for outdoor events.
- In hot weather, SEMS providers can expect dehydration and heat-related illnesses. Since heat-related illness is preventable, SEMS providers should consider measures to help prevent it.
- A dehydrated patient can rapidly deteriorate into heat exhaustion or even heat stroke. Though less common, dehydration can also occur in cooler weather. It is important that proper amounts of water are supplied to event attendees and participants.
- On cold and rainy days, SEMS providers can expect hypothermia, frostbite, and falls from slippery surfaces.
- Hyponatremia (an abnormally low level of sodium in the blood) is when an athlete takes in more water than the body can handle, diluting the electrolyte balance. This condition is more common in endurance events such as marathons and triathlons. Signs and symptoms include nausea, vomiting, lightheadedness, confusion, dizziness, and in severe cases, headache. Seizures, coma, and death can result from the pressure on the brain. Obtain a detailed patient history to help distinguish between hyponatremia and dehydration. Treatment varies by protocol, and severe cases will require transport.
- Road races, bike races, and marathons may be mega-events, requiring multiple first aid stations as well as hydration and cooling measures. Remember that these events might draw participants who are not well conditioned. Also remember that the windchill effect from bike riding can cause a cyclist to experience mild hypothermia.
- When preplanning SEMS coverage for any long-distance race, give special consideration to the best locations for rest stops and first aid stations. Rest stops and first aid stations should be placed at strategic points, considering the terrain and course.
- SEMS providers may work at events that involve water. The entire event may involve water, such as boat races, open swims, or polar bear plunges, or only a portion of the event may involve water, such as a triathlon.
- SEMS providers must always expect hypothermia at an event that involves water.
- River sports include white water rafting and river kayaking. Participants travel down a river's rapids. Participants are required to wear helmets, knee and elbow pads, and a personal flotation device.
- Riverboarding is an extreme water sport in which the athlete lies prone on the board while traveling down river rapids. The rider wears a wet suit and holds small fins for navigation. Flotation devices and helmets are worn. Riverboards are also used to rescue victims in water rapids.
- Open water sports include water sports held on the seas.
- Open swim is any swimming event that occurs on the open water. Dangers include riptides, injuries from marine animals, and drowning. Swimmers do not wear protective equipment. Injuries may range from muscle strains to cardiac arrest from either drowning or physical exertion.
- Open swim may be a component of a triathlon, an event that consists of a road race, a bike race, and an open water swim. Triathlon participants may become injured as a result of fatigue.
- Polar bear plunges are events in which participants jump into frigid water. These events are typically held in January and February when the water temperature is around freezing. Hypothermia can set in within minutes and can be fatal in 15 minutes.
- Surfing dangers include drowning, marine animal injuries, riptides, and collisions with other surfers, boards, or other objects. Surfers do not wear safety equipment or a personal flotation device.
- Free diving is an extreme sport in which divers hold their breath as long as possible while diving as long as possible. Free divers hyperventilate before an event to lower the level of carbon dioxide in their lungs and bloodstream. This may cause shallow water blackout or a deep water blackout. Most free divers wear a buoyancy belt.
- Scuba is an acronym for self-contained underwater breathing apparatus. There are no professional scuba competitions, but SEMS providers may work at other water-related events where scuba divers make up some of the rescue personnel and could become patients.

- The most common diving injuries are barotraumas. Ruptured ear drums and damaged sinuses result from pressure changes that are not dealt with while diving.
- Decompression sickness is another diving injury that results from the formation of gas bubbles in the body. This can occur when a diver ascends too quickly. Decompression sickness must be treated promptly; administer oxygen and transport to a facility with a decompression chamber. Take the diver's watch or dive chart with the patient to the hospital.
- Nitrogen narcosis may occur from diving. It is a state similar to alcohol intoxication and is found in divers who breathe high-pressure gas at depth. Nitrogen narcosis occurs quickly and the symptoms usually disappear rapidly during the ascent.
- Oxygen toxicity occurs when oxygen in the body exceeds a safe partial pressure (PPO_2). In extreme cases of this type of toxicity, the central nervous system becomes affected, causing a seizure. This seizure can result in the diver spitting out his or her regulator and subsequently drowning.
- Multi-venue water sports are sports that can be held either on rivers, lakes, or open oceans.
- Boat racing raises some particular concerns for SEMS providers because speedboats racing as fast as 160 mph may crash into crowds. These events are held near waterways that may have very limited access for EMS units. SEMS planners must perform an on-site inspection well before the event is scheduled and once obstacles such as spectator fences are in place.
- Hydroplane racing is a type of racing in which a specially designed watercraft with a jet-powered turbine engine is raced around a course.
- Water skiing may be done with water skis or barefoot (without skis). It may involve slalom racing, ski jumping, and trick skiing. A personal flotation device is worn, and sometimes a helmet is worn. Barefoot skiing requires higher speeds and is therefore more dangerous. Barefoot skiers wear a wet suit and may wear padded shorts.
- General issues for a SEMS provider at a water-based event include remaining safe around water and ensuring that very thorough preplanning has been conducted, including preplanning how to reach patients and how transport units will access the venue. Specialized rescue equipment will also be needed.
- Any SEMS provider working at an event involving water must be a capable swimmer. A personal flotation device for each provider is a must. In some cases, special training may be needed before working at these events.
- Preplanning measures for outdoor events include planning for a first aid tent (so extra shelter is provided) and possibly including more first aid stations than usual if more emergencies are expected.
- Outdoor terrain is another important factor when planning for an outdoor event. Consider the type of surface, the condition of the surface, whether or not it is level, and whether it affects your ability to view the entire event.
- A crucial step in preplanning for an outdoor event is researching the weather history.
- Weather will affect event attendees and also SEMS providers, so preplanning considerations should include both these groups. Consider all of your gathered weather information when arranging for staffing and ordering supplies.
- Review the weather history for the past 5 years to determine the average temperature for each day of the special event.
- Consider the heat index; the higher the humidity, the less the skin can cool itself with evaporative cooling.
- Check if a heat advisory has been issued. If a heat advisory is issued, the likelihood of a heat emergency will increase.
- Also research rainfall amounts, humidity levels, and potential inclement weather.
- Humidity affects respiration and a person's ability to cool down. Plan for more heat-related emergencies if humidity could be high.

- Consider windchill; the higher the wind speed, the greater the windchill will be and the colder it will feel.
- Prepare for extremes in temperature and weather. For example, a summer event may be hot during the day and cool at night.
- SEMS providers must consider the possibility of sudden changes in weather, including a thunderstorm, lightning strike, or tornado. Track any changes in the weather through the Internet or local weather reports during the event.
- If inclement weather does occur, information may need to be communicated to the crowd regarding suspending or evacuating the event. During preplanning, consider use of a loudspeaker or bullhorn in these cases, or a public address (PA) system for larger crowds.

Vital Vocabulary

barefoot water skiing A type of water skiing that is done without water skis and at higher speeds.

barotrauma Injury resulting from pressure disequilibrium across body surfaces.

decompression sickness A broad range of signs and symptoms caused by nitrogen bubbles in blood and tissues coming out of solution on ascent; also called the bends.

deep water blackout A loss of consciousness that occurs while ascending to the surface after a dive of at least 32 feet, and which is the result of a rapid drop in the partial pressure of oxygen on ascent.

free diving An extreme water sport in which divers hold their breath for as long as possible while diving, without using any device to assist breathing.

heat advisory A notice issued within 12 hours of the onset of extreme heat conditions, including a heat index of at least 105°F (40.6°C) but less than 115°F (46.1°C) for less than 3 hours per day, and nighttime lows remaining above 80°F (26.7°C) for 2 consecutive days.

heat index The apparent temperature of skin exposed to air with high moisture content.

hydroplane racing A type of boat racing in which a specially designed watercraft with a jet-powered turbine engine is raced around a course.

nitrogen narcosis A state resembling alcohol intoxication produced by nitrogen gas dissolved in the blood at high ambient pressure; also called rapture of the deep.

open swim Any swimming event that occurs on the open water.

open water sports Water sports held on the seas.

oxygen toxicity A condition that occurs when oxygen in the body exceeds a safe partial pressure (PPO_2); in extreme cases, the central nervous system becomes affected, causing a seizure.

polar bear plunge An event in which participants jump into frigid water.

relative humidity The ratio of the amount of water vapor actually in the air compared to the amount of water vapor the air can hold at a particular temperature and pressure.

riptide A current that runs perpendicular to the beach and that can pull a person out to sea very quickly.

riverboarding An extreme water sport in which an athlete lies prone on a board and travels down river rapids.

shallow water blackout A loss of consciousness that occurs while underwater in depths of about 15 feet or less, and which is caused by hypoxia from holding one's breath.

triathlon An event that consists of a road race, a bike race, and an open water swim.

windchill The apparent temperature of the air on exposed skin.

CHAPTER

Stadium Events and Mega-events 8

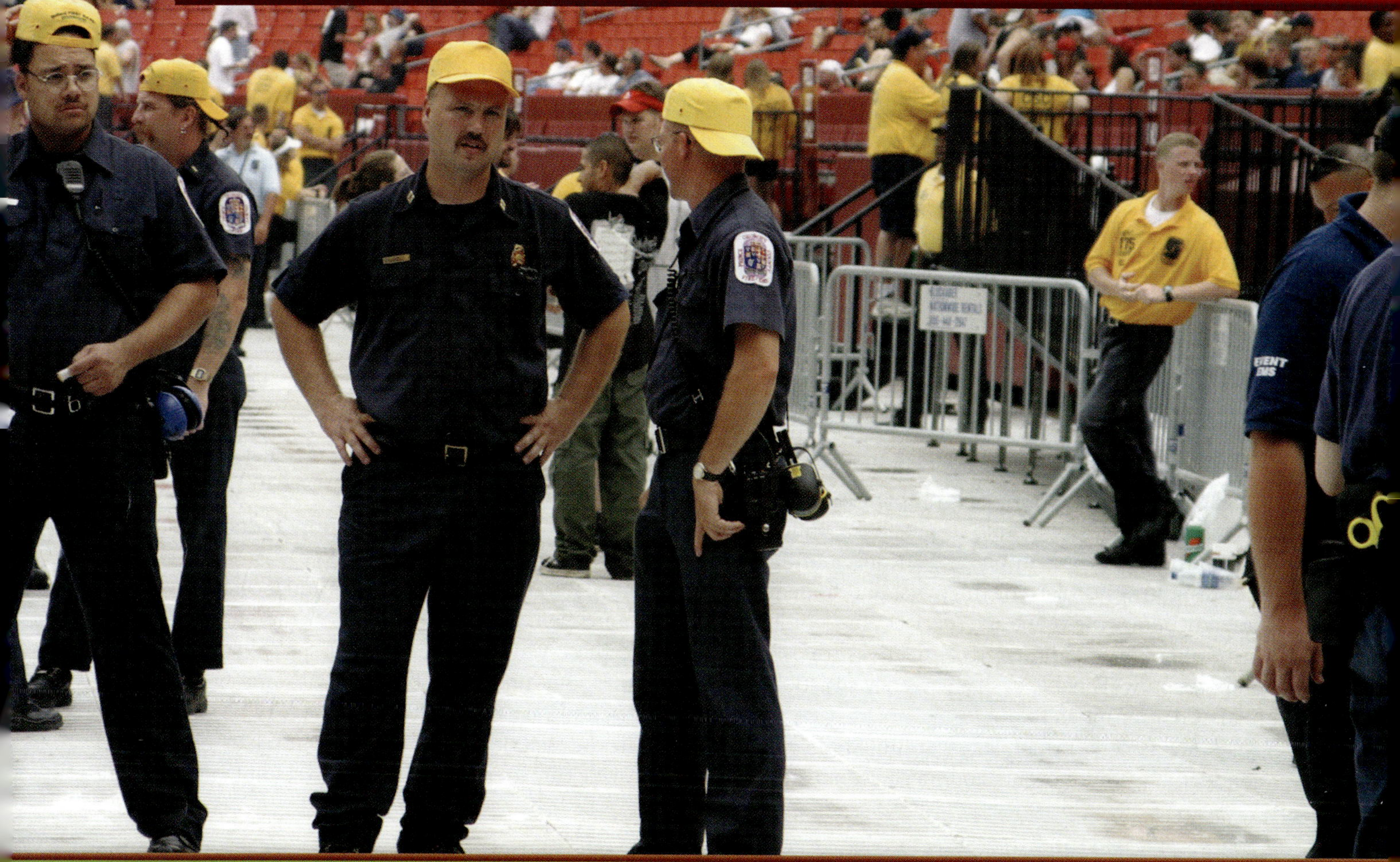

LEARNING OBJECTIVES

- Define the term *mega-event*.
- Define a stadium and design features that make it unique.
- Describe the first aid facilities that may be part of a mega-event.
- List general guidelines for staffing special events medical services (SEMS) providers at a mega-event.
- Define the term *mobile team* and describe its role at a mega-event.
- Discuss transportation considerations unique to stadium events and mega-events.
- Describe how operations may differ if an event is categorized as an event of national significance.
- Discuss preplanning considerations for a stadium event or mega-event.

Introduction

This chapter discusses stadium events and mega-events. These two types of events are often the same—a mega-event may take place at a stadium. However, a mega-event is defined by its size and therefore will not necessarily take place at a stadium. Regardless, stadium events and mega-events have much in common.

There are as many stadium response plans as there are stadiums, but the structure of a proper response plan is the same regardless of the facility for which it is designed. As any emergency medical services (EMS) provider knows, emergency situations can and do arise at any time. The goal is always to provide the best possible care as quickly and safely as possible. This chapter discusses how to adjust your preplan to full-scale stadium events or what we define as a **mega-event**—an event whose attendance exceeds 55,000 people.

Whether the venue seats 6,000 or 250,000, the SEMS principles are the same: preplanning, preparation, rehearsal, and execution. The preplan must address coverage strategies, operation sustainability, equipment, transport concerns, supply allocation, staffing, and reporting. Always plan for the worst and hope for the best. Encourage the venue and special event coordinators to implement accident-reducing measures. Proper preparation will enable each emergency situation to be managed appropriately.

A few general principles regarding SEMS provider conduct at stadium events and mega-events are worth mentioning. Often, these events involve celebrities. SEMS providers should never seek autographs. The provider's focus must be on providing emergency care and services at the event, as well as staying alert. If offered an autograph, the SEMS provider should decline. Similarly, SEMS providers should not take pictures of the celebrities and should not accept gifts from event participants or attendees.

Also, always keep Health Insurance Portability and Accountability Act (HIPAA) laws in mind when working at these events. SEMS providers may have access to celebrities; you are not to disclose what you see or hear. Remember that media may be present at these events and may try to obtain information from anyone, including SEMS providers. If anyone approaches you asking questions, remember that he or she could be a member of the media. It is best to say, "The situation is under control," and discourage further questions.

The Facility

A **stadium**, which can be indoor or outdoor, is home to a variety of special events Figure 8-1. Modern stadiums cost so much that taxpayers and local governments require them to produce a significant amount of revenue, and these venues therefore host special events all year round. Stadiums may be built with one type of event in mind, but once built, stadiums may become multipurpose facilities out of necessity. You may be called to provide care for a special event in a stadium that is being

You Are the SEMS Provider

CASE 1

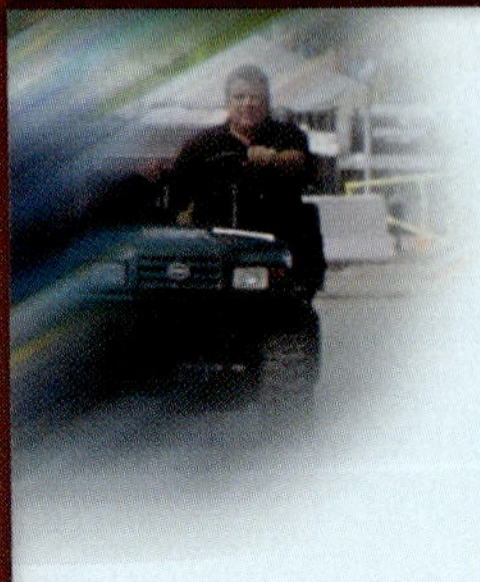

You are preplanning for a mega concert, which will take place in two weeks. After spending more than an hour discussing traffic patterns and the parking situation, you get the feeling that the stadium will be used to its limit. You schedule a follow-up meeting for the following week with both the fire department and hospital to discuss each organization's role for this special event. The special event has a maximum attendance of 60,000, but the special event organizers believe the turnout will be closer to 35,000 to 40,000. Your organization is replacing the service from previous years. Previously, at least seven ambulances had been used for a crowd of 35,000 people.

1. What is the optimal staffing level for this event?
2. Assuming there is one first aid facility currently in place at this stadium, how many additional first aid stations will need to be set up?
3. How will you address transportation issues to ensure that traffic and crowding do not prevent ambulances from having access and egress?

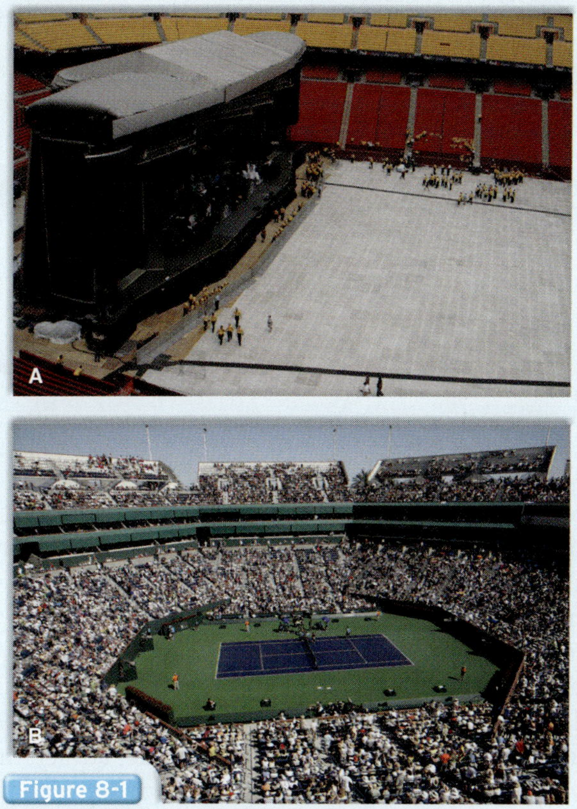

Figure 8-1

A. An indoor stadium. **B.** An outdoor stadium.

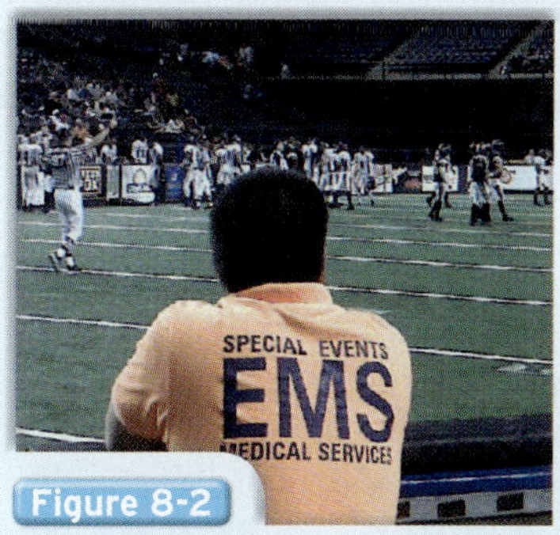

Figure 8-2

Most college and high school stadiums are designed to accommodate multiple types of sporting events.

used for a purpose it was never intended for such as concerts, religious revivals, and extreme sports.

Design Issues

Different sports require fields of different sizes and shapes. Some stadiums are designed primarily for a single sport while others, particularly ones with retractable seating, can accommodate different sporting events. Stadiums built for baseball or football games are the most common in the United States. Most college and high school stadiums are designed to accommodate multiple types of sporting events, such as football games, lacrosse games, track events, and other sports Figure 8-2.

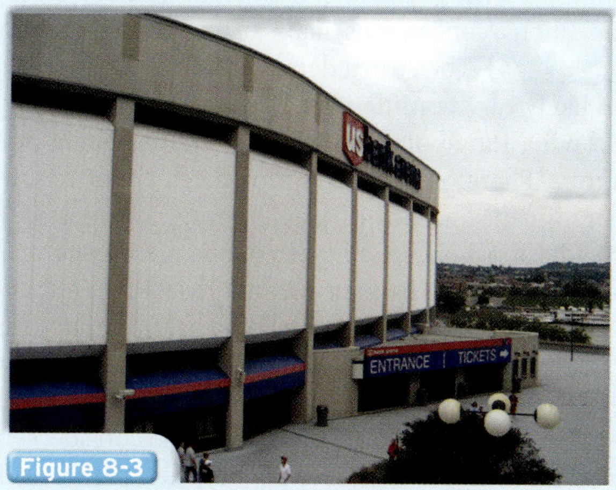

Figure 8-3

Events with festival seating are more dangerous because fans may rush to obtain front row seats, as with the December 3, 1979, Who concert at the Riverfront Coliseum in Cincinnati, Ohio (now called the US Bank Arena, shown). Eleven fans were killed and many more were injured.

Spectator Areas and Seating

Festival seating is mostly standing room only and is usually first-come, first-served. Many performers prefer festival seating because it allows the most enthusiastic fans to get near the stage and generate excitement for the rest of the crowd. This type of seating is dangerous and is tough to control, monitor, and access because fans may fight for seats toward the stage, which is what happened on December 3, 1979, at the Riverfront Coliseum in Cincinnati, Ohio. Eleven fans of The Who were killed and many more were injured in the rush for festival seating at the opening of a sold-out show Figure 8-3. After the tragedy, many indoor venues and some outdoor venues changed to assigned seating only. However, at many stadium events and mega-events, festival seating is becoming more common again.

The spectator areas of a stadium can be referred to as bleachers or grandstands. Many stadiums make luxury suites available to patrons. These suites can accommodate 10 to 30 people, depending on the venue, and of course are the most expensive seats in the stadium.

Types of Stadium Events and Mega-events

Stadium events and mega-events can include many different kinds of events, including concerts, sporting events, political events, theatrical shows, college graduations, conventions, rallies of many sorts, and more Figure 8-4. The crowd demographic at such an event will likely vary, considering that such events may appeal to a wide range of people regardless of age or other factors. Therefore, a stadium or mega-event requires a significant amount of preplanning, and the SEMS provider must expect all types of emergencies to occur at such an event. Patients can range from an attendee being trampled to an attendee being drunk and injuring himself or herself to an older person experiencing a heart attack. Always consider how this event is similar to other stadium or mega-events, but also consider what could make this event different. For example, consider whether there will be a higher incidence of drug use, a greater likelihood of intoxication, a potential increase in violence, or a higher average age of attendees.

Concerts often occur in a stadium. There are several factors that increase the need for medical services at concerts, including average age of attendees, presence of alcohol or drugs, type of music, and the crowd's mood. Some events may lead to serious trauma from factors such as violent accidents, tear gas exposure, riots, crowd crush, and activities in mosh pits during a stage rush. Each type of special event has its own unique aspects. Factors that can vary include venue setup, spectators, and weather, to name a few; they are as numerous as the events that SEMS protects. The duty of a SEMS provider is to ask the right questions, anticipate the answers, and then devise a means to meet the needs.

Music festivals and fairs are often mega-events. Music festivals are essentially large, multiperformance concerts and may be held in indoor and outdoor venues. Fairs include agricultural shows, carnivals, state fairs, flea markets, and specialty shows such as home shows and bridal shows. These events may take place at fairgrounds, public streets, or large private gardens. As with any special event, to create an effective response plan, SEMS providers must consider a number of variables such as anticipated crowd size, attractions, availability of food and drink, merchandise, vendors, performances, and social activities.

Many music festivals are annual events, which makes it easy to gather historical information about attendance, crowd demographics, and venue concerns. These events create a variety of unique challenges for SEMS providers. The more challenging events are the one-time, high-profile, high-energy special events such as rock festivals.

TIP

Budgeting for a mega-event should follow the same principles used for any event, but the numbers and costs will be higher. Total your costs, including fuel costs, supply costs, insurance costs, SEMS providers' paychecks, and any other special SEMS costs for the particular event. Be aware of any guidelines you need to follow. For example, government agencies may budget differently than private agencies.

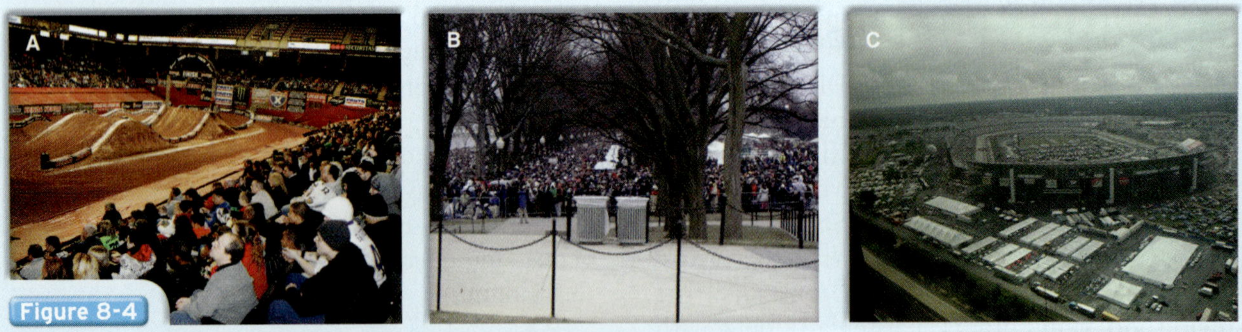

Figure 8-4

Stadium events and mega-events include many different types of events. **A.** A stadium event. **B.** A mega-event. **C.** A mega-event at an outdoor stadium.

SEMS Considerations at Stadium Events and Mega-events

Many of the considerations for providing emergency medical care at stadium events and mega-events build on concepts presented earlier in this book. Preplanning is always important but is absolutely crucial at these events. This section discusses considerations for providing emergency medical care at a stadium event or mega-event.

At these events, during the preplanning phase find out if there are minimum requirements for the event. For example, if the event is a sporting event, there may be specific medical staffing requirements or medical standby guidelines from organizations such as the National Collegiate Athletic Association or the National Athletic Trainers Association (NATA).

First Aid Facilities

Many modern stadiums have designated first aid rooms or treatment areas. In such facilities, you will not need to set up a first aid station, though you may still be responsible for stocking and restocking your supplies. However, you may need to set up additional first aid stations at other locations within the facility if you determine that the designated first aid room will not be sufficient. In contrast, many mega-events will be held at facilities that do not have a predesignated first aid area, for example, large outdoor parks, high school sports stadiums, or fairgrounds. As with stadium events, the SEMS provider will need to consider whether a mega-event requires additional first aid locations to accommodate the crowd size Figure 8-5. Finally, an event may have certain first aid stations dedicated to care of minor injuries and other stations for providing more advanced care.

If an additional first aid station or medical facility is needed, it must be equipped and staffed for first aid treatment and must be in a convenient location where all patrons have access. As always, on-site facilities must be clearly marked with signage directing people to the location Figure 8-6. Periodic announcements should be made alerting people that medical assistance is available and stating how to access it.

As always, the location of the first aid station is an important preplanning consideration. It may be wise to place SEMS providers near expected problem areas, such as the mosh pit at a concert. As always, make sure that spectators can easily see and access the first aid stations.

At larger special events with performers, provide a medical facility near the stage area. The path from the mosh pit to the first aid station or medical facility must be preplanned. In general, other medical facilities are situated in positions on the perimeter of the audience area enabling unrestricted access and exit for ambulances without entering areas occupied by the audience.

Remember, it is not good for the first aid station to be located too far from the center of the event. Also, if too many patrons surround you, you may not be able to move or be seen. Talk to the venue promoter and use previous experience to ensure that the first aid station is in the best possible position.

The front-of-stage area is frequently a problem because of the competition for limited space. This area poses risks of entrapment, crushing injuries, asphyxiation, and panic, as discussed in Chapter 5 Figure 8-7. SEMS providers may need to assist with issues that occur near the front of the stage and therefore must have a plan for how to access that area.

As discussed earlier, all guides must include a map with the first aid areas highlighted. All SEMS providers should have a copy of this map, and it should be available to event attendees as well. Also, before the event, ensure that all security staff, ushers, and other arena personnel are familiar with the first aid station locations.

Stocking Medical Supplies

At a stadium event or mega-event, SEMS providers will likely care for many different types of injuries and emergencies. They can certainly expect to provide basic first aid—caring for simple wounds, scrapes, and cuts, and providing cold packs for strains and bruises. Therefore, the first aid station should be staffed and stocked to the basic life support (BLS) level. First aid stations should also be available as comfort stations for those who need drinking water or a place to rest, cool down, or warm up.

Communication

Every first aid station must have communication devices to summon a higher level care if a situation warrants it. Communication plans at and during the event must

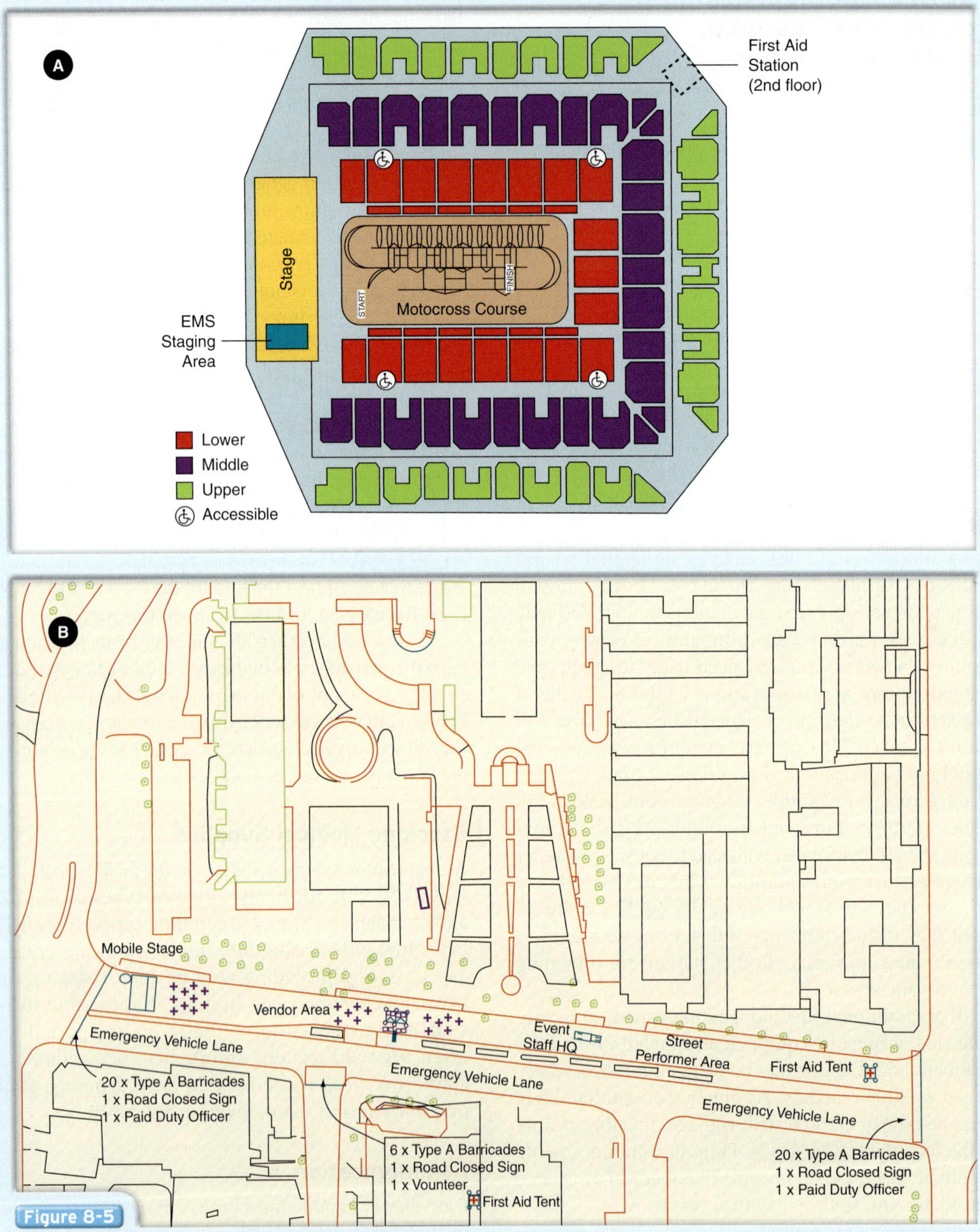

Figure 8-5

First aid station locations will need to be determined during preplanning, taking take into account many factors such as number of attendees, types of expected injuries, and access/egress. **A.** Map of a stadium layout. **B.** Map of a mega-event layout.
Modified from City of Toronto Economic Development and Culture Division, Toronto Special Events Planning Guide. *1 (2009): 30. Image produced by Matt Oates, Event Support Supervisor, Special Events.*

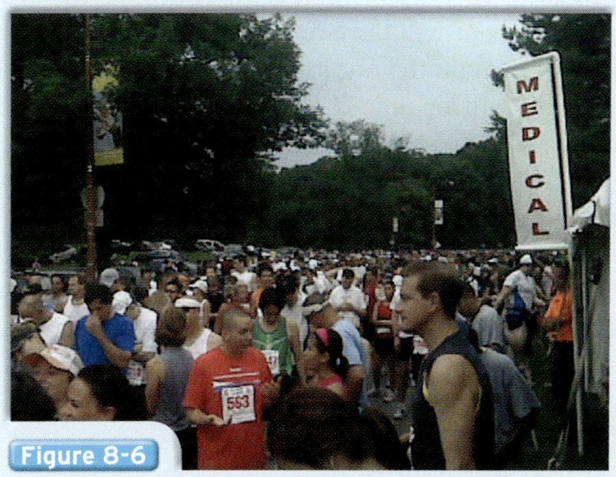

Figure 8-6

As with all events, first aid areas must be clearly marked at stadium events and mega-events.

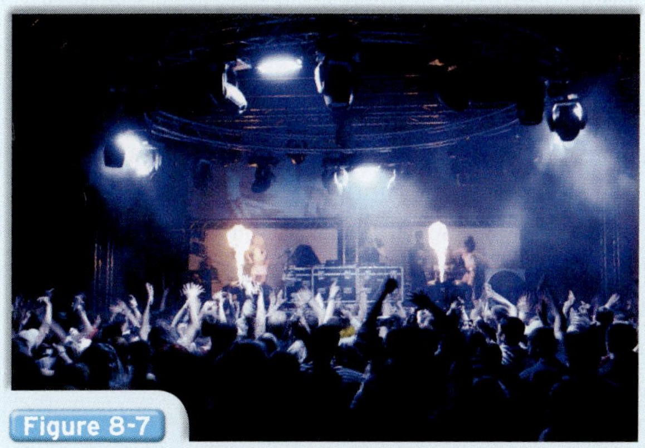

Figure 8-7

The area in front of the stage has an increased risk for injuries. Take this into consideration when planning first aid station locations and access/egress.

be clear. Prior to the event, it is crucial to review the emergency response plan with everyone who will be involved on Game Day. A clear communication system is key in making sure incidents run smoothly, should they occur. Ensure that the event staff has a method of communication to contact you for help and to guide you to an incident.

Staffing

Mobile Teams

A **mobile team** is used more often at stadium events and mega-events because of their size and complexity. This team of medical providers has a posted position to

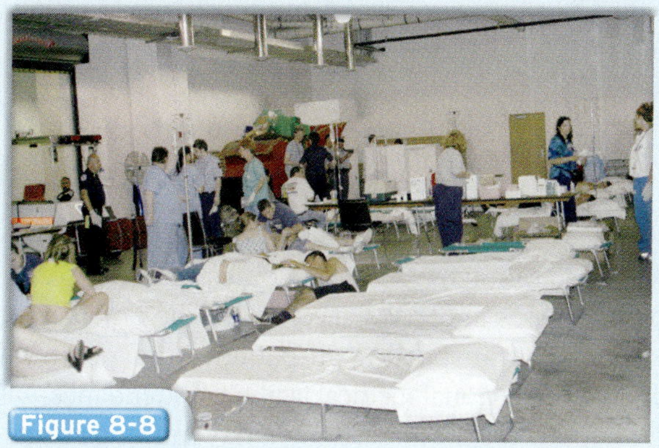

Figure 8-8

Large events may have ALS providers, nurses, and physicians on site. Note that the bed configuration in this photo does not allow for patient privacy and ideally would be arranged differently.

assist, assess, and, if needed, transport patients either to a first aid station or to a transport vehicle for further care and transport to a hospital. A mobile team should consist of three or more SEMS providers, the treatment supplies necessary for the providers' skill level, and communications capability with dispatch (whether dispatch is on site or stationed at a local dispatch center) and the main first aid station if one is being utilized.

It is important to maintain accountability of all staff at mega-events and stadium events. Working in teams (ideally of three SEMS providers) helps ensure that everyone is accounted for.

Determining the Number of SEMS Providers and First Aid Stations

As discussed in Chapter 2, at any event, it is always necessary to determine beforehand how many SEMS providers and medical teams will be needed. For example, will one ambulance per 10,000 people suffice? Are two physicians per 50,000 attendees too much? Not enough? Refer to the tables provided in Chapter 2 regarding staffing.

At larger events such as NASCAR races, National Football League games, and Major League Baseball games, first aid stations are staffed by advanced life support (ALS) providers and nurses, and most venues also have physicians on site Figure 8-8. The reasons that larger multiday events have ALS providers staffed at first aid stations are twofold. At these events, attendees may camp on site for 2 or 3 days. These people use first aid stations as their source of medical treatment for their entire stay. The second reason is that these events attract

TIP Most racing venues have designated landing sites for medevac helicopters. Prior to the event, SEMS providers must know these locations.

so many attendees that it becomes prudent to have on-site nurses and physicians to handle emergencies, rather than transporting all patients and potentially overloading regional medical facilities. Attendance-wise, motorsports are the largest single-day sporting events in the United States, with turnouts of more than 100,000 people. In such events, it has become essential that ALS providers, nurses, and physicians be on site to aid in patient assessment, care, and transport decisions.

It is worth mentioning that if the event will have on-site physicians or nurses, it is extremely important to involve them in the preplanning to determine their responsibilities versus those of the SEMS providers. As with any other agency working at the event, physicians and nurses need to know the details of the event, such as rendezvous points, the promoter's expectations, and transport arrangements.

Finally, if SEMS providers are not able to leave their assigned area, when planning staff rotation schedules, consider whether it is necessary to arrange for meals to be delivered to them.

Transportation Within the Event

A crucial part of preplanning a stadium event or mega-event is considering transport around the facility and to the scene of an incident. You must decide if you will use carts and at what level they will be equipped—first responder, BLS, or ALS.

You must also determine what type of on-site transport protocols you will employ. One such protocol is called "one out and one back." In this model, a team is sent to the incident, and the team has the ability to transport the patient. The advantage of this model is that the team will likely be able to handle the incident without requesting additional resources to that scene. The disadvantage is that it is extremely costly to equip a large number of teams with the ability to move patients. For example, if you have 10 teams of SEMS providers, you will need a minimum of 10 transport vehicles to furnish each team. The "one out and one back" protocol works best with small- to medium-sized special events requiring no more than four transport units to effectively service the facility.

Before working at the event, you must also find out if the event will have on-site physicians. If so, this will cut down on the number of transports because the physician will be able to evaluate and possibly treat patients on site. For example, if a patient is dehydrated, he or she may need only to be given intravenous fluids, and after reevaluation by the physician, the patient may be allowed to leave. Such treatment will eliminate the need for several transports at mega-events and is used quite often because it allows the paying customer to stay on site and enjoy the event.

Transportation to Outside Medical Facilities

When preplanning for a stadium event or mega-event, it will be necessary to decide whether transport units are needed on site. They may or may not be necessary depending on the event. For a very large event, on-site ambulances must be available. It may also be appropriate to have an ambulance on site at events that, based on your preplanning research, you expect to have a high percentage of emergency calls or at events where response times will be delayed due to the large volumes of people or traffic in and around the event.

EMS response times are one factor to consider when deciding whether on-site ambulances are needed. Other factors include crowd size, special circumstances, insurance regulations, and whether the number of potential transports from a particular event will put undue pressure on the local 9-1-1 service. Distance from the hospital is also an issue that cannot be overlooked. Does it take an hour by ground to get your transport units to the hospital? If so, you may need more units, strictly because of the amount of time it takes to return to the event site.

When determining on-site ambulance coverage and coordinating on-site ambulances, consider the capabilities of the venue. If you are working a high-risk special event and think an ALS unit would be appropriate, but the local jurisdiction cannot guarantee that the incoming unit will be ALS, it would be wise to arrange for a dedicated ALS ambulance on site during the event. If there is a need for specialized equipment that the local jurisdiction does not carry, an on-site ambulance should be considered.

If you decide that on-site ambulances are needed, you will need to determine the appropriate number. A good general guideline for determining this is provided in Table 8-1. For example, an event with 80,000 attendees would require six BLS units and two ALS units

TABLE 8-1 Guidelines for Determining the Number of Transport Units*

Number of Attendees	Number and Type of Transport Units
5,000-25,000	One BLS ambulance
25,001-55,000	Two BLS ambulances, with one additional ALS available if needed
More than 55,000	Three BLS units and one ALS unit, plus an additional three BLS units and an additional one ALS unit for every 25,000 additional attendees

*Note that the number of expected transports depends on a variety of factors. Adjust these numbers as needed to take all event factors into account.

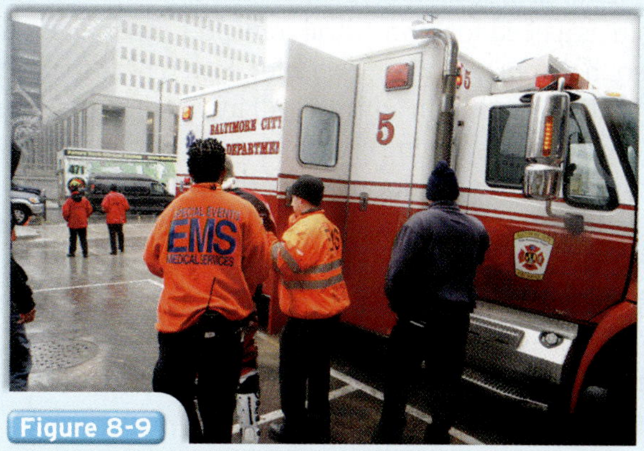

Figure 8-9

A predesignated rendezvous point should be determined and should be readily accessible to both the ambulance and the SEMS providers.

(three BLS units and one ALS unit for the first 55,000 attendees, plus an additional three BLS units and an additional ALS unit for the remaining 25,000 attendees).

Another guideline is that 25% of your transport fleet should have ALS capabilities if attendance reaches 55,000 or more, you expect attendees to be relatively active, and the temperature is above 72°F. When planning for standby ambulances, also be sure to consult local rules and regulations.

When determining the level of transport, you must also consult local protocols, national guidelines (if applicable), and accepted practices. Remember, ALS does not necessarily mean better life support. More is not better—having the SEMS response set up right is better.

If you have determined that an ambulance is required on site, there should be a predesignated rendezvous point that is readily accessible to both the ambulance and the SEMS providers Figure 8-9. Preferably, this rendezvous point should be isolated from the public and should be clear so that there are no problems entering and exiting the venue.

You Are the SEMS Provider

CASE 2

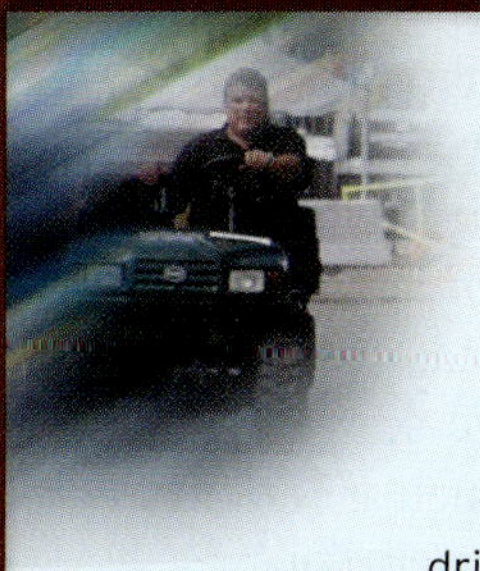

You are providing SEMS at a college football game with 4,000 attendees taking place at a large outdoor stadium. You receive a dispatch for an attendee with severe chest pain. He is located in section Q, row XX–one of the top-most rows in the stadium's bleachers, and on the opposite side of the stadium. You immediately head to your cart with the two other providers in your SEMS team, which include an emergency medical technician and another paramedic, and you take your ALS-level equipment with you.

You navigate the cart to the other side of the stadium, exit the cart, secure it, and climb the bleacher stairs with your equipment and the two other providers. By the time you have driven there and climbed all of the stairs, 10 minutes have passed. You and your colleagues quickly assess the patient and suspect that he is having an acute myocardial infarction. The designated third SEMS provider communicates with dispatch to arrange for a rendezvous with an ambulance at the predesignated rendezvous point, but there are crowds blocking the streets leading to this location.

1. What could have been done differently during the preplanning stage to cut down on the amount of time needed to reach the patient?
2. How can the issue of crowded streets be handled?

During preplanning you must also determine whether there is a need for air medical transport capabilities and if so, helicopter landing zones for each day of the event must be approved in advance. All involved parties must receive a map showing the approved sites so that SEMS providers know the locations of the landing sites.

If emergency medical transportation is not available on site during a special event, direct communication with the emergency medical system is necessary. Access to a working telephone or other telecommunications device, whether fixed or mobile, should be ensured.

Management of a Mega-event

Joint Operations Center Command Post

At a mega-event, because of its size, a **joint operations center (JOC)** may be necessary to manage SEMS and other event operations. The JOC manages the entire event operation. All event operations are run through this room. Each partner involved in the event will have its own representatives located here and will oversee all of its own operational needs from this location; for example, there will be a representative from the security personnel, fire personnel, SEMS personnel, etc. The JOC is a dispatch center and also an interactive location where all agencies can work together to ensure that the event runs smoothly and with as little impact as possible from the small emergencies that may arise. Should an incident arise, this room can quickly convert into a command post for managing the incident because all of the required agencies will already be in place and ready to participate. The **incident commander** is the coordinator of the event, ensuring that all operational needs are met and communicated.

As discussed in Chapter 4, remember that a mega-event will likely have a complex communications matrix with multiple channels and a dispatch center. Or, the communications matrix may involve multiple frequencies. During preplanning, it will be important to ensure that the designed communications matrix accommodates all of the groups that will need to be in communication during the event. A National Incident Management System (NIMS) 205 plan, Communications Plan, should be created. As a general rule, there should be a dispatcher for every three channels, or if there are high-volume channels, there should be one dispatcher for every two channels. A backup communication plan must be designed and ready to be implemented in the event that a failure of the primary communication arrangement occurs. For example, on-site communications vans may provide fail-safe communication backup if the primary communication system fails.

Multi-Tiered Response System

A **multi-tiered response system** is a staffing structure that can be expanded to meet the needs of even the largest event. With a multi-tiered response system, providers are divided into several teams. SEMS teams could be designated such names as the red team, blue team, green team, and go team. In this model, the red team is the largest group and responds first (usually on foot or bike) to the incident. The team is usually staffed with first responders or BLS providers, and they carry enough equipment to begin the care of a patient. The blue team staffs the transport carts and transports patients to either a green team location or to the go team location. Green teams are located at fixed, static locations such as a first aid room or first aid tent. Green teams remain at their location and can summon the red team, depending on SEMS procedures. Go teams (ambulance transport teams), which have the fewest staff, must be ready to assume care or to transport a patient. Depending on the size and expected patient load, a 3:1 ratio (three BLS teams for every ALS team) or a 5:1 ratio (five BLS teams for every ALS team) for BLS to ALS teams can be used.

Events of National Significance and NIMS

Planning for SEMS coverage of a stadium event or mega-event can take on a life of its own. Many of these events are classified as incidents of national significance by the Office of Homeland Security. This means the event has reached a level requiring the involvement of more than one federal department or agency because there may be a credible terrorist threat or a potential threat related to a high-profile, large-scale planned event. Most national sporting events such as National Football League games, Major League Baseball games, NASCAR races, and similar events are automatically placed in this category, allowing the venue to use the resources of the federal government to aid in both the preplanning phase and deployment of resources during the event itself. Major events such as the Super Bowl and major political national conventions are so large and deemed so high profile that the planning groups may involve more than 100 people from agencies all around the United States.

When an event is in this category, management of operations changes. The planning phase will usually occur for a whole year before the event, with meetings held more frequently as the event draws near. The planning committee's overall role is to ensure that the event runs smoothly from an operational standpoint. Members of this group may include:

- Law enforcement personnel (local, county, and state)
- Fire personnel
- EMS personnel
- Venue personnel (safety, operations, security, etc)
- Local emergency planning officials
- Public health officials
- Local utility officials (water, sewer, and power)
- Terrorism specialists
- Officials from federal partner organizations such as the Federal Bureau of Investigation; the Bureau of Alcohol, Tobacco, Firearms, and Explosives; and the Department of Homeland Security
- Private contractors involved in filling any of the above roles

All this input from outside parties does not mean you lose operational control of your individual discipline, but rather that you all work as a group to establish incident action plans that can be enacted during both normal event operational modes, as well as during an emergency incident.

The operational plan for normal event mode is basically to bring together each agency's standard operational plan and to make them work as one. In other words, law enforcement personnel follow their normal police standards and are responsible for handling crime, SEMS providers use their patient care protocols to treat patients, and so forth. While working independently, each group still has the goal of the operation running smoothly. However, the incident action plan is a tool that places all of the agencies under one umbrella to achieve the common goals of life saving, incident stabilization, and property preservation during an emergency incident. Under this plan, agencies still function in their discipline, but each supports the other. Police trained in triage may assist EMS in this function. Event security personnel trained in evacuation may assist police in clearing the stadium. Under your incident action plan, make sure to use the proper NIMS incident command system (ICS) forms to track all of your functions, resources, and plans. Required NIMS ICS forms include the following and are available at the Federal Emergency Management Agency Web site:

- ICS 201—Incident Briefing Form
- ICS 202—Incident Objectives
- ICS 203—Organizational List
- ICS 204—Division Assignment List
- ICS 205—Communications Plan

Each day of the event, your group should meet upon arrival to review the day's planned activities and discuss any new items. This is known as an operational period briefing. Information shared here is then passed down to the people actually performing the tactical functions at the event during their morning briefing period. The same meeting is used during an incident, although in this situation the incident commander is required by law to oversee all areas, even areas that are not normally part of his or her role. For example, a fire chief, law enforcement official, or local public safety official may be the incident commander and will ultimately oversee all incident operations, including SEMS operations related to the incident.

As you can see, the entire process is set up so that decisions are made by a group that is knowledgeable about the interworkings of the event, thus allowing the field staff to perform their duties as effortlessly and flawlessly as possible and to have all of the tools needed to complete their task.

Preplanning for Stadium Events and Mega-events

Many preplanning concerns have been mentioned throughout this chapter. This section highlights additional preplanning items to focus on.

Pregame Rehearsal

To borrow a saying from the military, "Slow is smooth, and smooth is fast." The point of this saying is that if you preplan slowly and thoroughly, the operation will ultimately progress faster because you have considered and resolved possible obstacles ahead of time so they do not occur or are well-handled when they do occur. Conversely, if you do not plan out slowly, the results will ultimately be slowed by problems that could have been addressed during preplanning.

The goal in providing SEMS is for operations to run smoothly. Rehearsals may be important at smaller special events, but at mega-events and stadium events, they are absolutely crucial. The day of the special event is not the time for SEMS providers to become oriented to the layout, study the communication procedure, and learn the egress route. If SEMS providers do not know the layout of the event, their job assignments, and all egress routes before they arrive, response time will be slow and cumbersome.

For all mega-events, do a detailed walk-through and orientation a week prior to the special event. It is advisable to perform mock scenarios to acclimate team members to the venue's layout, terrain variations (if outdoors), access issues, and protocols for treating and transporting patients.

Walk-through

The layout of the stadium will likely be unfamiliar to SEMS personnel unless they have worked at events in the facility several times before. Even if they have, it is necessary to refresh their memory of the details of the particular venue. During the rehearsal phase, familiarize your team with the floor plans for the day of the special event. Also be sure that outside agencies that may be involved have a layout of the floor plan.

Maps

Ensure that all SEMS providers have detailed maps of the stadium, grounds, parking lots, and any area directly or indirectly related to the special event. The map should show permanent routes and temporary routes for SEMS providers and ambulance access. If the special event takes place between more than one venue or on several acres, highlight routes between venues and any roads or intersections. Ensure that the maps denote any natural or man-made obstacles, such as fences or barricades.

Maps must be provided for all locations associated with the special event. These maps need to show surrounding streets with street names clearly marked.

TIP

At large events, you may need to work with many other event personnel. Make sure your event contact person has introduced you to other personnel and agencies who you will be working with at the event. If your role has been explained, the stage has been set for a smooth relationship. If your role has not been explained, you may need to explain your role and may need to work harder to build a relationship with personnel you will interact with at the event. In such cases, it is especially important to be professional and have a professional appearance so that you command respect from colleagues.

Security and limited-access gates and areas enclosed by fencing need to be clearly noted. At some venues, gates may be opened by security if needed for emergencies. In these cases, make sure during preplanning that the appropriate security personnel are in place and that they have the appropriate keys.

Documentation

It is always prudent to determine during preplanning what procedures will be followed for providing and documenting emergency care at an event. For mega-events, it is a good idea to establish ahead of time which patients need a written report. For example, will SEMS providers be expected to report every instance when medical items (such as bandages and cold packs) are handed out? Will SEMS providers need to note if alcohol was ingested? To whom will the data be communicated? The venue promoter may wish to know certain data, and SEMS personnel should work this out well in advance. Identify and communicate to SEMS personnel what the expectations are for documentation of emergencies that occur at the event.

Preplanning Checklist

As always, use the preplanning form that was shown in Chapter 2. This form is useful for preplanning any type of event but is especially crucial in preplanning for a stadium event or mega-event.

TIP At colossal events such as the Olympics, a political event, or a large festival, SEMS providers should use the same principles used for any other event. Preplanning is crucial, as always. It may be necessary to obtain resources in addition to those you would normally secure. This could even include recruiting personnel from neighboring states, if needed.

Finally, the following lists may assist in preplanning. Some of these factors are common for any event, and others may be specific to a stadium event or mega-event. General considerations include:

- How large is the event?
- How far is the event from the nearest medical facility?
- What are the other available medical resources?
- How will local ordinances affect SEMS coverage of the event?
- Will there be peak periods or special circumstances requiring additional staff?
- Are interpreters required?

Considerations relating specifically to SEMS providers include:

- Is the dress of SEMS providers and medical team members easily identifiable?
- Are medical team members appropriately dressed for the conditions?
- Have all SEMS providers and medical teams been provided with maps of the venue?
- Are there procedures in place addressing provider safety, such as how SEMS providers will be protected from violence and crowd crushes?
- How will SEMS providers and other medical staff be fed, hydrated, rested, and (if the event is outdoors) protected from the elements?
- What arrangements are in place for moving medical teams onto and off of the site?
- Do SEMS providers and medical teams understand the command structure and their role within it as well as the emergency activation system?

You Are the SEMS Provider SUMMARY

CASE 1

1. **What is the optimal staffing level for this event?**
On the basis of the tables presented in Chapter 2, an event with more than 25,000 attendees should be staffed with more than 4 providers. Because this event is expected to have 35,000 to 40,000 attendees, and maximum attendance is 60,000 attendees, you will need to have significantly more providers and first aid stations. For an attendance of 40,000, you would need 6 to 8 SEMS providers. If attendance reaches the maximum of 60,000 people, you may need as many as 10 to 12 SEMS providers. Because you sense that the stadium will be used to capacity, it would be prudent to plan for the maximum 60,000 attendees and staff at least 10 SEMS providers. You will also use the recommended number of on-site ambulances for an event with an attendance greater than 55,000 people: three BLS units and one ALS unit, plus an additional three BLS units and an additional one ALS unit for every 25,000 additional attendees. Using these guidelines, you could plan to have four BLS units and two ALS units. This would be a total of six ambulances, which is less than the seven ambulances used in the past at this event when the crowd size was 35,000. Be sure to discuss previous events with personnel who have worked at these events to determine the reason why this many ambulances were used at previous events. There could be a factor that makes it necessary to have more ambulances at this event, or they may have simply had more ambulances available than were needed.

2. **Assuming there is one first aid facility currently in place at this stadium, what additional first aid stations will need to be set up?**
According to the table in Chapter 2, an event with more than 25,000 attendees requires more than 2 first aid stations. Assuming there are 40,000 attendees, you would probably need 3 first aid stations. If attendance reaches the maximum 60,000, you would likely need 5 or 6 first aid stations. Because you sense that the stadium will be used to capacity, it would be prudent to plan for the maximum 60,000 attendees and set up at least 5 first aid stations dispersed throughout the stadium.

3. **How will you address transportation issues to ensure that traffic and crowding do not prevent ambulances from having access and egress?**
During preplanning for this event, it will be crucial to plan the access and egress route for ambulances and ensure that these routes remain free of traffic and crowds. You will need to ensure that the preplanned route is cordoned off in some way so that traffic and crowds do not use it. It may be necessary to use road blocks or arrange for assistance from law enforcement personnel. Also plan a secondary route that can be used should the main route become impassable.

CASE 2

1. **What could have been done differently during the preplanning stage to cut down on the amount of time needed to reach the patient?**
The best solution for cutting down on the time needed to reach this patient would have been for a second first aid station to have been placed on the other side of the stadium, if possible. Another option to consider during preplanning would have been having teams of SEMS providers stationed at various points throughout the event so that at any given time, a group of SEMS providers would have been relatively close to any potential patient. Depending on the event, you may consider having SEMS providers stationed with their cart at specific strategic locations at the event, even if a first aid station is not present at that exact location.

2. **How can the issue of crowded streets be handled?**
The crowded streets could be handled several ways at this point. The third designated SEMS provider should communicate with dispatch to alert them of the situation and call in backup resources to help disperse the crowds and traffic. Another option is to communicate with dispatch to determine a different rendezvous point. The best way would have been to preplan a route that would remain free of traffic crowds, which would likely have required security personnel to ensure that the routes stay clear.

Ready for Review

- Regardless of the facility for which a mega-event or stadium is designed, the SEMS response plan should be the same: preplanning, preparation, rehearsal, and execution.
- Stadium events and mega-events often involve celebrities. The SEMS provider's focus must be on providing emergency care and services at the event, as well as staying alert. SEMS providers should never seek autographs, should not take pictures of celebrities, and should not accept gifts.
- Remember HIPAA laws when working at events. Do not talk about what you see or hear. Media may be present at these events. If anyone approaches you asking questions, it is best to say, "The situation is under control," and discourage further questions.
- Stadiums can be indoor or outdoor. Some stadiums may be built with one type of event in mind, but once built, they can become multipurpose facilities.
- Consider seating and spectator areas when planning for a stadium event.
- Festival seating is a style of seating that is usually assigned on a first-come, first-served basis, rather than being preassigned. It is mostly standing room only and can be dangerous because fans may fight for seats toward the stage.
- The spectator areas of a stadium are referred to as bleachers and grandstands. Many stadiums offer expensive luxury suites that can accommodate 10 to 30 people, depending on the venue.
- When planning for a stadium event, consider whether the stadium was designed for the event. When a stadium is used for its designed purpose, there are usually sufficient seats for all spectators. However, when a stadium is used for a purpose for which it was not intended, there are often not enough seats.
- Because stadium events attract a varied crowd demographic, they require a significant amount of preplanning. The SEMS provider must expect any and all types of emergencies to occur. Patients may include an attendee being trampled or an older person experiencing a heart attack.
- Preplanning is always important but is absolutely crucial at a stadium event or mega-event. Always consider similarities and differences with other stadium events or mega-events.
- While modern stadiums have designated first aid rooms or treatment areas, the SEMS provider may need to set up additional first aid stations at other locations within the facility if the designated first aid room is not sufficient for the crowd size. However, many mega-events will be held at facilities that do not have a predesignated first aid area, such as large outdoor parks.
- At larger special events with performers, provide a medical facility near the stage area. The path from the mosh pit to the first aid station or medical facility must be preplanned.
- The front-of-stage area is frequently a problem due to the competition for limited space. It poses risks of entrapment, crushing injuries, asphyxiation, and panic.
- Additional first aid stations or medical facilities will need to be equipped and staffed for first aid treatment, and should be accessible. Clearly marked signs and maps as well as periodic announcements should be used to alert people that medical assistance is available and to tell them how to access it.
- At a stadium event or mega-event, the SEMS provider may care for many different types of injuries and emergencies. Because one can certainly expect to provide basic first aid, the first aid station should be staffed and stocked to the BLS level.
- First aid stations should also be available as comfort stations for those who need drinking water or a place to rest.
- Communication is imperative. Every first aid station must have communication devices to summon higher level care if needed. This communication is especially important if a mobile team is used.
- The number of SEMS providers and first aid stations will vary depending on the type of event. The number of SEMS providers and first aid stations will need to be adjusted to take into account special characteristics of the event that could result in more injuries and emergencies.
- Transportation around the facility and to the scene of an incident is a crucial part of preplanning. SEMS providers need to decide whether to use carts and to what level they will be equipped—first responder, BLS, or ALS. They must also determine what type of on-site transport protocols will be used.

- SEMS providers should find out if the event will have on-site physicians. The physician will be able to evaluate and possibly treat the patient on site and will therefore cut down on the number of transports.
- On-site ambulances are necessary for large events, high-risk events, or events where response times will be delayed. To decide whether to use on-site ambulances, SEMS providers should consider crowd size, special circumstances, insurance regulations, and distance from the hospital. Assessing the venue's capabilities is also important. For example, if there is a need for specialized equipment that the local jurisdiction does not carry, an on-site ambulance should be considered.
- Whenever on-site ambulances are used, SEMS providers must designate a rendezvous point that can be accessed by both the ambulance and the SEMS providers. This point should be isolated from the public and should be kept clear to ensure easy ingress and egress. If emergency medical transport is unavailable on site, direct communication with the emergency medical system is necessary.
- At a mega-event, a JOC is necessary to manage SEMS and other event operations. As the center of the entire event operation, the JOC serves multiple functions: all event operations are managed through this room; it is a dispatch center; it acts as an interactive location where all agencies work together to ensure that the event runs smoothly; and the room quickly converts into a command post for managing any incidents that arise.
- A multi-tiered response system is a staffing structure of multiple provider teams that expands to meet the needs of even the largest event.
- Many mega-events and stadium events are classified as incidents of national significance by the Office of Homeland Security. This means the event has reached a level requiring the involvement of more than one federal department or agency due to possible threats, such as terrorist threats.
- When an event is in the national significance category, management of operations changes because the National Incident Management System (NIMS) will be used. The planning phase usually occurs for a whole year before the event. To ensure that the event runs smoothly, each agency's standard operational plans are brought together to work as one.
- The goal in providing SEMS is to be quick. While rehearsals may be important at smaller special events, at mega-events and stadium events, they are crucial. Performing walk-throughs and mock scenarios are advisable to acclimate team members to the venue's layout, terrain variations, and access issues.
- All SEMS providers should have detailed maps of the stadium, grounds, parking lots, and any area directly or indirectly related to the special event.

Vital Vocabulary

festival seating A style of seating that is usually assigned on a first-come, first-served basis, rather than being preassigned.

incident commander The overall leader of the incident command system to whom commanders or leaders of incident command system divisions report.

joint operations center (JOC) The central location from which all operations of a large-scale event are managed.

mega-event An event that has an on-site attendance of over 55,000 people at any given time.

mobile team A group of medical providers that leaves a posted position to assist, assess, and if needed, transport patients to either a first aid station or to a transport vehicle for further care and transport to a hospital.

multi-tiered response system A type of staffing structure that can be expanded to meet the needs of even the largest event.

stadium A facility that consists of a center where an event takes place, which is surrounded by rows of seats or bleachers on all sides; may be home to a variety of special events.

CHAPTER

Equestrian Events and Rodeos 9

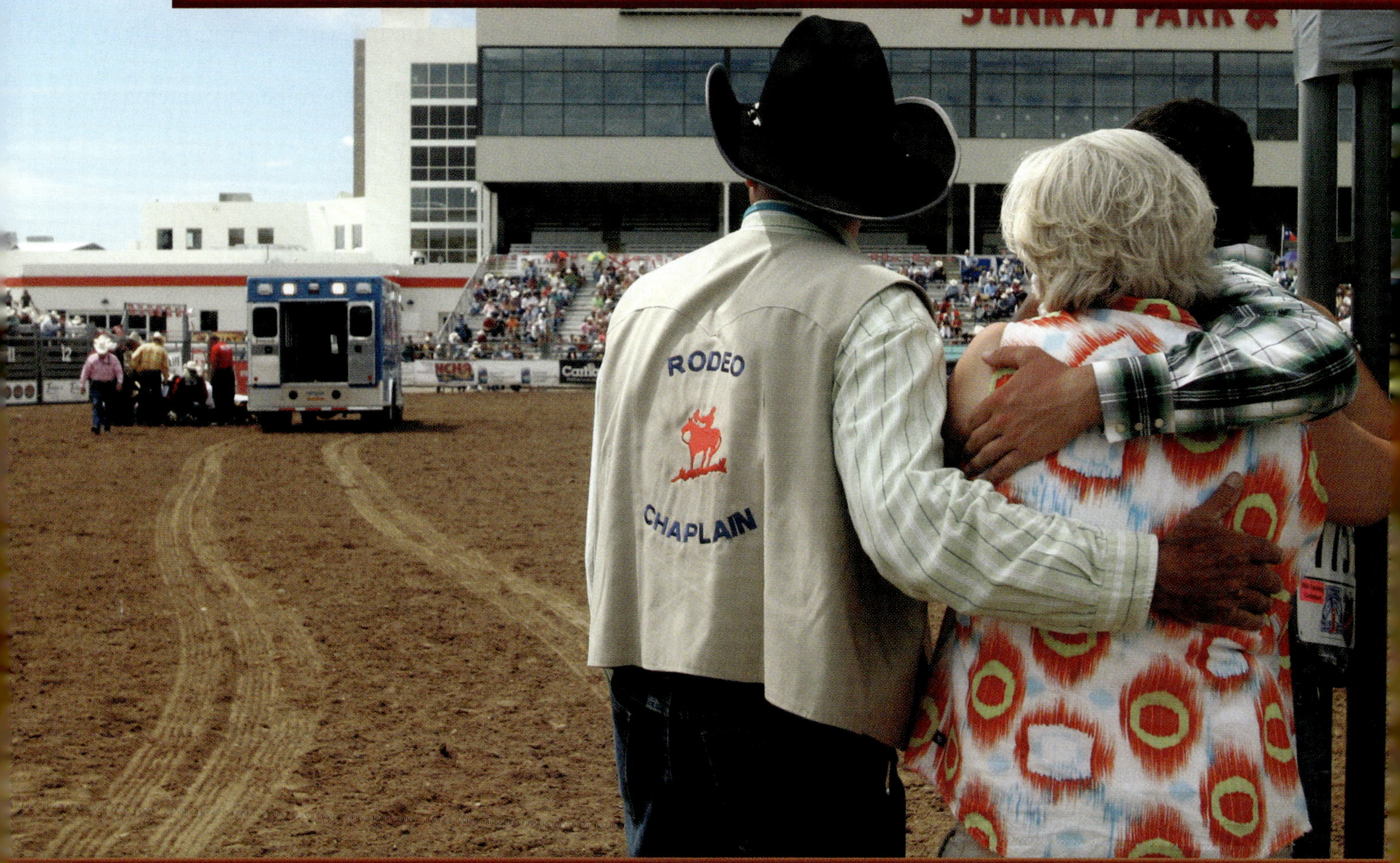

LEARNING OBJECTIVES

- Be familiar with the different types of equestrian events.
- Understand how the differences between types of horses can affect an event.
- Recognize the equipment associated with the different types of events.
- Understand typical safety measures that should be put into place by the event sponsors.
- Understand and be able to anticipate the different kinds of injuries that are most likely to occur at equestrian events.
- Distinguish the specific steps in preplanning that are most pertinent to equestrian events.
- Know how weather impacts equestrian events.
- List specific questions to consider during the preplanning stage for an equestrian event.
- Discuss rodeo events, their associated gear and equipment, and special considerations related to the following types of events:
  - Rodeos
  - Bull riding
  - Stunt riding
  - Saddle bronc/bareback racing
  - Barrel racing
  - Steer wrestling
  - Calf roping
  - Cutting

Introduction

As with any event, when working at an equestrian event, it is important to be prepared. Each type of equestrian event presents its own set of unique challenges to SEMS providers. Rodeo events can be challenging as well. This chapter will offer an overview of the different types of equestrian and rodeo events and the types of injuries a SEMS provider should expect when working at these events. In addition, this chapter will cover preplanning for an equestrian event. Preplanning meetings and walk-throughs are absolutely essential to ensuring that the event is successful and completely understood by every member of the SEMS team.

SEMS providers may be responsible for providing emergency care to both event attendees and participants, may only be hired to care for event attendees, or only to care for event participants. There may also be variations from event to event regarding which services will provide transport; in some cases, the SEMS providers may treat event attendees, but are only responsible for transporting event participants (or vice versa). These considerations should be determined long before the event, as they will affect the number of SEMS providers to staff, the amount of supplies to have on hand, and what injuries to expect. For example, if covering an equestrian event on a hot day, the SEMS provider should anticipate heat-related emergencies in the crowd and event-specific injuries among the riders.

Equestrian Events

Equestrian events include racing, jumping, and eventing, which is a combination of events that will be described in detail in the next section. As mentioned, it is important to be familiar with the event's format, the language specific to the event, and the types of emergencies and injuries likely to be encountered at the event.

Racing Events

Thoroughbred Racing

Thoroughbred racing (also called flat racing) is a race that occurs on a flat track Figure 9-1. This race is a

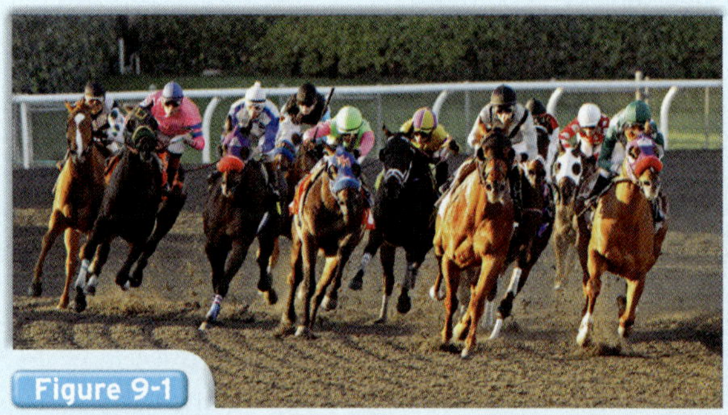

Figure 9-1

A thoroughbred race.

You Are the SEMS Provider

CASE 1

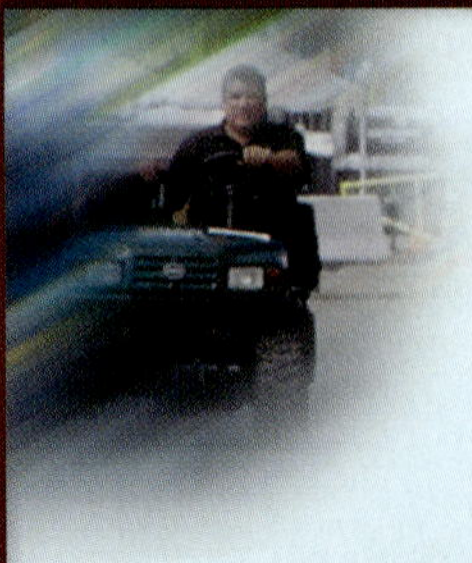

It is a warm April afternoon, and your EMS crew is standing by at an annual benefit steeplechase race. It is the fifth race, the 3-mile timber (a track that contains rails made of solid timber over which the horses jump). You casually watch as the riders gallop by your static post. The first four horses pass, then two more, and lastly, three stragglers that have fallen off the pace.

You hear the track announcer call the race, "Horse 1 and Horse 2 battle for the lead." The announcer calls that Rider 1 is up and over, and that Rider 2 is up, meaning that Rider 1 has completed the jump and Rider 2 is now jumping.

Then the announcer says over the loudspeaker, "The rider is down." You spring to attention and are preparing to respond when you hear on the outrider radio that you have a horse running with the pack but no rider. Where is the rider?

On your radio, dispatch states, "We need an ambulance at fence 12." Fence 12 happens to be the farthest away and the most difficult fence to access.

1. How should you have preplanned for this event, and how would you put the plan into action?

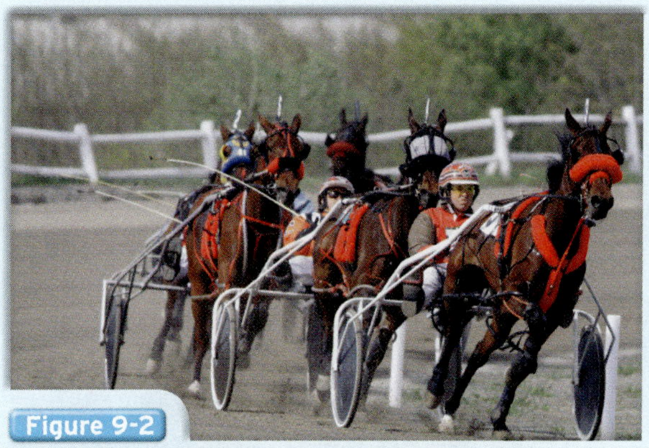

Figure 9-2

A harness race, in which a horse pulls a sulky.

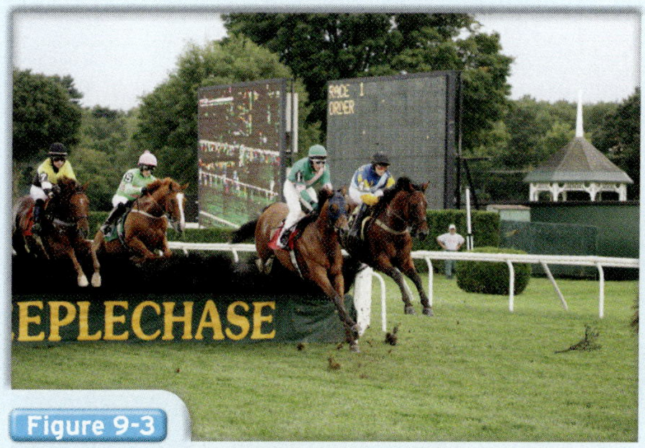

Figure 9-3

A steeplechase event.

test of a horse's speed and a jockey's ability to maneuver the horse. The track is a set length of usually less than 2 miles, and the track material is typically made of turf or a synthetic material.

Harness Racing

In **harness racing**, the horse pulls a cart called a **sulky** (pronounced sool-key) while racing in a certain gait Figure 9-2. The sulky is a lightweight cart with two wheels. It is sometimes called a bike. Harness races are usually 1 mile in length.

In a harness race, the horses can be required to trot or pace. When trotting, a horse's front leg and opposite back leg (for example, left front leg and right back leg) hit the ground at the same time. When pacing, a horse's front leg and back leg on the same side hit the ground at the same time. Trotting is slower than pacing. The majority of harness races in North America involve only pacing, though they may involve both trotting and pacing. With the exception of the United Kingdom, harness races in Europe only involve trotting. This distinction is significant because pacing is faster than trotting; therefore, injuries at races involving pacing will be affected by higher speeds.

Harness races usually begin with the horses behind a gate. This gate may be attached to a vehicle that drives the horses to the point where the race will begin. The vehicle drives away from the horses at the start of the harness race. In thoroughbred racing, the gate is moved after the horses start. The gate is important for SEMS providers to note because it can cause dangerous situations. Horses may run into the gate, injuring the driver. Also, if the gate malfunctions (for example, it fails to open), this can cause injuries.

Steeplechase

Steeplechase horse racing is essentially the same as thoroughbred racing, except it includes obstacles. It originated in England and Ireland when church steeples were used as the end point of a race because they could be seen from a distance. Over time, these events evolved from the simple idea of a chase to the steeple to the sport we know today.

Steeplechase courses require the rider to jump and maneuver around a variety of obstacles. The obstacles are not seen by the rider until he or she is close to them and therefore require horse and rider to think and adjust quickly as they race. Steeplechase courses are designed to include obstacles such as water, stone walls, brush fences, and timber rails Figure 9-3. The length of a steeplechase race is 2 to 4 miles, and the pace is slower than some other races due to the longer distance. The crowd is centralized in one location to watch the event. One consideration for SEMS providers would be the danger of a number of horses (perhaps as many as 20) attacking an obstacle simultaneously. Riders are often thrown into obstacles, crushed by overturned horses, and trampled in the pits near the obstacle.

Hurdling is a form of steeplechase racing often used to train horses for more challenging courses Figure 9-4. This race is generally shorter than steeplechase races, normally totaling no more than 2 miles, and is a fast race due to the shorter distance. Obviously, this race includes hurdles; they are transportable fences made of a steel frame with plastic "brush" screwed into the frame. These hurdles are 1 to 2 feet lower than the obstacles on a steeplechase course. It is important to note the height of an obstacle, as this

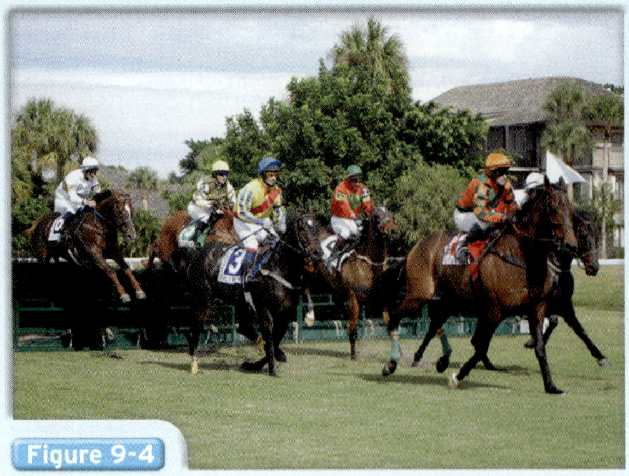

Figure 9-4

A hurdling event.

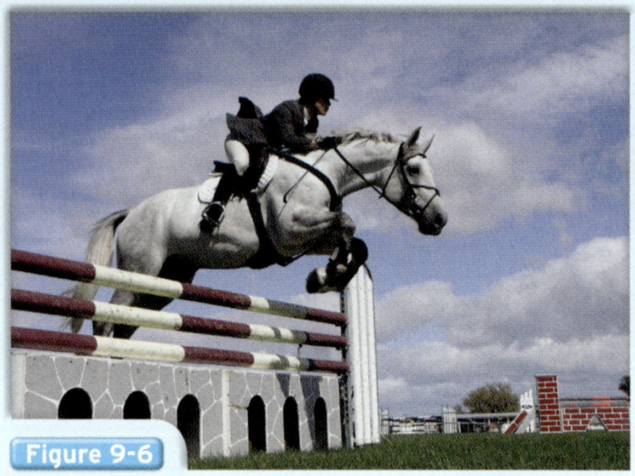

Figure 9-6

A show jumping event.

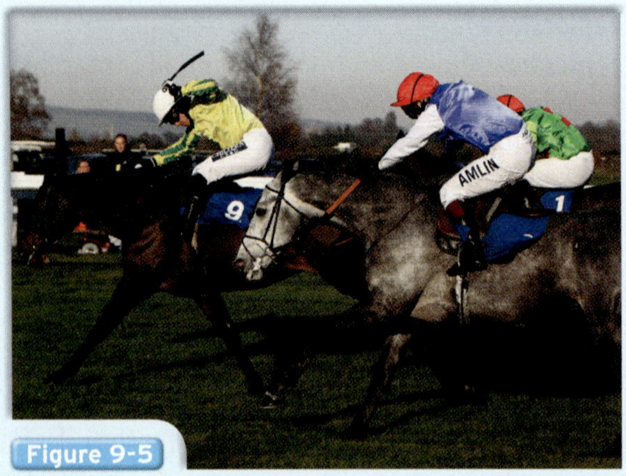

Figure 9-5

A point-to-point race.

determines the height a horse is required to jump and therefore how far the rider can potentially fall.

Point-to-point racing is an amateur type of steeplechase race in which hunting horses race in a straight line from a starting point to a finish point, jumping a certain number of fences Figure 9-5. Point-to-point races are the most dangerous type of equestrian sport simply because the contestants are amateur riders. According to Jockey Club statistics, point-to-point racing results in a fall in 1 in 7 rides and injury in 1 in 42 rides. The Jockey Club is an equestrian organization involved in many equestrian initiatives and is the registry for thoroughbred horses in the United States, Canada, and Puerto Rico.

Show Jumping

There are two primary types of **show jumping**, show hunter classes and jumper classes. These two types differ in how they are judged. Hunter events test factors such as the horse's style, manner, and gait against a set ideal. Jumper events test the horse's ability to jump, and a score is given based on three criteria: whether the horse attempts to jump the obstacle, whether the horse successfully jumps the obstacle, and whether the horse finishes the event in a specified time. Jumper events are more complex than courses at hunter events and may include colorful obstacles or designs Figure 9-6.

Eventing

Eventing is an event that consists of three phases that test a rider's accomplishment in various areas of equestrian sport. The three phases are: show jumping, dressage, and cross-country. The show jumping phase is the same as the event previously described.

Dressage is a component of eventing and usually occurs first. Dressage requires horse and rider to perform a sequence of movements in an arena Figure 9-7. Judges give scores based on the horse's obedience as well as stylistic factors such as balance and rhythm. Note, dressage is itself a distinct riding discipline, and dressage competitions can occur independent of eventing competitions.

Cross-country equestrian jumping tests the horse's endurance, speed, and jumping ability. It also tests the rider's ability to pace the horse. Horses are started at

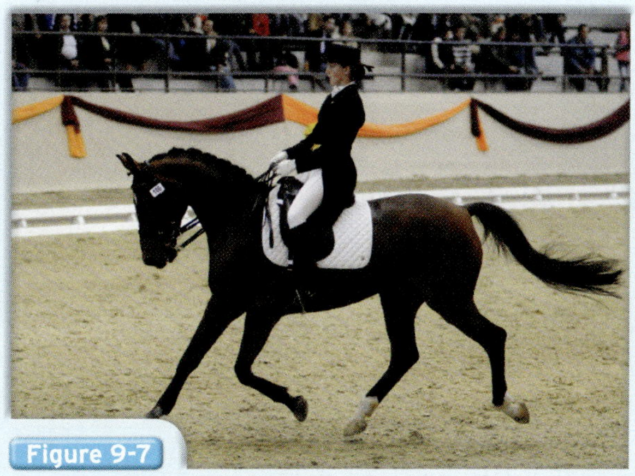

Figure 9-7

Dressage.

different times and do not compete with one another to clear an obstacle. The course is designed over a 2- to 4-mile stretch of land, spread over a landscape (rather than a flat track), and contains a variety of obstacles, some of which may be natural (such as logs, water, etc). Like dressage, cross-country competitions can occur independent of eventing competitions.

Eventing has two main formats: the 1-day event and the 3-day event. Other variations of eventing are sometimes referred to as militaire, horse trials, or combined training.

One important consideration for SEMS providers is that spectators at a cross-country event are not contained to one area; they can walk from jump to jump—even crossing the course at times. Therefore, it will be important to preplan how to access any part of the course in the event of an emergency.

Types of Horses

Though extensive knowledge of types of horses is not required of a SEMS provider, it is important to know some basic facts. Thoroughbred horses are purebred horses and are known for their superior speed and stamina as well as their sensitive and difficult personalities.

The most important thing for providers to remember is that horses in general are very sensitive and can react suddenly without warning. This is especially true of thoroughbreds and horses involved in harness racing (those pulling sulkies). Basic knowledge of how to behave around horses is important for the SEMS provider to have if providing EMS coverage at an equestrian event. Some basic rules include:

1. Never approach a horse from the rear.
2. When approaching a horse, it is best to approach from the side, then pat the horse as you move toward its rear. These pats keep you in frequent contact with the horse's body so it knows where you are and that you intend no harm. The pats should not be too hard or too gentle; they should not be a slap, but they should also not be so light that the horse does not notice them.
3. Horses are sensitive, perceptive creatures. They will sense your fear. It will benefit you to develop confidence and assurance working around horses. If you work at many equestrian events, it may be a good idea to become familiar with horses and riding in your spare time to help develop techniques and confidence.
4. Always expect a horse to kick or rear (raise up on its hind legs), and be prepared to quickly move away or protect yourself.

It may not always be possible to follow all of these guidelines. For example, if a patient is behind a horse and the provider needs to get to the patient quickly, the provider may have to approach the horse from the rear. However, providers should follow these rules when possible and use them to help anticipate and prevent problems.

Another important factor for SEMS providers covering an equestrian event is a horse's height. Horses used for show jumping tend to be tall—their backs are usually over 5 feet high (over 15 hands)—while other breeds may be shorter. Horse height is measured in hands. One hand equals 4 inches. As part of becoming familiar with horse lingo, providers should familiarize themselves with horse measurements so they understand what equestrian attendees and participants are saying. Some common heights are as follows:

- 4 ft = 12 hands
- 5 ft = 15 hands
- 6 ft = 18 hands

Ponies may also participate in some equestrian events and are generally less than 5 feet in height, so falls do not occur from as great a height. However, pony riders tend to be children, so a SEMS provider covering an event involving ponies should refresh his or her knowledge of pediatric anatomy and physiology, as well as assessment and management of pediatric emergencies Figure 9-8.

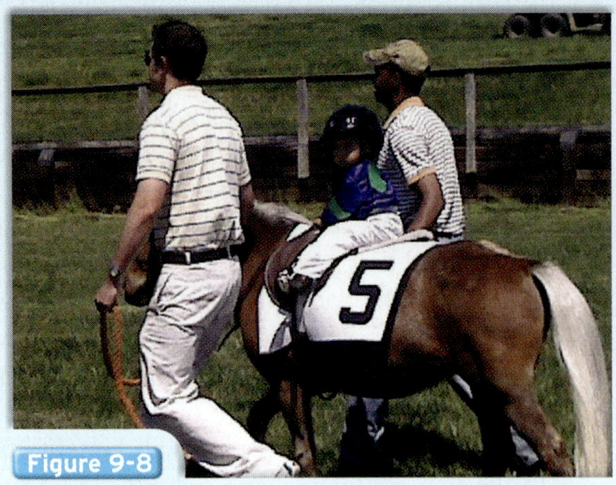
Figure 9-8
Events involving ponies usually have pediatric participants. Refresh your knowledge of pediatric emergencies before such an event.

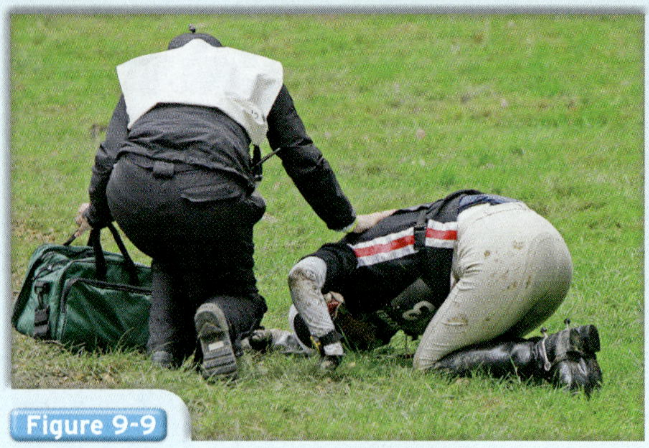
Figure 9-9
Injuries are likely in point-to-point racing and jumping.

TIP Riders sustain more injuries when in a pack of horses because they are stepped on or accidentally kicked by horses to the side and behind. Sometimes things happen so fast that a horse cannot help trampling a rider who is thrown underfoot.

Injuries

Today, equestrian courses are designed with safety in mind. For example, jumps may be designed so that a horse can be maneuvered around them if the horse refuses to jump. Fences can be constructed to easily collapse should a horse collide with them. Also, the area between the horizontal posts of a jump can be filled so that the horse's legs do not become trapped between the posts.

The inclusion of an inside rail in race tracks has been eliminated in favor of flexible pylons that allow horse and rider to maneuver past the edge of the course if necessary (without crashing into a solid railing).

Despite these measures, horse riding is a dangerous sport. Several factors affect the type and severity of equestrian-related injuries, and certain types of events lend themselves to certain types of injuries. This section will discuss the types of injuries that can be expected at equestrian events.

In an overall review of horse riding injuries, head injuries outnumbered spinal injuries at about 5:1. The majority of the injuries result from the following; these are ordered from most common to least common:

- Falls from a mounted position on a horse
- Crushed as horse falls
- Strike obstacles while mounted on the horse
- Injured by entrapment of the reins

Statistically, approximately 20% of equestrian-related injuries involve the head and face. Of these, about half involve a concussion or possible concussion. The remaining half of the injuries are not serious enough to prevent the rider from completing the event. The most frequent injuries are to the shoulder region and most often involve fractured clavicles or shoulder separations.

Injuries are more likely to occur in point-to-point racing and jumping than in thoroughbred racing or in social riding Figure 9-9. Of all horse riding activities, jumping is the most likely to produce a spinal injury.

Finally, equestrian-related injuries involve more women than men, although this may just be a reflection of the fact that there are more female riders. Women riders are also more likely to sustain serious injury.

Injuries While Mounted

When a rider is mounted, his or her head can be 13 or more feet from the ground. Obviously the height of the horse is a factor in how far the rider will fall. Speed is also a factor; a horse can travel as fast as 40 miles per hour. Mass and force are other factors; a horse can weigh more than 1,000 pounds. This weight combined with speed can create a force in excess of 2,000 pounds when the horse is falling. Therefore, when a rider falls, there are many factors that contribute to the severity of the injuries he or she receives.

Injuries While Dismounted

A large percentage of injuries occur while the rider is dismounted (standing near the horse, rather than riding it). Horse kick injuries can occur while in a horse's stall, while applying or removing bandages to a horse's legs, while leading a horse, while walking past a tied horse, or while trying to catch a loose horse. Horse kick injuries can range from very minor bruising to paralysis to even death. An article published in the *Emergency Medical Journal* in 2002 gauges that the average horse kick exerts over 10,000 newtons, which is over 2,000 pounds of force. A horse is a very powerful animal and, depending on a number of variables, the SEMS provider could encounter patient injuries such as lacerations, broken bones, neck and spine injuries, crush injuries, or even traumatic cardiac arrest. Other injuries include being run over by a horse, stepped on by a horse, or bitten by a horse.

Collisions

Certain types of events are more prone to collisions, such as jumping fixed obstacles. If a horse hits one of these obstacles, either the rider, the horse, or both may fall. During eventing, warm-up areas for the jumping phases are another area where injuries are likely to occur. Dressage accounts for only 1% of injuries. The jumping phases account for 86% of injuries. Injuries that occur in the stable account for the remaining 12% of equestrian-related injuries during eventing. The remaining 1% is attributed to miscellaneous injuries during the cross-country phase.

Fall Injuries

In equestrian-related injuries, lumbar and thoracic fractures are much more common than cervical fractures; this is likely due to falling on the buttocks or being thrown against obstructions. Rearing horses and tree branches can unseat riders and cause them to fall backward.

There is speculation in the equestrian community as to whether riding style affects the probability of injury. There are two dominant methods of riding:

- **Jockey style** (cross-country position) with the head forward, in which the rider would be more likely to sustain a cervical injury accompanied inevitably by a head injury Figure 9-10.
- **Classical style**, in which the head is held high and the rider would be likely to fall onto the buttocks Figure 9-11.

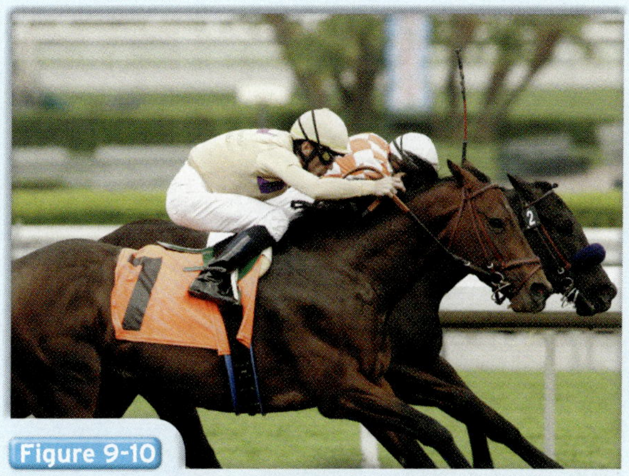

Figure 9-10

Jockey style is when the rider's body is angled forward, essentially parallel to the horse's neck.

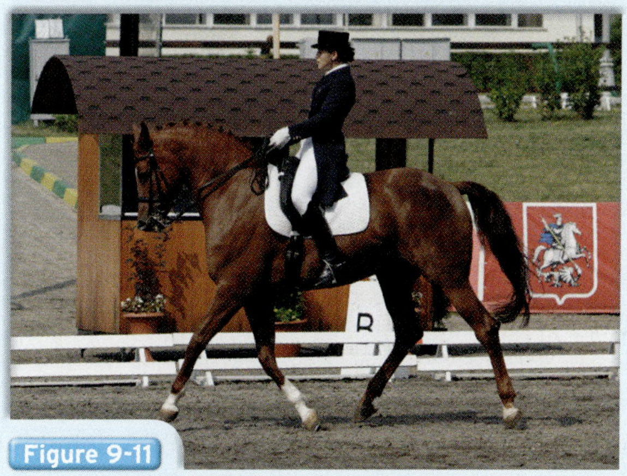

Figure 9-11

Classical style is when the rider's body is essentially perpendicular to the horse's back.

The speed of falling is considered relevant to the likelihood of serious injury, as slow falls sometimes result in the most severe injuries. Here, a slow fall refers to a fall that does not happen instantaneously; instead, the rider begins to fall and at least partially recovers, but then ultimately has an accident anyway.

When a rider falls from a horse and is within proximity of other horses, the downed rider is likely to receive more significant injuries from being kicked or trampled. Additionally, recent fatalities in eventing have frequently involved the horse falling on the prone rider. The rider can use a tuck-and-roll technique to reduce the severity of his or her injuries. This specialized technique is taught to equestrians to use as they become aware they are falling.

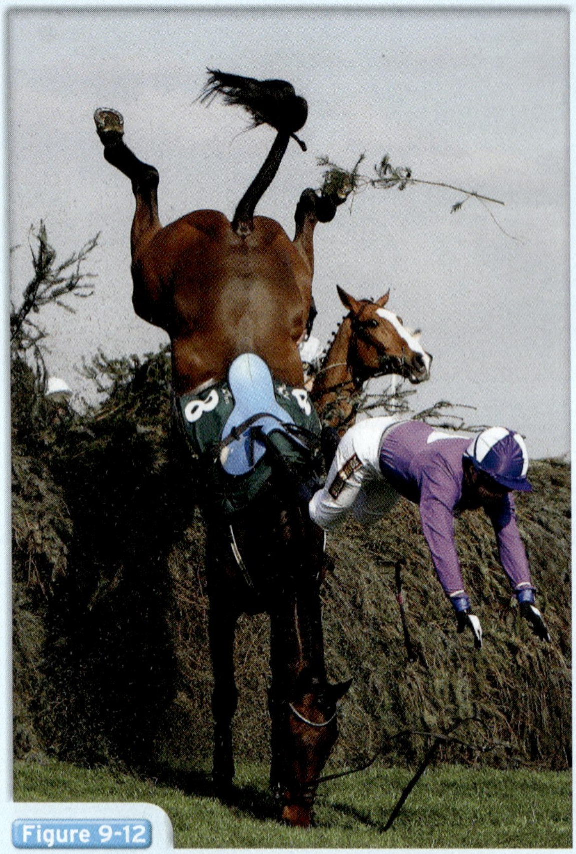

Figure 9-12

Any fall from a horse should be considered a significant injury.

Any fall from a horse regardless of proximity to other horses should be considered a significant injury due to the distance of the fall (Figure 9-12). Neck and back injury should be suspected immediately, and the patient should be promptly immobilized using proper equipment and techniques.

When providing SEMS for an equestrian event, EMS equipment must include spinal and other splint equipment/supplies, considering the types of injuries likely to occur.

> **TIP**
> Depending on the organization sanctioning the event, a jockey may be required to have pertinent medical information on his or her armband. This armband may include information that is important to the SEMS provider should the jockey become a patient, such as blood type and medical history. However, other events such as steeplechase events do not always require this.

> **TIP**
> SEMS providers may cover many dangerous events. It is always important to be familiar with the gear and equipment participants will be wearing. For example, equestrians wear significantly less protective equipment than motocross performers.

Catapult Injuries

Severe injuries can occur in harness races because the sulky can become caught beneath the horse's feet, resulting in falls. The lightweight cart can also launch like a catapult over the horse and rider, injuring them when it lands. Harness races can span long distances that tire the horses and make such accidents and **catapult injuries** more likely.

Another consideration related to harness racing is that jockeys are supposed to be strapped in, but they do not always comply with this precaution. A jockey who is not strapped in is unrestrained and can therefore sustain greater injuries.

Somersault Injuries

The most severe injuries in equestrian events occur when a horse somersaults over a fence or obstacle. **Somersaulting** happens when a horse's chest collides with a fence or object. The force causes the horse to flip over. If the rider is thrown, he or she may suffer head and fall-related injuries and may also subsequently be crushed by the horse. If the rider stays mounted, he or she can be crushed while still mounted when the horse lands. A somersaulting horse can be fatal for the rider; the force from the horse falling can be as much as 2,000 pounds. The SEMS provider should consider the height of fences and obstacles, as well as the height of the horses participating in the event, to help predict where on the course a horse could be likely to somersault.

Equestrian Equipment

Rider Attire

Rider attire varies depending on the event. Some events, such as show jumping and hunter events, require formal and traditional dress. Tall boots are required and are usually black. Per riding tradition, spurs are optional, but commonly used. Other events, such as steeplechase races and thoroughbred races, require less formal, more functional clothing. Breeches (also known as silks) are the pants worn by riders and are made from lightweight fabric, usually nylon, typically with elasticized lower legs. Traditional colors for breeches are white, tan, or

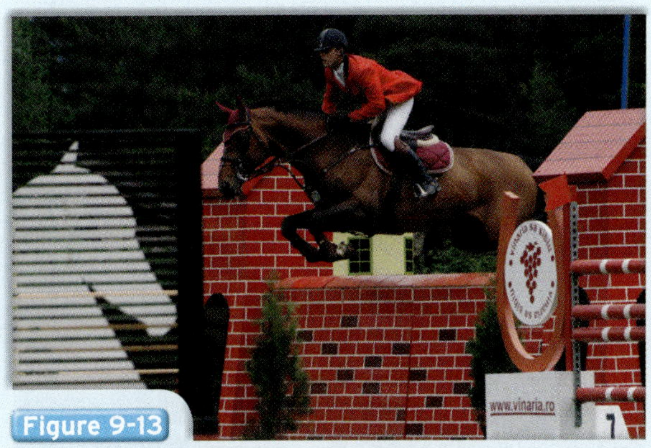

Figure 9-13

An equestrian grand prix uniform.

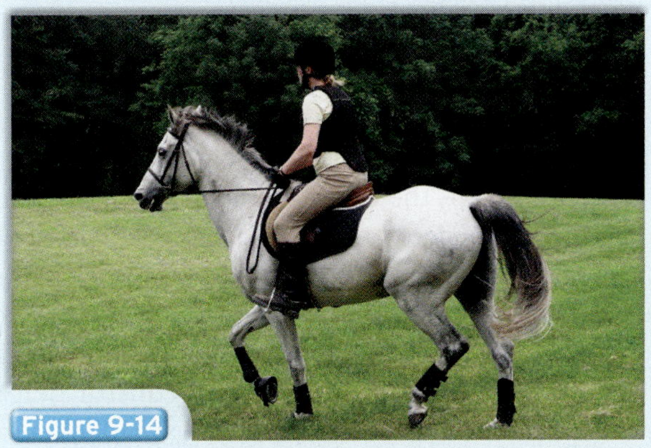

Figure 9-14

An equestrian safety vest.

beige. A dark or tweed coat or a short-sleeved shirt (depending on the season and event) is worn, and gloves are optional. Riders at the grand prix level of jumping usually wear red jackets and more formal attire Figure 9-13. At international events, riders will sometimes have a national emblem to help identify them. This could be important in some cases when identifying a patient.

Finally, riders in equestrian events must wear a safety vest during certain events, such as those that involve jumping Figure 9-14.

Helmets

Equestrian helmets are an important component of a rider's outfit and are particularly relevant to SEMS. Helmets are required in most equestrian events and are always required for riders under the age of 18 years. Certain states in the United States have specific laws requiring helmet use. Helmets must meet ASTM/SEI standards. ASTM/SEI stands for the American Society for Testing and Materials and Safety Equipment Institute. ASTM is an organization that writes standards for a variety of equipment, including sporting equipment. SEI is an organization that adopts the standards and certifies that the manufacturer has met the criteria. It is also important that the buckle be fastened; if it is not, the helmet may not serve its intended purpose of protecting the rider's head.

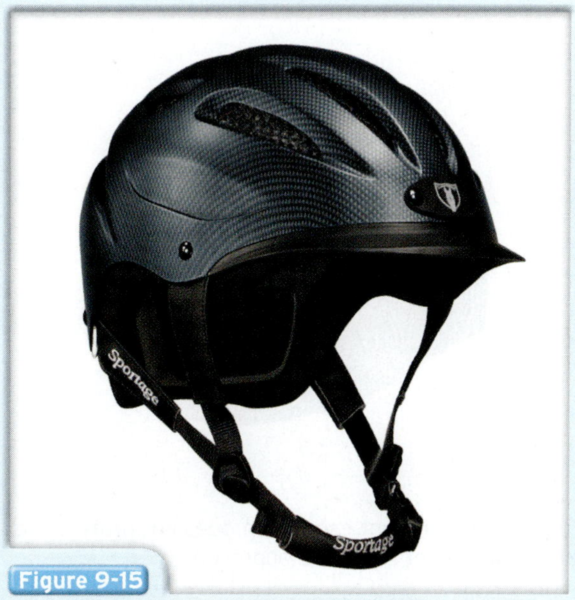

Figure 9-15

An equestrian helmet.

An equestrian helmet should consist of protective padding inside an outer durable plastic shell Figure 9-15. It contains a brim of a more flexible material that can move if needed upon impact. Equestrian helmet designs may or may not include ventilation and extra padding for comfort and a cloth outside the shell for aesthetic purposes.

Hunt caps were worn in the past, but these are no longer considered to provide enough protection and are not approved by ASTM/SEI Figure 9-16. They do not include the protective padding or design required for ASTM/SEI approval.

When responding to an equestrian-related emergency, providers should always note the type of helmet the rider was wearing, which can help indicate the extent of injury. If a rider wears a hunt cap, he or she has virtually no head protection and will likely have more severe head injuries than a rider wearing an approved equestrian helmet. Providers should note any damage to the helmet, as they would when responding to any other EMS incident involving a patient wearing a helmet, such as a motorcycle crash.

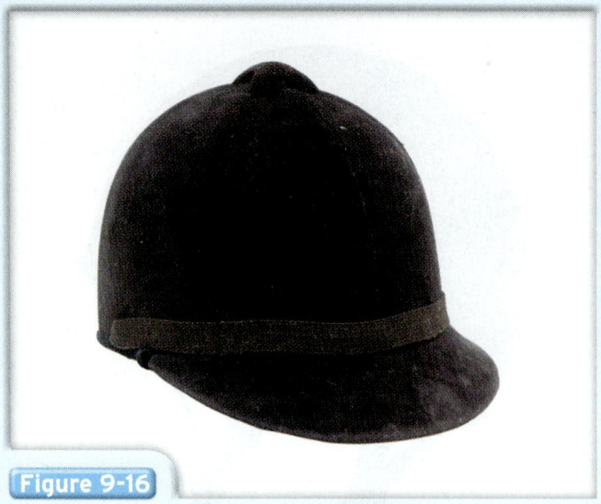

Figure 9-16

An equestrian hunt cap, which does not protect the head and is not ASTM/SEI approved.

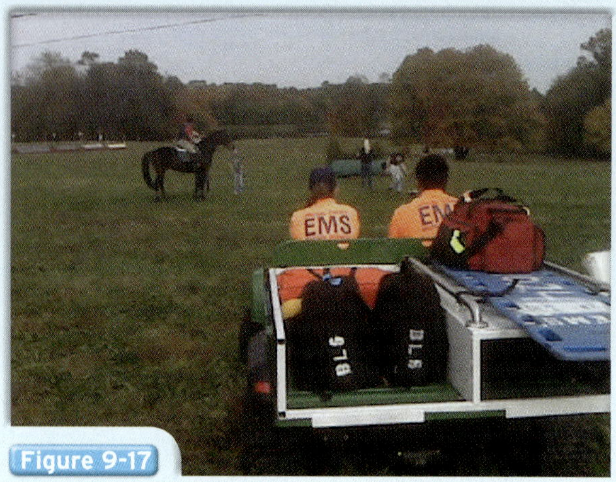

Figure 9-17

Providers must consider all objective factors during preplanning, such as the type of event, length of the course, and number of participants.

TIP

There are specially designed head immobilizers that are used by athletic trainers to stabilize the head of a patient with the helmet still in place during backboarding, but these products tend to be unknown within EMS. An example of one is the Helmet Hugger Head Immobilizer manufactured by Medco Sports Medicine. Such immobilizers are sold through sports medicine suppliers.

The procedure for removing helmets in the equestrian setting is the same as helmet removal procedures outside of the equestrian setting. Providers must consider the benefits of helmet removal versus the risk for causing potential additional spinal injury when removing the helmet. A helmet may be left on the patient during assessment and management unless it interferes with airway assessment and management, interferes with spinal immobilization, interferes with addressing management of life threats, or allows excessive head movement. A helmet should always be removed from a patient who is in cardiac arrest.

Removing a helmet is at least a two-person job; however, the technique depends on the actual type of helmet worn by the patient. One SEMS provider should provide constant in-line support. This is done by holding the helmet between the forearms while stabilizing the neck. While the first provider is holding in-line support, the second SEMS provider removes the helmet.

It is important to note that removing a helmet actually moves the c-spine even while the helmet is being held, unless the original space occupied by the helmet is filled. Therefore, if SEMS providers decide to remove the helmet, padding should be placed under the head to maintain the position the spine was in prior to the helmet's removal. Local protocols may require providers to consult with medical control before removing a helmet; providers must always follow local protocols.

Preplanning

The success or failure of SEMS in handling emergencies in an equestrian setting will be greatly affected by preplanning. To successfully preplan, providers will need to do research. As mentioned in Chapter 2, objective and subjective information are required. Objective information includes facts such as the type of event, the length of the course, and the number of participants Figure 9-17. Subjective information is information gathered from event personnel and those who have provided EMS at previous similar events.

Objective information that pertains specifically to equestrian events includes:

- How many races are scheduled?
- What types of races will occur?
- What is the distance of each race?
- What is the total number of participants?
- How many participants will there be in each race?

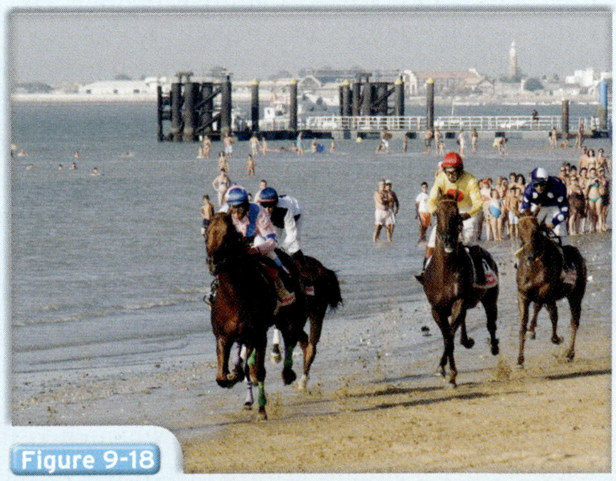

Figure 9-18

Providers must consider the terrain of the course when preplanning for an equestrian event.

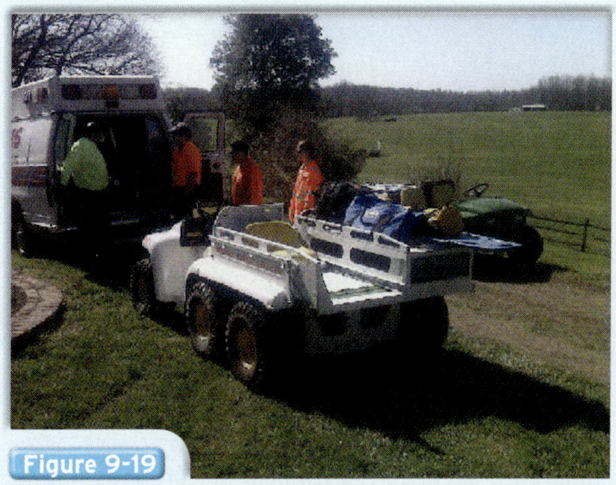

Figure 9-19

It is crucial to plan a practical way to access the track or course.

- What is the skill level and experience of individual riders in each race?
- How large is the facility?
- How big is the track?
- How can providers access the different regions of the usable track?
- What is the exact placement of the obstacles?

The terrain of the course is an important factor to consider during the preplanning stage Figure 9-18. Objective factors related to the terrain include:

- At what type of facility is the race being held?
- How much area (possibly measured in acres) does the track cover?
- What is the layout of the entire facility?
- What is the layout of the course(s)?
- What are the entrance and exit points for the course and facility?
- What type of surface will the event occur on?
- What is the condition of the surface?
- Are there areas that cannot be easily viewed?
- Where is the best vantage point?
- Where are the spectators located?
- How are the spectators contained?
- How far from the track are the spectators?
- Are there any areas of the track that are not accessible to emergency vehicles, and if so, how will SEMS providers access this part of the track?
- How long is the event?
- Will more than one shift of SEMS providers be required to cover the duration of the event?

It is crucial to plan a practical way for SEMS providers to access the track or course Figure 9-19. Considerations include the layout of the track and the longest distance that SEMS providers may need to travel to reach an emergency incident. Because the event normally continues while SEMS providers are handling an emergency incident, getting off the track safely with the patient can be even trickier than getting onto the track. Providers should never cross a track in front of the horses and should always wait until the horses have passed, then quickly cross the track behind them.

Also before the event, a map of the course should be devised. This can be used for reference at the event, and should include all pertinent areas, such as the track or course, stable areas, parking areas, surrounding streets, and first aid station locations Figure 9-20.

Upon arrival at the event, SEMS providers should conduct a walk-through of the course or track before the event begins, to ensure that no access points have been closed off or locked. It is possible that an uninformed party could lock or block preplanned access points.

TIP

There are different options for how to best reach incidents at an equestrian event. In some events, an ambulance trails behind the race. Many different options must be considered when preplanning how SEMS providers are going to reach patients.

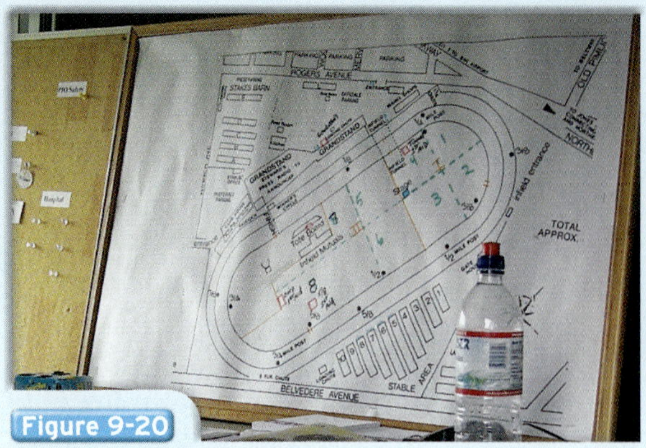

Figure 9-20

Before the event, devise a map of the grounds, noting all pertinent areas.

Performing a walk-through immediately upon arrival at the event will identify such problems and give the SEMS provider the chance to fix them in advance of emergencies occurring.

When considering subjective factors, providers should consider attendability (ie, how likely people are to attend the event and how important the event is to the attendees) and crowd mentality. Crowd mentality at equestrian events will differ depending on the type and size of event.

First Aid Station

It may be helpful to think of an equestrian event as two events in one: the race or event, and an outdoor fair or festival occurring around that race or event. The first aid station location depends on which groups SEMS providers are contracted to care for. If SEMS providers are providing emergency care for event attendees only, then it is wise to place a first aid tent in the spectator area and ensure that it is easy for spectators to see and find. If SEMS providers are also providing care for event participants, a first aid station may also be needed inside the course or track to allow quick access to sick or injured participants. Of course, a first aid station located within a course or track area must be in a safe location where horses will not likely collide with the station.

Weather

As with any event, when preplanning for an equestrian event, weather must be considered. Providers should research the weather history for the region and for the exact date of the event. This will give them a reasonable idea of the type of weather to expect and will help them determine the appropriate action. If it is traditionally hot and dry during the time when the event is to take place, providers should plan and equip their first aid station for warm or hot weather (see Chapter 3).

Another important consideration related to weather is how the weather will affect the ground. If the weather is expected to be hot and dry, the ground will likely be dry and hard. This will result in a faster race, thereby possibly creating an increase in falls and subsequent injuries. If the weather is wet, then the ground will be softer. If there has been a significant amount of rain, the ground may be sloppy. Though the race will be slower than if it were on dry ground, sloppy ground will likely cause horses to slip.

Weather is always a consideration when choosing vehicles. Vehicles should always match the terrain, weather, and conditions. As a general rule providers should never drive an ambulance onto uneven soft surfaces, and carts can also be difficult to maneuver on such surfaces. To decide what type of vehicle to use at an event, consider all factors, including the potential distance to be traveled, the terrain, and the types of emergencies likely to occur.

Communication

As always, it is important to consider communication during the preplanning stage. SEMS providers must have a baseline understanding of equestrian language.

Perhaps the most important phrase to understand at equestrian racing events is "close the gate." This is the phrase the SEMS provider should use when directing event personnel to divert other horses around the emergency site. For example, "Close gate 3" means that the incident occurred near gate 3 and that the horses must be diverted around that area. Specifically, as soon as an emergency incident occurs, the SEMS provider should tell the outrider which "gate" to close. The outrider is the referee at an equestrian event and rides along with the event. The outrider is an important point person for the SEMS provider.

Also, at equestrian events, personnel may signal to SEMS providers by waving a jacket. Of course this must all be established before the event, so SEMS providers know how they will be signaled when they are needed.

TIP

Remember that communication during the event is crucial. Prior to the event, be sure to review the emergency response plan with everyone involved in the event. Also be sure everyone knows the location of the ambulance rendezvous point and the helicopter landing site, if applicable.

Rodeos

Rodeo began in the American west around the early 1800s as a way for cowboys to demonstrate skill with handling livestock. Today, rodeos are a popular form of entertainment and have evolved into a sport around the world. Rodeos may include a number of different types of events that show cowboy skills such as riding, roping, and working with livestock Figure 9-21.

Riding events include bull riding, stunt riding, saddle bronc/bareback riding, mutton busting, and wild horse racing. In these events, the performer generally needs to stay on for 8 seconds. Racing events include barrel racing and pole bending. Other types of rodeo events include steer wrestling, calf roping, and cowboy poker, all discussed later in this section.

At these events, keep in mind that many of the participants have a cavalier attitude toward injury (for example, they may believe it is the "cowboy way" to tolerate injury). This is also true of participants of extreme sports, which are discussed in Chapter 10. While this should not affect the care provided by SEMS, it is important for SEMS providers to expect this attitude and be prepared with strategies to deal with it. Also, during the preplanning phase, it is important to determine with the event organizers who will decide if an injured participant can continue. You may even wish to establish ahead of time which specific injured patients will be allowed to continue and which will not.

Finally, like many events, rodeo has its own language. It is always advisable to learn the terminology of the event before the event begins.

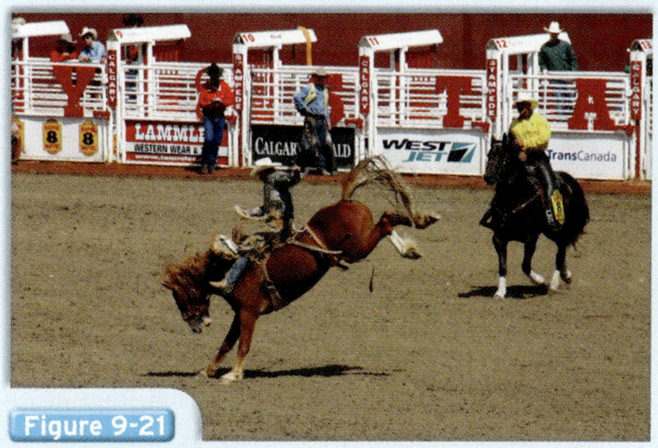

Figure 9-21

Rodeos include many different types of events that showcase skills related to riding and working with livestock.

TIP Because of the presence of livestock, it is not uncommon to have an on-site veterinarian at rodeos. SEMS providers may be asked for equipment or assistance if the veterinarian needs it.

Environment

The rodeo environment is as varied and multifaceted as the participants and livestock. A rodeo can be outdoors, with exposure to the sun and elements, or in a large indoor arena isolated from the local weather. The effects of exposure to heat, dust, dirt, and manure can create all types of respiratory problems, as well as secondary infections if traumatic injuries occur.

The work site itself consists of a large ring or arena with multiple pens that hold the livestock. Often, this area is set up and taken down rapidly. Usually there is a consistent layout that is known by the staff that travels with the rodeo.

SEMS providers must preplan procedures for entering the ring. When entering an arena, always gain clearance from the arena director, pick-up man, or bullfighter (and it is best to designate during preplanning which of these will signal SEMS). When an emergency occurs, SEMS providers must pay special attention to all livestock in the ring. SEMS providers will also need to preplan access and egress from the site; at many of these events, the roads in and out of the area are not well organized. It will be up to SEMS providers to take the initiative to ensure that they have clear paths for transport in and out of the event. Preplanning the event with the promoter is a key to ensuring a successful event.

At rodeo events, there are often physicians and athletics trainers on-site to care for the participants. SEMS providers may be responsible for the care or transport of injured participants, or for providing emergency care for sick or injured attendees in the crowd.

Gear and Equipment

Many of the participants in rodeo have little to no padding or head protection. Jeans, cowboy hats, and cowboy shirts are usually the standard. Some participants who have had an injury may wear braces, helmets, tapes, Elastic bandages, or custom items that they have made or had made.

TIP Rodeos may require a higher level of care for the riders than the crowd. Determine well in advance whether your service will be responsible for caring for the participants, the crowd, or both.

Other equipment relates to the animals. **Rigging** is used in some of these events. For example, in bareback riding, the rigging includes a handle that goes around the horse and allows the performer to hold on. Other standard equipment can include saddles, spurs, chaps, lassos or lariats, and **bull ropes**. If it is the SEMS provider's first rodeo, he or she should talk with the event promoter about which events will be part of the rodeo and the equipment involved.

Common Injuries and Conditions

Common injuries occurring at rodeos include sprains, strains, dislocations, lacerations, concussions, and crush injuries from being stepped on, rolled on, or pinned between the animal and the barrier/ground. There are also many overuse injuries (injuries that occur as a result of repetitive stress) from competitors being thrown from livestock. Repetitive stress from working with livestock and training causes injuries as well. Although not common, puncture wounds also occur during the bull riding events.

As mentioned, many competitors will not seek medical assistance, preferring to "tough it out" or "suck it up." The SEMS provider should be prepared to obtain signed refusals from those participants. It is also important that the provider be able to explain to the athlete the benefits of treatment and the consequences of not being treated. Also, at an event, an otherwise mild form of trauma could suddenly aggravate existing injuries that have previously gone untreated. The SEMS provider needs to take all of these issues into account when assessing any patient.

One phrase used at rodeo events is "Cowboy up!" (or "Cowgirl up!"). This is a common motivational phrase used by rodeo participants to encourage each other to tolerate injuries and keep going. For example, it is used when a participant is injured and participating anyway.

The next sections cover events that may be part of a rodeo or may be an event in and of itself. At these events, SEMS providers may need specialized knowledge of what occurs during these events, the language of the event, and what injuries to expect.

Bull Riding

In **bull riding**, a rider attempts to sit on a bull for 8 seconds while the bull attempts to buck the rider off. Bull riding is a dangerous rodeo sport **Figure 9-22**. Bulls typically weigh more than 1,000 pounds, behave unpredictably, and buck with great force and energy. Riders are often thrown off the bull and may be injured from the fall or may be run over or hit by the bull (the bull is said to "**camp on**" a rider). Even if the rider is able to stay mounted for the 8-second duration, he or she must dismount the bull safely, a task that requires special training. Dismounts often focus on getting clear of the bull rope, which is a rope that wraps under the

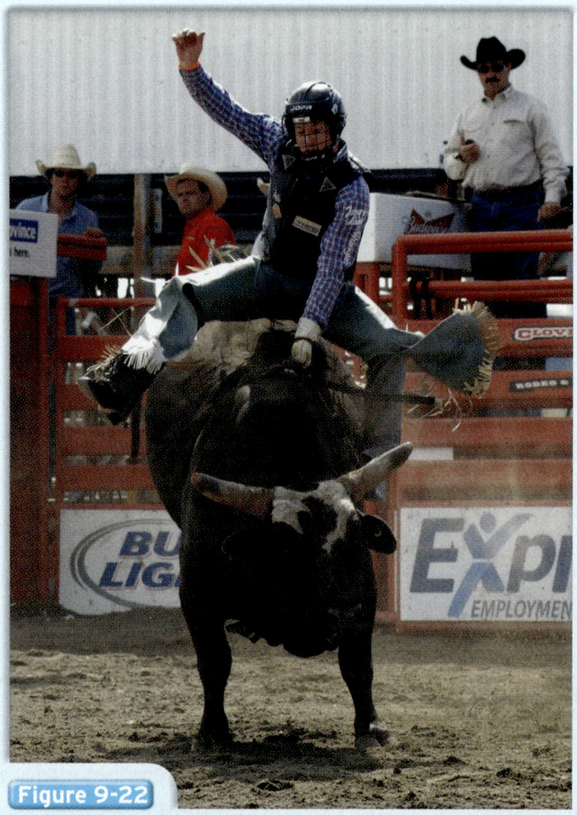

Figure 9-22 Bull riders commonly experience concussions and shoulder and groin injuries.

TIP Keep in mind that event promoters may be your best source of information, or they may choose to withhold certain information from you to prevent leaks of poor publicity. Include other sources when researching the type of event during preplanning; the event promoter should not be your only source.

bull behind its front legs. **Hanging up** is a major factor in a rider dismounting a bull. Hanging up occurs when a bull or horse continues to buck after the rider begins to fall off, but has not gotten loose from the rope or saddle. Many injuries can occur as the bull (or horse) continues to stomp and crush the rider who is hanging, and sometimes pulled under the **well** (the area beneath the bull).

As always, it is a good idea to be familiar with the language of your event. A **rank bull** is a bull known for trying to injure riders. A bull may try to **kiss the rider**, which means it will use its head and horns to throw the rider and draw him or her into the well.

Bull riding may take place at an indoor arena or outdoors at a ranch. The ground is usually covered in clay and at least 3 inches of dirt in the bull ring. To protect spectators and athletes, the arena is entirely enclosed by metal gates so the bull cannot escape. If a person is in the arena when a bull charges, the person can jump on top of the gates for safety **Figure 9-23**.

Before and after the bull ride, bulls are kept in a staging area (**pens**) and are separated from one another and restricted from moving by metal railings. When a bull is ready, rodeo workers push the gates back to allow the bull to move to the mounting area called a **chute box**. In the mounting area, the bull can only stand and cannot move as the rider mounts it. Each bull is in its own chute box, and sliders separate the bulls from each other. The rider holds the bull rope, which is wrapped around the bull's chest. Another strap, called the **flank strap**, wraps around the bull's underside to provoke the bull to buck more.

When the rider is mounted and ready, he or she nods or yells "outside," the gate opens, and the rider attempts to ride the bull for 8 seconds. The bull spins, bucks, twists, turns, kicks, and runs during this time. Riders are only permitted to have one hand on the bull and may be disqualified if the other hand touches the bull. Depending on the judges, a rider may or may

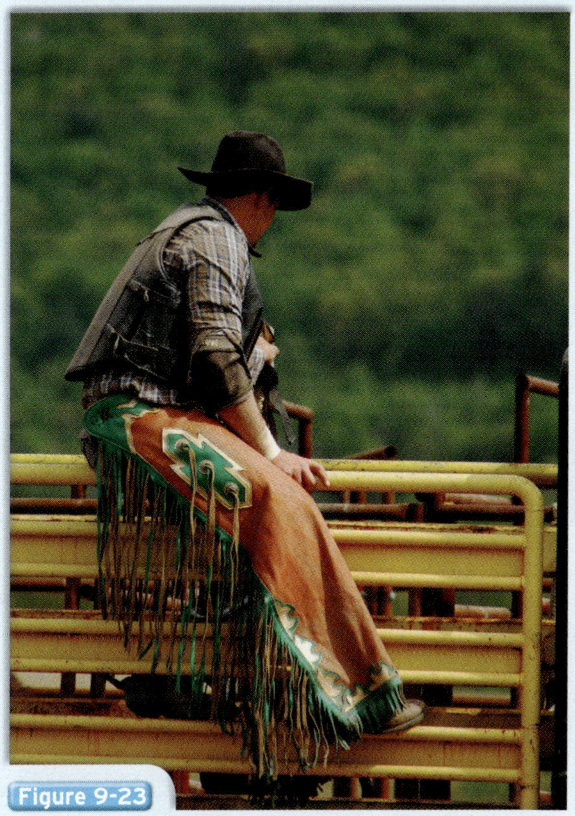

Figure 9-23

A person in a bull riding arena may jump on top of the gates for safety.

You Are the SEMS Provider

CASE 2

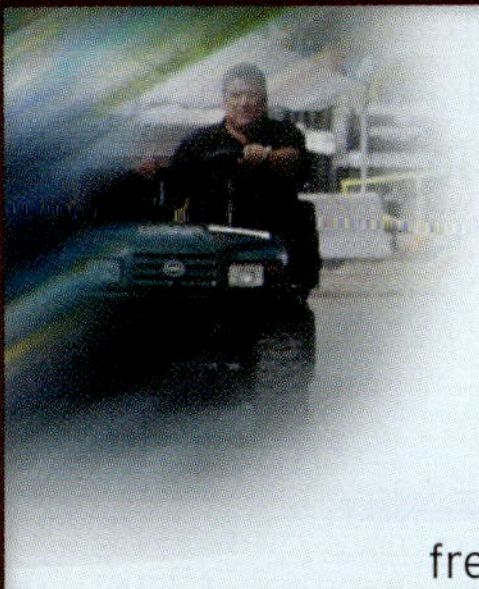

You are working at a bull riding event. A physician is on-site to provide care to the bull riders, but you are responsible for providing emergency care for the crowd and transporting participants, if needed.

As you watch, you see a rider having a particularly difficult ride on a rank bull. He suddenly gets hung up and pulled into the well. You see the arena director look at you and wave a jacket in your direction.

Two pick-up men attempt to free the rider from the bull. The rider receives several blows. You see the on-site physician waiting to enter the arena. The pick-up men finally manage to free the rider. A bullfighter guides the bull to the separate exit area, and the physician enters the ring. After a few moments, the physician waves to you.

1. When should you enter the ring?
2. What injuries should you expect in this patient?

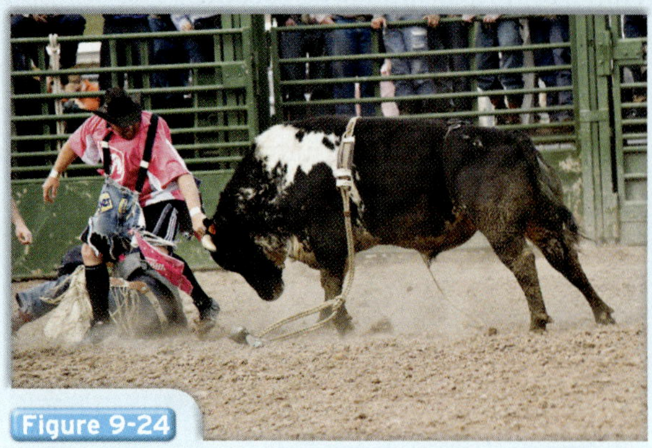

Figure 9-24

Bullfighters round up the bull after the performance.

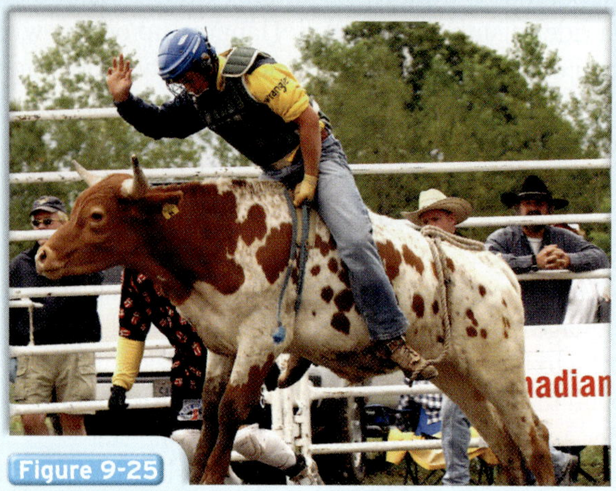

Figure 9-25

A bull riding helmet.

TIP Bull riders stand a high chance of being injured. Be sure to plan for more injuries than usual at a bull riding event.

not opt to re-ride the bull in an attempt for a higher score. Once the performance is over, **bullfighters** round up the bull to the exit chute, which is then closed so that the bull may not reenter the arena Figure 9-24. Most bulls are conditioned to return to the **outgate** (the gate through which the bulls are supposed to exit the arena). If the bull will not leave the arena, a rider on a well-trained horse lassos the bull into the exit chute.

Bull riders wear various pieces of protective equipment, including a vest to disperse shock over the body when the bull bucks and to protect the chest and ribs if a bull steps on a fallen rider. They also wear leather gloves to maintain a firm grip on the bull rope. Some riders wear cowboy hats, while others wear helmets with a hard outer shell and an insulated foam interior. These helmets are spherical and bulky and include a face guard with thin pieces of the outer shell arranged in a cage appearance Figure 9-25. Helmets may interfere with vision and balance. Riders often wear thick, durable denim pants and leather chaps. The chaps may protect the skin but are worn mostly for show. Bull riders also wear cowboy boots, usually made of leather with attached stirrups. They may wear spurs on their boots to help with grip; these spurs cannot puncture the animal.

Concussions are the most common bull riding injury, caused by head trauma from hitting the bull's head or falling off the bull and hitting the ground. Shoulder injuries (eg, dislocations, muscle tears, sprains, and strains) are the second-most commonly occurring injury, as the rider's free arm flails around wildly during the ride. After many rides, the shoulder may be worn down and weakened, requiring surgery.

Groin injuries are seen in nearly all bull riders at some point in their career. Because this area is in full contact with the bull during the performance, muscle pulls and tears are very common. Bulls have wide torsos over which riders must stretch to sit. Sitting in this position repeatedly can weaken the rider's groin muscles. Riders with groin injuries should be transported on a stretcher or stair chair, given ice for the injury, and, if they will agree to it, transported to a local hospital. Less commonly, riders may experience internal organ damage including pneumothoraces and fractured ribs. However, though they may accept ice and a wrap, bull riders will rarely agree to be transported to a hospital to receive care for a groin injury.

TIP To be safe, responders should not enter the arena until livestock is secured.

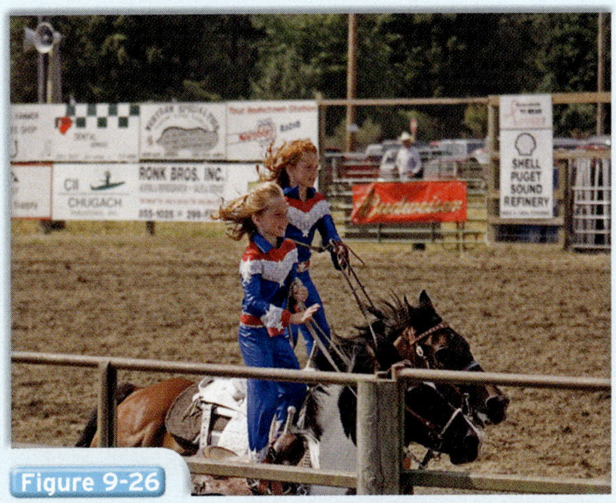

Figure 9-26

Stunt riders use a variety of gear and equipment.

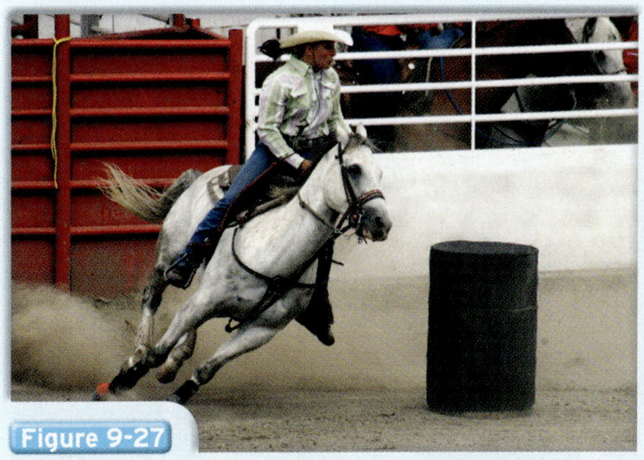

Figure 9-27

Barrel racing involves a horse and rider maneuvering in a cloverleaf pattern around three barrels without knocking any over.

Stunt Riding

In **stunt riding**, a rider performs acrobatic moves while riding a horse around an arena. It is very dangerous. For example, if the stunt rider falls, the horse can fall on top of him or her.

Stunt riding gear is often customized for a rider. Often, additions will be built onto standardized equipment such as saddles and rigging. Stunt riders may use a trick saddle. Other gear can include chariots, buggies, tables, barrels, and whatever the stunt rider and his or her staff can come up with Figure 9-26.

As with many rodeo events, stunt riding commonly causes overuse conditions from repetitive strains and insufficient healing time between shows, as well as strains, sprains, bruises, and lacerations.

Saddle Bronc and Bareback Riding

In a **saddle bronc** (bronco) event, a rider rides a horse with a saddle, and the horse bucks around the arena until the rider is thrown or falls off. As with bull riding, the horse bucks because a strap is buckled too tightly around its belly. The horse continues to buck until the strap is loosened by one of the **pick-up men**. Pick-up men are professional cowboys on horses who assist the rider if he or she is thrown, needs to be removed from a bucking horse, or after dismounting the horse. Also, in bull riding events they may rope a bull to assist it in exiting an arena. **Bareback riding** is the same as saddle bronc, except the rider is on the horse's back without a saddle. Instead, there is a rig that the rider can hold onto.

To score points, the rider must stay on for the total 8 seconds and must mark the horse out. This means the rider's spurs must touch the animal above the point of the horse's shoulder on its first jump out of the chutes. Failure to do so results in a penalty.

The standard gear and equipment for saddle bronc and bareback riding events include saddles, riggings, gloves, boots, and sometimes protective vests and helmets.

Common injuries resulting from saddle bronc or bareback riding include sprains and strains to the arm from trying to hold on. The shoulder and surrounding structures may also be injured. Bruises and dislocations from being thrown off the animal are common. Occasionally a rider can become hung in the rigging, meaning the rider's hand gets stuck and does not release. This is a real danger because the rider is dragged around the arena until he or she can be freed from the rigging.

Barrel Racing

Barrel racing is a timed event in which a horse and rider maneuver in a cloverleaf pattern around three barrels placed in a triangle Figure 9-27. In this event, one horse and rider perform at a time (as opposed to several racing at once). The goal is to complete the race in the shortest time possible. Time penalties are given if a barrel is knocked over or the pattern is not completed. This sport is often completed in less than 25 seconds. Speed is a factor in injuries at these events; the horse and rider enter the ring at full gallop and try to maintain the highest possible speed throughout the ride without losing control.

Pole bending, also called equine slalom, is a timed event as well. It involves five posts or poles placed in

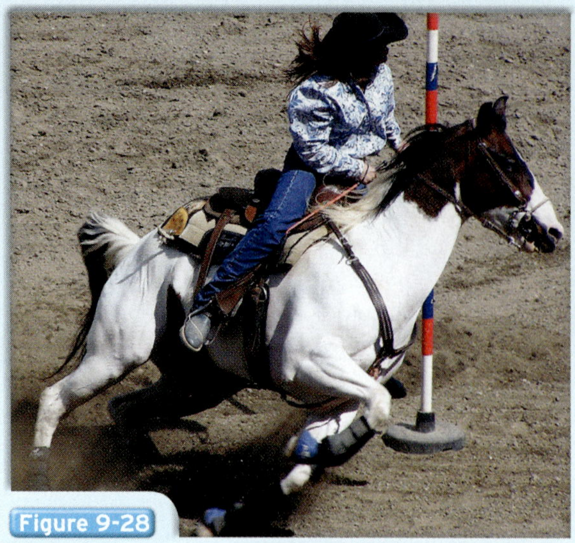

Figure 9-28

Pole bending involves a horse and rider moving in a slalom or serpentine pattern around poles without knocking any over.

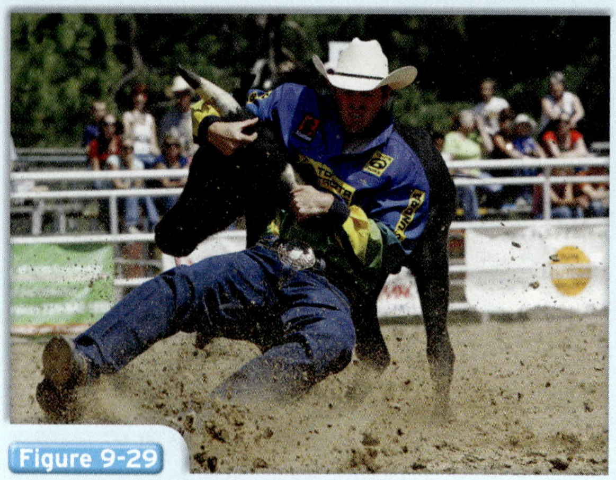

Figure 9-29

In steer wrestling, a rider approaches alongside a steer, jumps off the horse, and tackles the steer with the goal of rolling it over.

a straight line. One horse and rider perform at a time. The horse and rider must move around the poles in a slalom or serpentine pattern without knocking any over Figure 9-28. The horse and rider must race to one end of the course, then turn around and race back through to the starting point. Again the shortest time wins.

There is no specialized equipment at a barrel racing or pole bending event except the saddle and barrels or poles.

Sprains, strains, and contusions to the lower legs occur from striking the barrels or poles while maneuvering around them. Back injuries may also occur. Horses may spook, causing the rider to fall off. The somersault and catapult injuries discussed in the equestrian section of this chapter are also possible.

Steer Wrestling

Steer wrestling begins with two cowboys pursuing a steer that has been released from a pen. There is a string barrier similar to a trip wire that the cowboy cannot break until after the steer is out of the chute. If the cowboy breaks this barrier, a time penalty is assessed to the run. After the steer leaves the chute, the cowboy approaches alongside the steer. The rider then attempts to jump off the horse and tackle the steer with the goal of rolling it over onto its back by twisting its head and neck Figure 9-29.

The only gear sometimes worn in steer wrestling is gloves.

Like many rodeo athletes, steer wrestlers sustain bruises, bumps, and lacerations. Specific injuries in their sport occur when they jump off the horse and tackle the steer, causing strains and sprains to the ankle, hip, and knee. They may also receive injuries to the shoulder when throwing or twisting the animal.

Calf Roping

The purpose of **calf roping** is to simulate the old practice of roping a calf before branding. This is achieved by the cowboy and a partner pursuing a calf that has been released. As with steer wrestling, there is a string barrier that the cowboy cannot break until after the calf is out of the chute. The cowboy attempts to lasso the calf. Once the calf is lassoed, the cowboy must roll the calf over and tie at least three of its feet together. To score a time, the calf must stay tied for at least 6 seconds.

Gear and equipment used in calf roping include a calf rope used to catch the calf and a small section of rope, usually carried in the cowboy's teeth, used to tie the animal's feet. Gloves are sometimes worn to prevent rope burn.

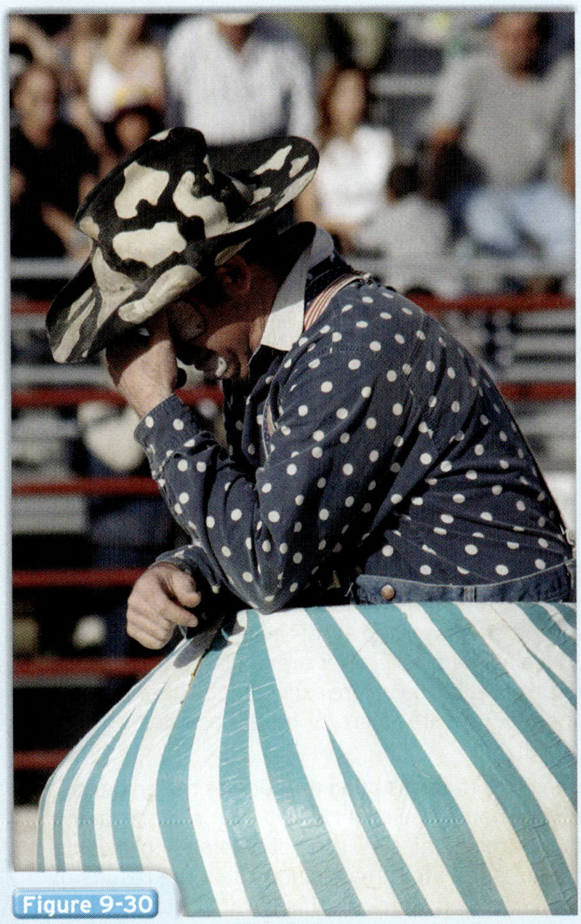

Figure 9-30

A barrel man provides an island of safety for a bull rider.

As with steer wrestlers, ropers have to dismount their horse and wrestle the calf onto its back. This can result in injuries to the knees and ankles as well as the shoulders. Injuries such as tendonitis and bursitis are common.

Cutting

Cutting is an event in which a horse and rider attempt to separate an animal from a herd. The animal separated in this event is usually a cow. The rider must keep the animal separated from the herd for a certain amount of time, and the horse is responsible for much of the task, without the assistance of the rider. Injuries at these events are not common. SEMS providers will likely only care for minor bumps and bruises.

Rodeo Clowns and Barrel Men

In addition to the riders, there are other performers at rodeo events. These may include **rodeo clowns**, a **barrel man**, or a bullfighter. A rodeo clown and a barrel man both perform acts to entertain the crowd and keep the rider safe, but a barrel man uses a padded barrel that he can jump into if protection is needed Figure 9-30. Often they will place themselves between the livestock and an injured rider. They will assist however they can and are often the best extra set of hands you have in the ring outside of your staff. It is always important to meet with these performers and to include them in planning. They have a wealth of knowledge about the sports and participants, as they see them many times throughout the tour or rodeo season.

Gear and equipment worn by these performers vary. Some will use pyrotechnics in their act, while others juggle objects. Many wear a radio microphone headset on their clown or bullfighter outfit. The outfit usually includes oversized clothing and whatever else they can dream up. They may wear braces and padding to help protect them from livestock impacts.

As with other rodeo performers, injuries include sprains, strains, bruises, dislocations, lacerations, and concussions.

Additional Rodeo Events

Other events at a rodeo can include **wild horse racing**, in which a team of cowboys has to catch and ride an untamed horse for 8 seconds. **Bull poker**, also called cowboy poker, another rodeo event, is not for the faint of heart. It usually involves four to six participants sitting around a card table that is set up in the ring. A bull is released into the ring, and the last person to flee from the table wins. This event can result in some exciting showmanship. Often a participant becomes airborne as a result of not getting up quickly enough. Another event held at some rodeos is **money the hard way**. In this event, a pouch containing a $100 bill (or higher dollar amount) is tied around the horn of a bull. Participants attempt to grab the pouch off the horn.

Some rodeo events involve children as participants. Two such examples are mutton busting and calf scramble. In **mutton busting**, a child, usually between ages 6 and 10 years, climbs atop a sheep and holds on for as long as possible. These children usually wear a chest protector and helmet. Another youth event is a **calf scramble**, in which something is tied to a calf and the child who pulls it off wins a prize.

You Are the SEMS Provider SUMMARY

CASE 1

1. **How should you have preplanned for this event, and how would you put the plan into action?**
First and foremost, you must never cross a track in front of the horses. Wait until the horses have passed, then cross the track behind them. Once on the scene, you complete a rapid size-up of the patient and realize that he will require transport. Because this patient is closer to the secondary patient exchange location determined during preplanning, you alert the ambulance to meet you there rather than at the primary patient exchange location. You may or may not remove the patient's helmet depending on local protocol. This patient would, however, need a cervical collar to be placed, which would likely necessitate removing the helmet. After stabilization is addressed, you load him onto your mobile transport unit, and then slowly and methodically move him to the secondary patient exchange location. Finally, the patient is transported to the local trauma center.

CASE 2

1. **When should you enter the ring?**
Hopefully during preplanning, the event promoters and SEMS providers agreed upon the signal to use for calling SEMS to a scene. In this case, it is not clear whether the arena director is calling you to the scene. If you are unsure, you should not rush in. Also, since there is an on-site physician at this event, he or she would likely be the one called to provide initial care to the rider. Usually, the physician or arena director will signal you to approach once they determine whether your services are needed. If you are expected to approach, you must check if it is safe to enter, and then proceed with caution. Always stay alert for other hazards.
2. **What injuries should you expect in this patient?**
A rider who was hung up may have injuries to the part of the body that was hung up, such as the ankle, leg, or wrist. Considering that the rider received several blows, you should also expect head injuries and trauma to other parts of the body, such as extremity, chest, and abdominal injuries. If responsible for providing care to riders, you will need to perform a full assessment, address all life threats, and expect the results of trauma: sprains, strains, fractures, head injuries, internal injuries, and shock. In this particular case, since there is an on-site physician, you would likely wait for the physician (or designated official) to signal you to approach, then you would approach with equipment needed to immobilize, backboard, assess, treat, and transport this patient.

Ready for Review

- Each type of equestrian event presents its own set of unique challenges to SEMS providers. It is important for providers to be familiar with the type of event they are working at.
- Equestrian events include races, jumping events, and eventing.
- Racing events include steeplechases, hurdling, thoroughbred racing, point-to-point racing, and harness racing.
- Thoroughbred racing occurs on a flat track and is usually less than 2 miles. This race is a test of a horse's speed and a jockey's ability to maneuver the horse.
- In harness racing, the horse pulls a cart called a sulky while racing in a certain gait, either trotting or pacing. The sulky is a lightweight cart with two wheels. It is sometimes called a bike. Harness races are usually 1 mile in length. Harness races usually begin with the horses behind a gate.
- Steeplechase events require the rider to jump and maneuver around a variety of unforeseen obstacles. These races are 2 to 4 miles in length.
- Hurdling is a form of steeplechase racing often used to train horses for more challenging courses. This race is generally no more than 2 miles.
- Point-to-point racing is an amateur race in which hunting horses jump fences. This is the most dangerous type of equestrian sport because it involves amateur riders.
- Show jumping is divided into two primary types, hunter classes and jumper classes, that differ in how they are judged. Hunter events test factors such as the horse's style, manner, and gait against a set ideal. Jumper events test the horse's ability to jump, and a score is given based on whether the horse attempts to jump the obstacle, whether the horse successfully jumps the obstacle, and whether the horse finishes the event in a specified amount of time.
- Eventing is an event that consists of three phases (show jumping, dressage, and cross-country) that test a rider's accomplishment in various areas of equestrian sport.
- Dressage is a component of eventing that requires horse and rider to perform a sequence of movements in an arena. Scores are based on the horse's obedience and style.
- Cross-country equestrian jumping tests the horse's endurance, speed, and jumping ability, as well as the rider's ability to pace the horse. The course length is usually around 2 to 4 miles and contains a variety of obstacles, some of which may be natural.
- Horses can be very sensitive and can react very suddenly. Basic knowledge of how to behave around horses is important when providing EMS coverage at an equestrian event. Providers should remember to never approach a horse from the rear, always expect a horse to kick or rear up, and be ready to protect themselves.
- When providing EMS coverage at an event involving ponies, participants may be pediatric. Before the event, providers should refresh their knowledge of pediatric patients as well as their assessment and management.
- The majority of the equestrian-related injuries result when riders fall from their mounts, are crushed as their horse falls, strike obstacles while mounted, or are injured by entrapment of the reins.
- The most frequent injuries are fractured clavicles and shoulder separations.
- Injuries are more likely to occur in point-to-point racing and jumping than in thoroughbred racing or in social riding. Of all horse riding activities, jumping is the most likely to produce a spinal injury.
- In equestrian-related injuries, lumbar and thoracic fractures are much more common than cervical fractures. Rearing horses and tree branches can unseat riders and cause them to fall backward.
- Injury patterns may be related to riding style. Jockey style (cross-country position) is the position in which the rider's head is forward and his or her body is essentially parallel to the horse's neck. Classical style is the position in which the rider's head is held high and his or her body is essentially perpendicular to the horse's back.
- When a rider falls from a horse and is within proximity of other horses, the downed rider is likely to receive more significant injuries from being kicked or trampled.
- Any fall from a horse regardless of proximity to other horses should be considered a significant injury due to the distance fallen. Neck and back injury should be suspected immediately.

- When providing SEMS for an equestrian event, EMS equipment must include spinal and other splint equipment/supplies. A basic jump kit without splints or long backboards will not suffice.
- When caring for a participant of an equestrian event, providers should check the rider's armband for medical information. Some events require jockeys to have pertinent medical information on their armbands.
- Severe injuries can occur in harness races when the sulky becomes caught beneath the horse's feet or when the sulky catapults over the horse and rider.
- The most severe injuries in equestrian events occur when a horse somersaults over a fence or obstacle. This can cause the rider to fall, resulting in head and fall-related injuries, and the rider can also subsequently be crushed by the horse. Providers should consider the height of fences and obstacles, as well as the height of the horses participating in the event, to help predict where on the course a horse could be likely to somersault.
- Rider attire depends on the event, but riders should always wear an approved ASTM/SEI equestrian helmet with a harness. Jumping riders at the grand prix level usually wear red jackets and more formal attire. Riders must wear a safety vest during certain events, such as those that involve jumping.
- Hunt caps do not provide enough protection and are not approved by ASTM/SEI. When responding to an equestrian-related emergency, providers should always note the type of helmet the rider is/was wearing, to help gauge the extent of injury. They should also note any damage to the helmet.
- The procedure for removing helmets in the equestrian setting is the same as helmet removal procedures outside of the equestrian setting. A helmet may be left on the patient during assessment and management, unless it interferes with airway assessment and management, interferes with spinal immobilization, interferes with addressing management of life threats, or allows excessive head movement.
- Preplanning is a crucial part of all SEMS events; equestrian events are no exception. Providers should consider both objective and subjective factors. Objective factors include the type of event, distance, number of participants, and accessibility of the track, among others.
- The terrain of the course is an important factor that should be considered during the preplanning stage.
- It is crucial to plan a practical way for SEMS providers to access the track. Considerations include layout and the longest potential distance that SEMS providers may need to travel to reach an emergency incident.
- Providers should never cross a track in front of the horses. They should always wait until the horses have passed, then quickly cross the track behind them.
- Always conduct a walk-through of an equestrian course or track immediately upon arrival at the event to ensure that no access points have been closed off or locked.
- Providers should research the weather history for the region and for the exact date of the event and plan for the expected weather.
- Providers should consider how the weather will affect the ground. Dry, hot weather results in a hard ground and a faster race. Rain causes slippery ground.
- Providers should consider weather when choosing what type of vehicles to use at the event.
- Providers should learn the language of the event. The phrase "close the gate" is used in racing events to divert horses around the emergency site. The outrider is the referee at an equestrian event and is an important point person for the SEMS provider.
- Rodeos showcase events that display cowboy skills such as riding, roping, and working with livestock. Types of events include riding events, racing events, and other entertainment.
- Many rodeo performers have a cavalier attitude toward injury. SEMS providers should expect this and be prepared with strategies to deal with it.
- During preplanning, determine with the event organizers who will decide if an injured participant can continue. You may even wish to establish ahead of time which specific injured patients will be allowed to continue, and which will not.
- Rodeos may occur outdoors or indoors, in a large ring or arena. SEMS providers must preplan procedures for entering the ring. When an emergency occurs, SEMS providers must pay special attention to all livestock in the ring.
- SEMS providers must preplan access and egress from the event site; at many of these events, the roads in and out of the area are not well organized.

- Many rodeo performers wear little to no padding or head protection. The standard outfit includes jeans, cowboy hats, and cowboy shirts.
- Other equipment relates to the animals, such as saddles, rigging, and ropes.
- Discuss with the event promoter which events will be part of the rodeo and the equipment involved.
- Common injuries occurring at rodeos include sprains, strains, dislocations, lacerations, concussions, and crush injuries. There are also overuse injuries and stress injuries.
- Bull riders attempt to sit on a bucking bull for 8 seconds at an indoor arena or outdoors at a ranch.
- SEMS providers should know the terminology associated with rodeos and bull riding before working at a rodeo event.
- The most common bull riding injuries are concussions and injuries to the shoulder, groin, and internal organs.
- Stunt riding is performing acrobatic moves while riding a horse. Stunt riding gear is often customized and may include a trick saddle.
- In a saddle bronc (bronco) event, a rider rides a horse with a saddle, and the horse bucks around the arena until the rider is thrown or falls off. As with bull riding, the horse bucks because a strap is buckled too tightly around its belly.
- Bareback riding is the same as saddle bronc, except the rider is on the horse's back without a saddle. There is a rig that the rider can hold onto. If a rider becomes stuck in the rigging, he or she may be dragged around the arena until he or she can be freed.
- Barrel racing involves a horse and rider maneuvering in a cloverleaf pattern around three barrels placed in a triangle without knocking over any barrels. Speed is a factor in injuries at these events.
- Pole bending (equine slalom) involves a horse and rider moving around five poles placed in a straight line. Horse and rider must race to one end of the course, then turn around and race back to the starting point.
- In rodeo racing events, injuries similar to those in equestrian events can occur.
- Steer wrestling involves a cowboy jumping from a horse onto a steer and wrestling the steer onto its back.
- Calf roping involves a cowboy riding a horse, lassoing a calf, and tying at least three of its feet together. The rope for tying the calf's feet is often carried in the cowboy's teeth.
- Cutting is an event in which a horse and rider attempt to separate an animal, usually a cow, from a herd. Usually only minor bumps and bruises occur at these events.
- Rodeos usually have performers to provide entertainment and protect the riders. These performers include rodeo clowns, barrel men, funny men, and bullfighters. They may be willing to assist SEMS providers and are an important source of knowledge.

Vital Vocabulary

bareback riding An event in which no saddle is used to ride a bucking horse until the rider is thrown or falls off.

barrel man A rodeo performer who entertains the crowd, works to keep riders safe, and uses a padded barrel for protection if needed.

barrel racing A race in which a horse and rider maneuver in a cloverleaf pattern around three barrels placed in a triangle.

bull poker An event in which four to six participants attempt to be the last one sitting around a card table while a bull is in the ring.

bull riding A sport in which a rider attempts to sit on a bull for 8 seconds while the bull attempts to buck the rider off.

bull rope In bull riding, a rope that wraps under the bull behind its front legs.

bullfighters People who round up the bull to move it to the exit chute in bull riding.

calf roping An event in which a cowboy attempts to lasso a calf, roll it over, and tie at least three of its feet together.

calf scramble A rodeo event in which something is tied to a calf and children compete to pull it off.

camp on The term in bull riding for a bull throwing a rider off and running him or her over.

catapult injury A type of injury unique to harness racing in which the cart, or sulky, launches over the horse and rider, causing injury when it lands.

chute box The area where the rider mounts the bull.

classical style A rider position in which the rider's head is held high and the rider's body is perpendicular to the horse's back; in this position, the rider is more likely to fall onto his or her buttocks.

cross-country equestrian jumping A riding event that tests endurance and includes obstacles such as water, logs, and fences that the horse must jump; horses are started at different times and do not compete with one another to clear an obstacle; a component of eventing.

cutting A rodeo event in which a horse and rider attempt to separate an animal, usually a cow, from a herd for a set amount of time.

dressage A riding discipline in which horse and rider perform a sequence of movements and are scored on specific criteria such as style and obedience; a component of eventing.

eventing A type of equestrian event that includes three phases: cross-country, dressage, and jumping.

flank strap A strap that wraps around the bull's underside to provoke the bull to buck more.

hanging up A situation that occurs when a bull or horse continues to buck after the rider begins to fall off, but has not gotten loose from the rope or saddle.

harness racing A type of horse racing in which the horses pull a type of cart called a sulky, and the horses race in a specified gait.

hurdling A type of steeplechase racing often used to train horses for more challenging courses; it involves jumping hurdles.

jockey style A rider position in which the rider's body is relatively parallel to the horse's neck and the rider's head is forward; in this position, the rider is more likely to sustain cervical injury accompanied by head injury.

kiss the rider In bull riding, when the bull uses its head and horns to throw the rider and draw him or her into the area beneath the bull.

money the hard way A rodeo event in which participants attempt to grab a pouch of money that is tied around the horn of a bull.

mutton busting An event in which a child, usually between ages 6 and 10 years, climbs atop a sheep and holds on for as long as possible.

outgate In bull riding, the gate through which the bulls are supposed to exit the arena.

pens The areas where bulls are held to separate them from each other before a bull riding event.

pick-up man In rodeo, a professional cowboy on a horse who assists the rider if he or she is thrown or needs to be removed from a bucking horse, or after dismounting the horse; may also rope a bull to assist it in exiting an arena.

point-to-point racing A type of amateur horse racing that involves hunter horses jumping fences.

pole bending A race in which a horse and rider move around five poles in a slalom or serpentine pattern; also called equine slalom.

rank bull A bull known for trying to injure riders.

rigging The rope used in rodeos that allows the performer or rider to hold on.

rodeo A type of event that showcases cowboy skills such as riding, racing, roping, and working with livestock; includes a number of subevents.

rodeo clown A rodeo performer who entertains the crowd and works to keep riders safe.

saddle bronc An event in which a rider rides a saddled, bucking horse until he or she is thrown or falls off; also called bronco.

show jumping A type of equestrian event in which horses jump obstacles and are judged on different criteria depending on whether the event is a hunter event or a jumper event; a component of eventing.

somersaulting A dangerous situation in which a horse's chest collides with a fence or object, causing the horse to flip over, either taking the rider with it or causing the rider to fall off.

steeplechase horse racing A form of horse racing that involves obstacles such as fences, water features, and jumps.

steer wrestling An event in which a cowboy attempts to jump from a horse onto a steer and wrestle the steer onto its back.

stunt riding An event in which a rider performs acrobatic moves while riding a horse.

sulky A two-wheeled cart that is pulled behind a horse in harness racing.

thoroughbred racing A type of horse racing that occurs over a flat, even track; this race is a set distance.

well In bull riding, the area beneath the bull.

wild horse racing An event in which a team of cowboys attempts to catch and ride an untamed horse.

CHAPTER

Extreme and Combat Sports 10

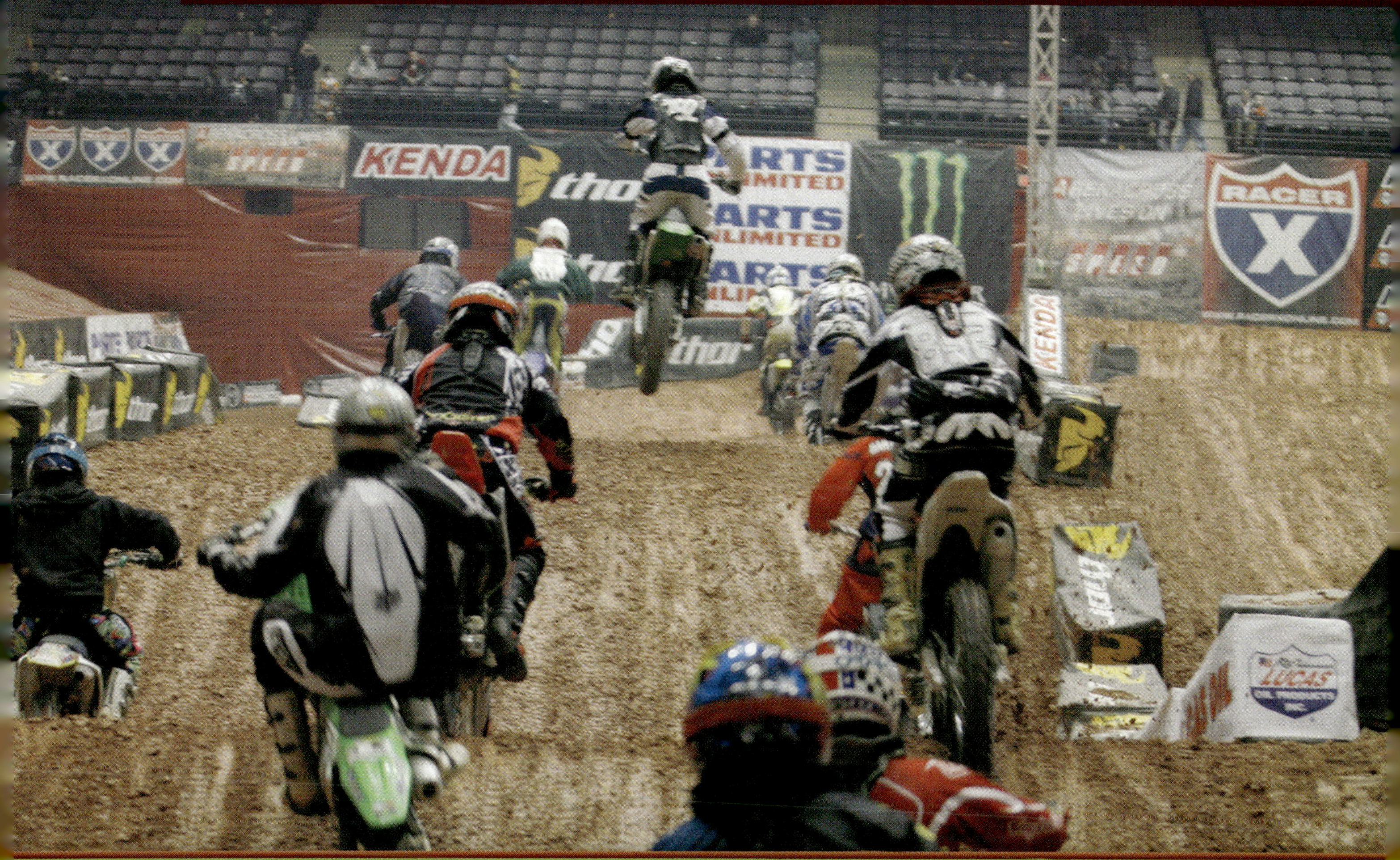

LEARNING OBJECTIVES

- Describe preplanning efforts necessary for extreme or combat sporting events.
- Identify the following extreme sports, their environments, and associated gear and equipment: skiing, snowboarding, skateboarding, in-line skating, bicycle motocross (BMX), motocross, and rock climbing.
- Identify the following combat sports, their environments, and associated gear and equipment: boxing, fencing, wrestling, and martial arts.
- Outline typical injuries and conditions associated with various forms of extreme and combat sports.
- Discuss dangers and injuries specific to cheerleading.
- Discuss injuries specific to paintball.
- Understand SEMS considerations for treating conditions and injuries commonly associated with extreme and combat sports, such as heat injuries, hypothermia, dehydration, hyponatremia, closed head injuries, spinal injuries, sprains, and fractures.
- Discuss considerations for effectively preplanning for an extreme or combat sport event.
- Consider transportation options and complications at special events that involve extreme or combat sports.

Introduction

Extreme sports involve dangerous and high-risk sport activities that include a significant risk of injury such as snowboarding, in-line skating, rock climbing, and bicycle motocross (BMX) Figure 10-1. **Combat sports** involve two fighters competing in a contact sport according to a set of specific rules, using striking, grappling, or weapons Figure 10-2.

Each of these sports and the injuries commonly associated with them is discussed in the following sections. In general, SEMS providers will be required to treat a wide range of injuries from extreme and combat sports including spinal cord injuries, fractures, dislocations, groin injuries, eye injuries, cuts, and concussions. Appropriate treatment depends on the situation and the patient's presentation. With any incident, SEMS providers should be cognizant of the

TIP The treatment of any injury or condition should be in accordance with established protocols and best practices.

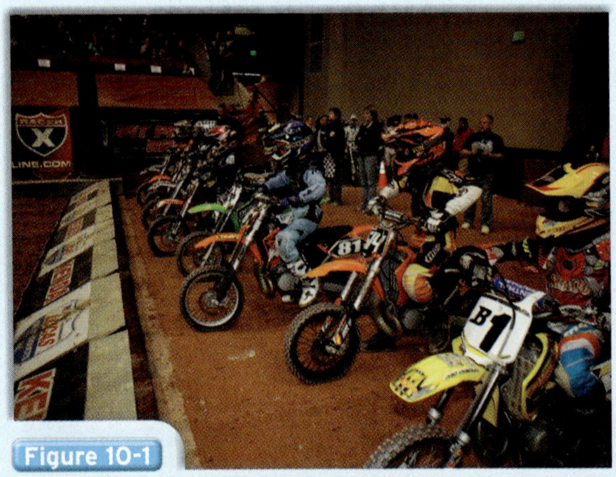

Figure 10-1

Motocross is an example of an extreme sport.

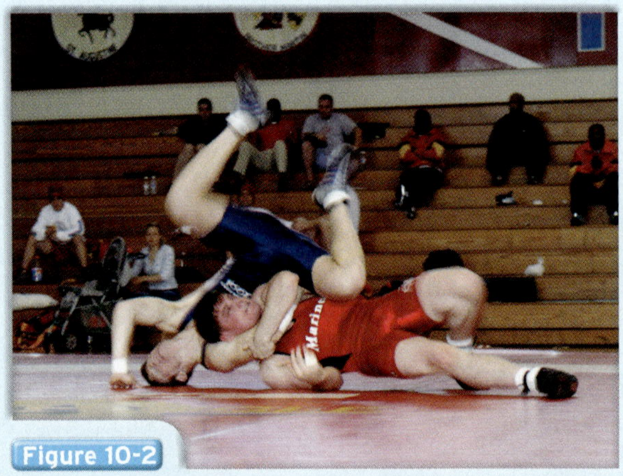

Figure 10-2

Wrestling is an example of a combat sport.

You Are the SEMS Provider

CASE 1

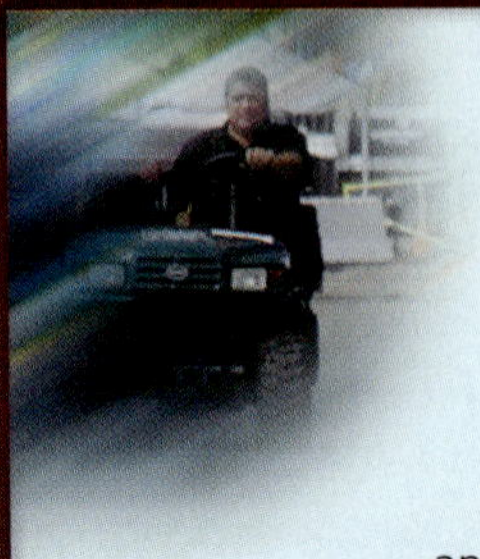

At a motocross competition in a stadium, an athlete is thrown from his bike while landing a jump. He lands on his head and cervical vertebrae. He is wearing the standard motocross outfit and protective gear, including a motocross helmet. SEMS providers quickly arrive at the athlete's side. One provider maintains cervical spine precautions, while others assess airway, breathing, and circulation. The patient is not breathing and does not have a pulse. SEMS providers remove the helmet per local protocol and then begin CPR. Other SEMS providers prepare to move the patient onto a backboard for transport to the closest trauma center. This traumatic event was witnessed by other athletes, spectators, and sports broadcasters, and a crowd of onlookers has gathered around.

1. How do you manage the scene, keeping the crowd calm and controlled while ensuring that the patient receives necessary and adequate care?
2. What should SEMS providers do to increase the patient's chance of survival?

mechanism of injury and relay this information to any medical personnel who assume care for the patient after transport.

Extreme and combat sporting events provide an adrenaline rush for both spectators and performing athletes. Spectators are often excited by the high energy of the event and may react to an injured athlete with shock or anger. In these events, you must treat the athlete—working with the physician, athletic trainers, and referees—and possibly assist security personnel to maintain crowd control, usually simply by serving as a professional presence and setting an example. At these events, it is important to work out roles and responsibilities of the various medical providers (ie, physicians, athletic trainers, and SEMS providers) before the event and to determine the communication procedures these providers should follow during the event.

At extreme and combat sporting events, SEMS providers may also be hired to treat event attendees. These events are very popular with teenagers and young adults. This audience presents some unique challenges because members may be unaware that they require medical attention or be reluctant to seek or receive help. SEMS providers are often not notified of an injury or a condition until it is serious. For example, a teenager may be suffering from heat exhaustion but feel peer pressure not to seek help, suppressing symptoms until he or she goes into shock. Because of this tendency, prevention efforts are crucial. Take steps to inform event-goers of the medical conditions they may experience, and remind them to eat, drink, and seek warmth or shade as appropriate. It may be beneficial to post signs around the venue to encourage such behavior and to provide audio announcements as reminders.

As mentioned in Chapter 8, find out during preplanning if there are specific medical staffing requirements or medical standby guidelines from organizations such as the National Collegiate Athletic Association (NCAA) or the National Athletic Trainers Association (NATA).

TIP Teenagers may mask the signs and symptoms of shock due to compensatory mechanisms until they reach a very late stage of shock. Prevention is the key to ensuring that young participants and spectators remain healthy throughout an event.

Preplanning for Extreme and Combat Sports Events

SEMS providers should be specially trained for each type of sporting event. Proper preplanning is essential; as with most events, the success or failure of a SEMS service to handle emergencies at extreme and combat sporting events is determined well before personnel set foot on the event grounds. As part of preplanning, SEMS providers should consider:

- What types of events/competitions will be taking place?
- How many events/competitions are scheduled?
- What is the distance or duration of each event/competition?
- What is the total number of participants for the entire event?
- What is the total number of participants per event/competition?
- What is the skill and experience level of participants?
- What are the type, size, and layout of the facility?
- What are the type, size, layout, and condition of the performance area?
- How can providers access different regions of the facility?
- If the event includes obstacles, how will they affect access and egress?

Timeline

Once this information is gathered, SEMS providers should create a detailed timeline of the event including every planned action that will occur over the course of the event. This way providers can ensure they are in the right place at the right time. The timeline should note:

- Move-in time for vendors
- Move-in time for equipment
- Start time of the event
- Start time for each race/subevent
- Arrival time for event staff
- Arrival time for SEMS staff
- Arrival time at first aid station or standby location
- Gate time (when participants must be at their starting gates)
- Departure time for SEMS staff post event

Note: The term "gate time" may mean different things at different events. It may be the time when participants

TIP Always find out what special event officials expect from your service, and explain to them what can reasonably be provided in the given circumstance.

must be at their starting positions, or it may mean the time when the contest begins. Be sure to clarify this prior to the event.

In many cases, SEMS providers will be among the first personnel to arrive at the event and among the last to leave. However, this may not always be the case. For example, SEMS providers may not be required to stay while the stage is being broken down. As always, determine arrival and departure times with event organizers before the event.

Spectators

Spectators should also be considered. For example, consider the following questions:

- Who will provide care for the spectators?
- How will providers be notified when a spectator requires care?
- Will there be a separate first aid station for spectators, and if so, where will it be located?
- Will alcohol be served at the event? If so, how will it be dispensed?
- What is the crowd management plan?
- Who will provide security/law enforcement?
- How is the crowd seated or arranged?
- Where are spectators located?
- How are spectators contained?

Like many events, at extreme and combat sporting events, SEMS providers may need to respond to emergencies involving the participants or emergencies involving the crowd. Alternatively, at some extreme or combat sporting events, SEMS providers may be hired to provide care to only the attendees; the athletes may have their own medical team. This varies from event to event. Regardless, it is important to have a specific plan in place for responding to any kind of emergency, whether it involves a participant or a spectator. SEMS providers will need to plan access and egress routes to various parts of the venue, considering how to access the performance area (stage, ring, course) and how to access any area within the crowd.

As always, it is wise to consult with other SEMS providers who have worked at similar events and to consider this information during preplanning.

First Aid Facilities

As in any event, it is important to identify the best location for the first aid station or first aid tent. Note the best vantage point at the event. Considering event size, determine how many first aid stations will be needed, and plan personnel and equipment appropriately. Review the discussion of first aid stations in Chapter 2. The station will need to be kept away from the center of crowds, usually on the boundaries where vendors are. As always, first aid stations should be easily accessible and easily seen.

Remember that at some sporting events, there may be separate medical teams for spectators and participants. There must be separate personnel and first aid areas for the spectators, especially because in several venues spectators are relatively far away from the event area and cannot be easily reached from the performance area.

Keep in mind that extreme sports events tend to be held in extreme weather conditions that may range from cold weather or snowy conditions to hot weather and events involving water. These events will present a variety of issues that you will need to consider when preplanning and designing first aid station locations. These factors will also affect the configuration of the station itself. Will it need to be heated or cooled? Will it require a temporary floor to insulate it from the elements?

For outdoor events, an open tent can serve as the first aid station, providing coverage from precipitation and the sun for patients and SEMS providers. The larger the crowd, the larger the tent will need to be. Without shade, providers are bound to get sunburns in these conditions; SEMS providers should be sure to apply sunscreen regularly and wear proper protective gear such as a hat with a wide brim. In cold weather, providers should be dressed warmly enough for the conditions.

Working at indoor events is tiring for SEMS providers, who must constantly remain alert, travel quickly to patient locations, carry equipment, and carry patients. Working at an outdoor event can be even more tiring. Walking at the special events may seem manageable for a few hours, but once temperatures

TIP An automated external defibrillator (AED) should be immediately available at every event. At youth sporting events, such as lacrosse and baseball games, remember that a child hit in the chest can experience sudden cardiac arrest. Pediatric patients have been found to respond very well to AEDs in such cases.

and weather set in, provider exhaustion is a huge risk. Special events may last up to 14 hours in a day and extend over several days. It is necessary to travel quickly and safely over what may be a vast area. Patients may be spread across a variety of locations at the venue, such as on the east side of an arena, for example, or in a parking lot on the west side. It is vital to preplan first aid stations effectively to prevent SEMS providers from becoming patients.

Stocking Medical Supplies

Equipment for extreme and combat sporting events includes typical BLS and ALS equipment.

The stretcher and bulky equipment (eg, AED, backboard, head blocks, blankets, and straps) should be stored next to an easily accessible area between the ambulance and performance area **Figure 10-3**. Some EMS equipment at sporting events will remain in one location, while other equipment will need to be carried to and from emergency scenes. When responding to a call, consider what equipment you will need. For example, you may consider securing equipment that is not immediately necessary at the station, since bringing it could result in it getting stolen. However, never let theft concerns override the need for adequate patient care.

If a security team is at the special event, let them know where the extra equipment will be located, and ask for their assistance in helping you get this equipment if a performer is injured.

Communication

SEMS providers must know how they will be alerted to respond to an emergency. Designating communication methods should occur during the preplanning phase, as with any event. As usual, the communication matrix will also need to be planned to accommodate the many different groups and personnel that may need to be in communication during the event.

In many extreme and combat sporting events, hand signals or symbols will be used for communication, instead of communicating verbally. This is sometimes a necessity due to the noise level. Be sure you know how SEMS providers will be called to a scene.

Remember that due to extreme weather conditions, extreme sporting events may require equipment designed to be more rugged. Also, it may be a good idea for SEMS providers to wear radio headsets if possible; they not only protect hearing but also allow communications to be heard despite ambient noise.

Staffing

Staffing levels will vary depending on the size of the event and on whether the SEMS team will be providing care for the spectators, participants, or both. During preplanning, determine whether BLS will suffice or whether ALS providers are required. BLS may be sufficient for spectators, but sport participants may need ALS care.

Also, in some states, at certain extreme sporting events such as boxing and mixed martial arts events, a physician must be present per state law or sporting regulations. Find out beforehand whether nurses and physicians will be present, and predetermine how your role will be affected by them. Involve them in preplanning if possible.

Transport Considerations

As always, there must be a plan for who will transport the patient. Will SEMS providers also provide transport

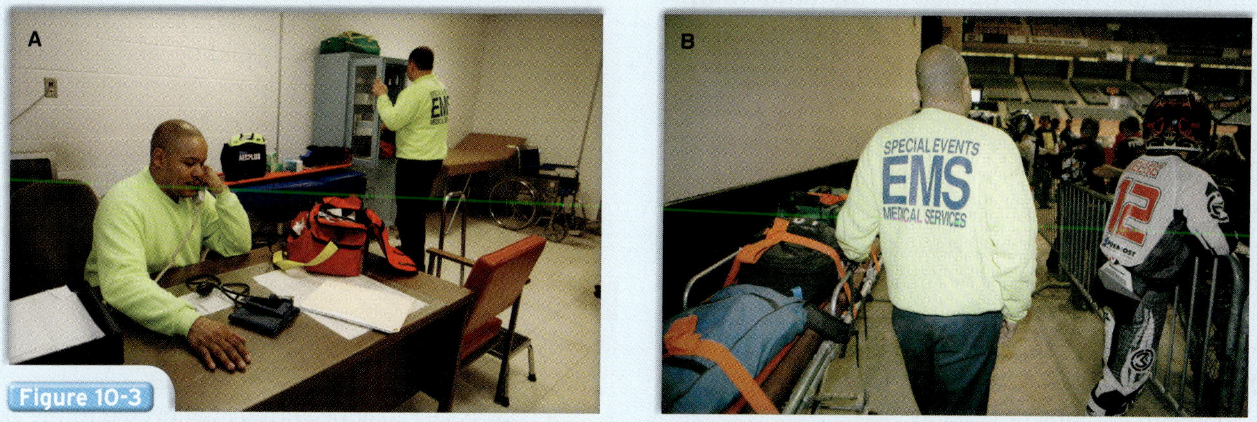

Figure 10-3

(**A**) Some equipment may be stored in a first aid room, if one is available on the premises. (**B**) Other equipment is best kept close at hand.

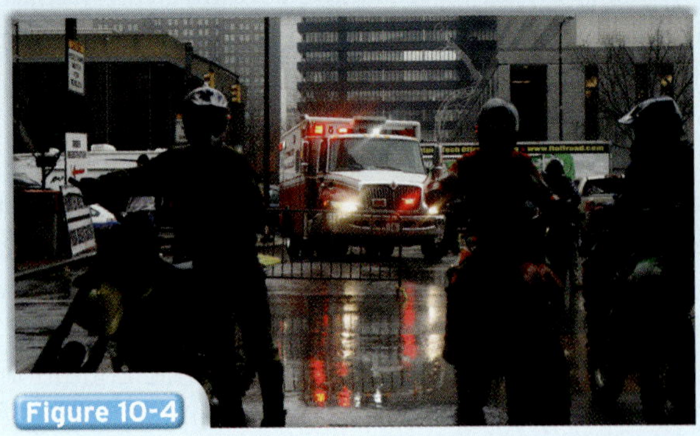

Figure 10-4

During preplanning, always determine whether the transport unit will be on site or requested once the emergency occurs.

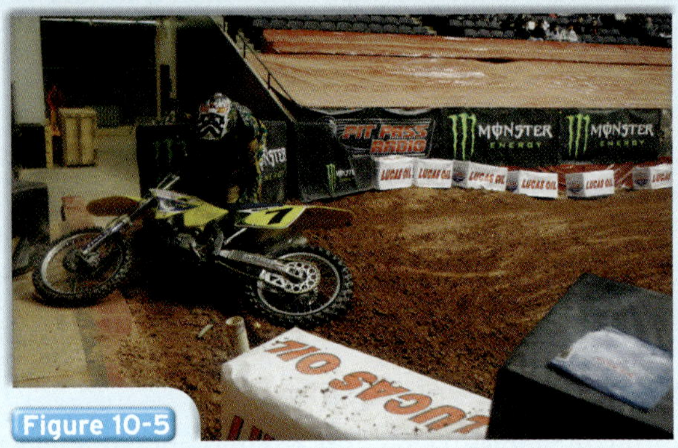

Figure 10-5

Examine the environment and ensure that potentially unsafe conditions are taken care of properly.

to the receiving facility? Or will SEMS providers package the patient and hand off to a transport unit? Will the transport unit be on site, or will it need to be requested once an emergency occurs Figure 10-4? Many of the considerations discussed in Chapter 8 may apply to extreme and combat sporting events, as they often occur in a stadium setting.

Always factor the crowd into transportation decisions. Many extreme or combat sporting events are held at arenas or in stadium parking lots. Most arenas are small enough to walk from one side to the other in less than 5 minutes. For larger arenas, it may be necessary to consider using EMS carts, such as gators, or motorized carts to move around outside the arena. This means leaving the inside to travel faster around the outside and avoid most of the crowds and commotion. As discussed in earlier chapters, egress routes and modes of transportation should be determined during the preplanning phase.

When athletes are backstage or in the performance area, they will not be injured in the crowd. Still, providers must get through the crowd to access them. Many performance areas are surrounded by fences or steep slopes. Only powered vehicles can be used at these locations, such as the ones discussed in Chapter 3. EMS gators with proper tires for the terrain or carts made specifically for EMS outdoor events will work best in these areas. For motocross events, there will be dirt and small hills; these can easily be maneuvered on foot with equipment in hand. For skateboarding, in-line skating, and BMX events, ramps and concrete courses may be where an athlete is injured. These too can be managed on foot with equipment in hand.

Consider how to best access a patient in a crowd. Consider using a battery-powered or small fuel-powered vehicle to respond to calls and transport patients, instead of maneuvering equipment and backboards by hand through a crowd, which can be difficult and unsafe.

Game Day

Continue preplanning on the day of the event by examining the environment carefully to prevent any unnecessary injuries from occurring. Ensure that any damaged equipment, loose objects, or unsafe (eg, slippery, sticky, or poorly lit) areas are taken care of properly Figure 10-5. Point out any problems you may find to the referees, officials, or the location manager.

Extreme Sports

The following sections discuss common extreme sports, their environment, gear and equipment, and frequently associated injuries or conditions. Another category of extreme sports is aerial extreme sports, such as sky diving, bungee jumping, hang gliding, and parasailing. SEMS providers may work at events involving these activities, but they would likely be stationed on the ground and would likely only respond to a catastrophic event should one occur on the ground. Therefore, these activities are not covered here.

Skiing

SEMS providers may be called upon to provide medical care at skiing events.

A skier's feet may be entirely connected to the skis as in downhill skiing or only partially connected as in cross-country skiing where the top portion of the boot touches the skis Figure 10-6. In downhill skiing, the

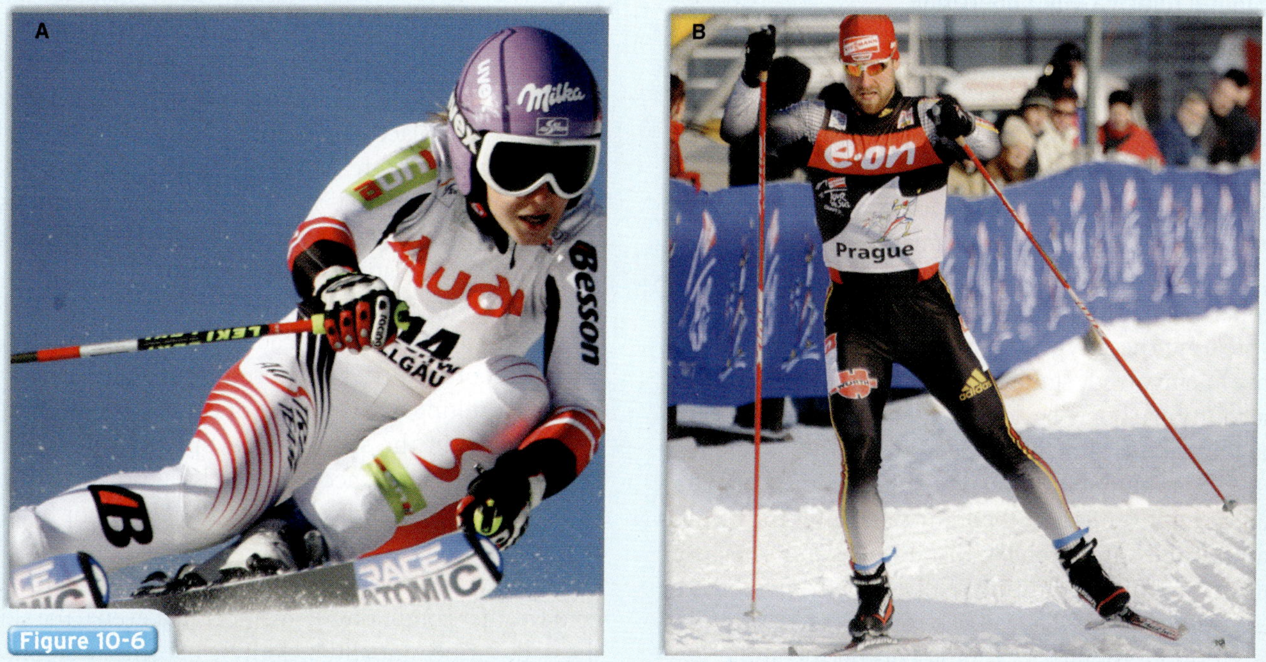

Figure 10-6

Skiing includes downhill (**A**) and cross-county (**B**) racing.

skier races down a snow-covered hill. In cross-country skiing, an athlete or team races to reach the finish line first across snowy flat ground or mild slopes.

Environment

As an outdoor, winter activity, skiing takes place in a cold, snowy area. Ski courses may be long paths through the countryside, requiring supervision for miles by event personnel on skis, sleds, four-wheelers, or snowmobiles. In this environment, helicopters may also be necessary to ensure that skiers are properly supervised along their entire journey, not just at the start and finish lines. Downhill skiing competitions may take place at ski resorts with slopes of varying lengths, width, and steepness or on special slopes that feature ramps and obstacles for tricks and jumps.

First aid stations should be positioned both at the summit and the end of the slope to access injured skiers. When there is a low number of participants in these events, one to three first aid stations may suffice, depending on the course length.

Obviously, it is easier to travel downward to access the patient than to climb up the slope against gravity and snow. However, at downhill events, ski patrollers will likely be present to provide initial medical care and transport patients from the course to SEMS providers. SEMS personnel must interact and work with the ski patrol. They are experts when dealing with injuries resulting from skiing and snowboarding. Also, it is a good idea to work out SEMS and ski patroller roles in advance.

At cross-country skiing events, SEMS providers will also need to preplan how to reach injured skiers; options include sleds, four-wheelers, and snowmobiles. The easiest path of travel should be decided before the special event. It is always important to have a way to transport the patient off the event course to an appropriate treatment center. Most venues use snowmobiles with specially adapted sleds or a specialized track vehicle to extricate and transport injured skiers.

Gear and Equipment

Skis vary in length and size but are generally long and narrow. Bindings secure the skier's boots firmly to the skis so they do not fall off. Boots vary greatly depending on the use and type of event (jumping, downhill skiing, or cross-country skiing); the padding and outer shell of the boots are softer or harder depending on the type of skiing to be performed. Additional ski equipment includes:

- Poles
- Wrist guards
- Gloves
- Jackets
- Pants
- Goggles
- Helmets or hats

Helmet use is highly recommended for both skiing and snowboarding.

Common Injuries and Conditions

The most common injuries and conditions associated with skiing are knee and thumb injuries, trauma, and hypothermia.

Skiers often experience knee injuries when their bodies twist, because motion of their lower legs is restricted in the ski boot. Knee injuries may range from tearing the anterior cruciate ligament (ACL) in the knee, fracturing the patella, or dislocating the entire knee. Proper extremity immobilization, as follows, is the key to treating these types of knee injuries. If a joint (eg, knee) is involved, stabilize the bone above and below the injury. If a bone (eg, lower leg) is injured, immobilize the joint above and below the injury.

Proper immobilization will reduce additional pain, decrease movement of the injury, and prevent further damage. Be sure to check distal pulse and sensation before and after splinting. Note that in most cases, it is advisable to leave the boot on, as it provides stabilization, though local protocols on this topic may vary. Of course, you should always gently remove the ski from the patient's boot so it does not get in the way and cause additional problems.

After stabilizing the site of injury, transport the patient quickly. Also remember to consider treating the patient's pain per local protocol, as these injuries can be very painful. If included in your skill level, pain management through medication administration would be appropriate, especially considering the terrain and distance that may need to be traversed to extricate the patient from the location of the incident to definitive care.

Thumb injuries are the second most common skeletal injury for skiers. A skier may grasp the poles the wrong way, or they may be pulled away from the hand, causing tears and sprains. Skiers with thumb injuries should stop skiing to receive proper treatment; further problems may result if they ignore the injury thinking it is not very severe; if severe enough, the skier may lose control or feeling in the thumb.

The thumb should be wrapped and stabilized, individually or against the rest of the hand, depending on the site. Ski gloves may not fit over the bandage used for stabilization. Due to the concern of a cold injury from the elements, SEMS personnel must protect the hand after bandaging. A trauma dressing or burn towel can be used in place of the glove if the glove will not fit over the bandaged area. In certain cases, the glove can be left on if the thumb is not as painful and warmth is a concern. The skier must make sure not to use that hand until further evaluation by a physician.

> **TIP**
>
> Though a wound would normally need to be exposed in order to be assessed, when treating skiers with knee injuries, you may need to partially remove clothing to assess the injury. However, after assessment it may be useful to keep the patient's pants on for padding, warmth, and stabilization; it is not necessary to completely remove clothing to wrap the knee with bandages, as doing so may cause more pain.

Skiers may be going so fast that they hit obstacles or fall onto their heads or backs, causing trauma such as spinal cord injuries or closed head trauma. Spinal injuries resulting from extreme or combat sports should be managed in the same way as spinal injuries from any other cause, and according to local protocols. This would include the indications and methods for helmet removal.

Finally, skiers may experience hypothermia due to cold weather conditions. Remember that even if the skier dressed warmly initially, if clothing becomes wet, SEMS providers will need to secure dry clothing. Be sure to have plenty of blankets available. Rescue blankets are relatively inexpensive and are an important item to stock for any event in the winter and also at other times when the weather may become cool, such as in the evening.

Snowboarding

In snowboarding, both feet are mounted on the board, and snowboarders (also called riders) stand with one foot ahead of the other and the body turned sideways. Snowboarding events may be races or obstacle-course competitions. They may be judged based on time (racing) and in some cases the number of tricks performed in the shortest amount of time (freestyling).

Environment

Snowboarding events may take place at ski resorts with varying terrains rated by difficulty of steepness, obstacles, and level of skill required to safely maneuver. Courses may include flags to be avoided or ramps or **half-pipes** (special U-shaped ramps) to perform tricks Figure 10-7. By using simple gravity, the natural sledding potential of snow, and speed, a snowboarder can perform such tricks as flips, jumps, and other aerial acrobatics.

As with downhill skiing events, SEMS providers will likely work with ski patrollers at snowboarding events. Determine access and egress routes, rendezvous points, and roles and responsibilities well in advance of the event.

Gear and Equipment

Snowboards vary in size, color, width, and length. Snowboards are longer than they are wide, extending only a few inches beyond the snowboarder's boots. Specialized snowboard boots are required to keep both feet on the board. Boots usually have a hard shell and soft padding on the inside Figure 10-8. Alternatively, they may have a softer outer shell, a harder shell in the middle, and then padding on the inside.

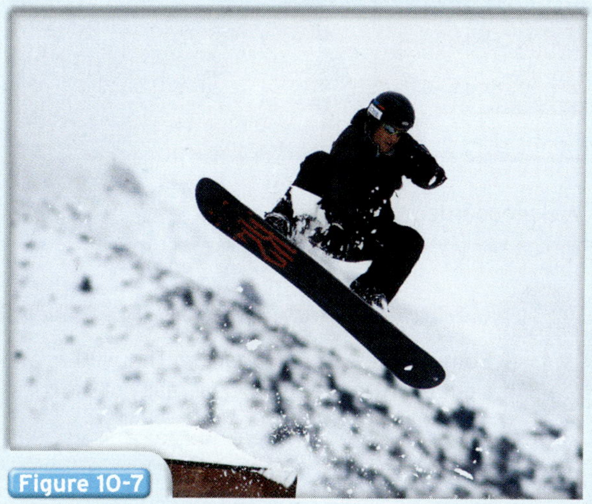

Figure 10-7

Snowboarders may perform flips, jumps, or tricks in a half-pipe.

Boots are strapped onto the board. This means that the athlete falls with the board and cannot lose it during tricks and jumps. Bindings keep the boots on the snowboard.

Snowboarders may wear goggles to protect their eyes from snow and sun. Helmets for this sport are specialized to include padding but also ventilation to prevent the head from becoming too cold or hot. Additional cold-weather gear includes specialized jackets and pants to insulate the body and keep the snow and cold air out. Hats and gloves are worn for the same purpose. Hands are used for balance and to hold the board during certain tricks, so it is important that they are protected so the fingertips will not freeze. Underneath the gloves, wrist guards may be worn to prevent tears, strains, or sprains.

Common Injuries and Conditions

Wrist, knee, and ankle injuries are the most common skeletal issues occurring on the slopes. Wrist damage may happen if a snowboarder falls on his or her side. Sprains or fractures are common if the snowboarder lands incorrectly. Proper immobilization and transport are critical when dealing with joint injuries. As with skiing injuries to the lower leg, if a snowboarder has an ankle injury, it may be better to use the boot as an

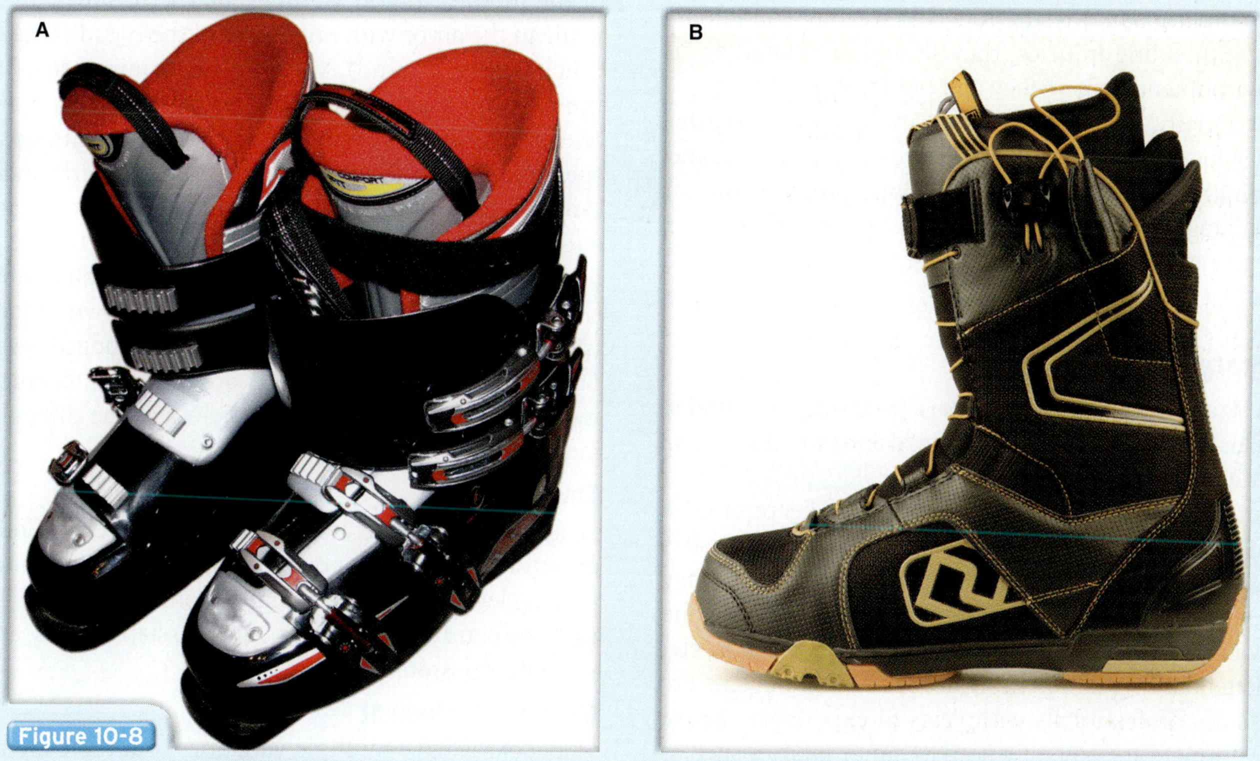

Figure 10-8

Ski boots (**A**) and snowboarding boots (**B**) may have several layers to protect the foot from injury and cold.

TIP In cold weather environments, only remove the clothing necessary to assess and treat life-threatening injuries. Additional injuries may be treated once the patient is inside a controlled-temperature environment. The exception to this rule is situations where the patient has wet clothes and must be transported a long distance; in such cases, it would be prudent to remove the wet clothes and warm the patient.

immobilization tool than to attempt to remove the boot. The boot will keep the leg stable and warm, which are both of high concern.

When snowboarders fall backward, they land on their buttocks and often hit their head against the ground or an obstacle such as a tree, fence, or rock. The head is also vulnerable during flips that are not finished, possibly causing the snowboarder to fall onto his or her head. In both cases, closed head injuries are common. The patient will need to be treated based on the injuries and symptoms presented. Snowboarders may experience head injuries or face trauma from falls onto metal ride rails or boxes used to perform tricks. Head injuries may also occur from hitting obstacles such as poles or trees.

Internal injuries may occur when snowboarders are not able to slow or stop properly and hit obstacles. Hypothermia may result from cold weather conditions. As with skiing injuries, they should be treated as an environmental emergency and per local protocol.

Finally, remember that an injured snowboarder or skier may be located anywhere on the course, and bringing a patient down a ski slope presents special challenges. SEMS providers must be properly trained in using the equipment they will need for moving the patient.

Skateboarding

In skateboarding competitions, athletes perform tricks, turns, and flips on a wooden board less than 2 feet long with a pair of wheels on each end Figure 10-9. When riding the skateboard, the skateboarder keeps at least one foot on the skateboard while the other foot pushes against the ground, though during competitions they may jump off the board, perform tricks with only one foot on the board, hold the board with their hands, etc. Skateboarding competitors at these special events are usually professionals with years of experience. These performers are generally used to minor injuries such as scrapes and bruises from falls. However, as their tricks increase in difficulty, so does the potential for serious

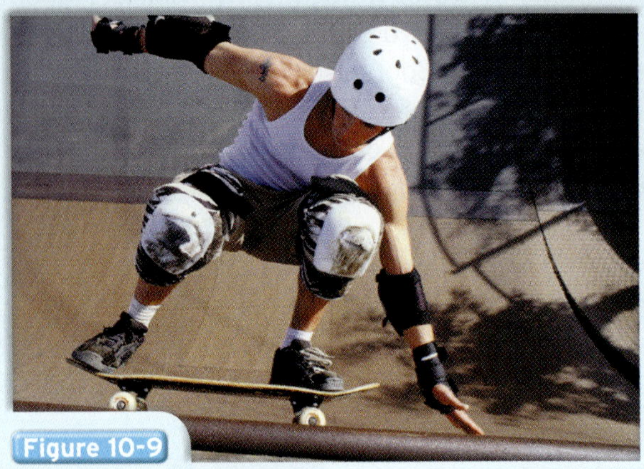

Figure 10-9

A skateboarder.

TIP Some athletes snowboard in the winter and skateboard in the summer, as many of the tricks and skills are the same.

injuries. An example is the incident that occurred on national television on August 2, 2007, when Jake Brown fell over 40 feet onto the ramp while performing at the ESPN X Games.

There are several styles of skateboarding. Some of the more common are freestyle (performing tricks while in the air or with only some of the board's wheels touching the ground), vertical (performing tricks in the air from a half-pipe), "big air" (performing tricks after racing off a very high ramp, and finishing at a specific end point/finish line), "flatground" (performing skateboard tricks on a flat surface rather than in the air), and street luge (lying down on a skateboard to race at top speed). These styles are sometimes combined in a skateboarding event. Each of these has its own unique tricks, stunts, and hazards. Some types are judged based on time or speed, while others are based on technical merit—that is, the number of tricks and the difficulty in performing them.

Environment

Skateboarding competitions are held indoors or outdoors either on a flat course or on ramps in arenas, skate parks, parking lots, or stadiums. Competitions may include flat obstacle courses with ramps, railings, steps, curbs, and miscellaneous objects.

Gear and Equipment

Skateboards have multiple variations, but there are no specific design changes that would cause injuries of different types.

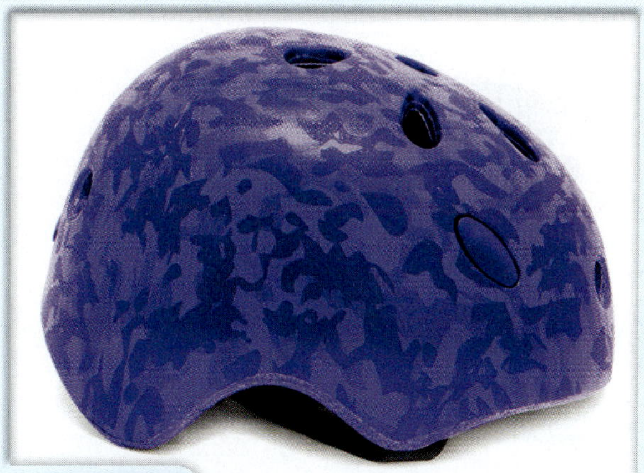

Figure 10-10

A skateboarding helmet.

Skateboarders wear a few pieces of equipment to lessen the severity of their falls. Helmets are required for major competitions. Skateboarding helmets sit on the forehead above the brow line and cover the top and most of the back of the head Figure 10-10. Supportive gloves and wrist braces are often worn to protect the wrists. Skateboarders may wear knee, elbow, wrist, and hand pads. Jackets and shorts with padding are available but are not commonly worn because they are perceived to inhibit mobility.

There are no specific safety-oriented shoes worn for skateboarding. Footwear is closed-toe and slip-resistant to improve surface contact on the ground and skateboard.

Common Injuries and Conditions

Skateboarding injuries stem from speed, complex ramps, and high jumps unique to each type of competition. While skateboarders do not go very fast, they can get quite high off the ground. According to the American College of Surgeons, any fall over 15 feet is a significant mechanism of injury. Likewise, any fall over three times the patient's height would require treatment as a priority trauma case. High-fall injuries may result in extremity trauma, spinal cord injury, closed head injury, and internal injuries.

In-line Skating

In-line skating (also called rollerblading) involves racing or doing tricks while wearing rollerblades (hard-shelled boots with four or five wheels on the bottom) Figure 10-11. As with skateboarding, this type of sport has different judging criteria depending on the event. In-line speed skating is judged on time, while artistic

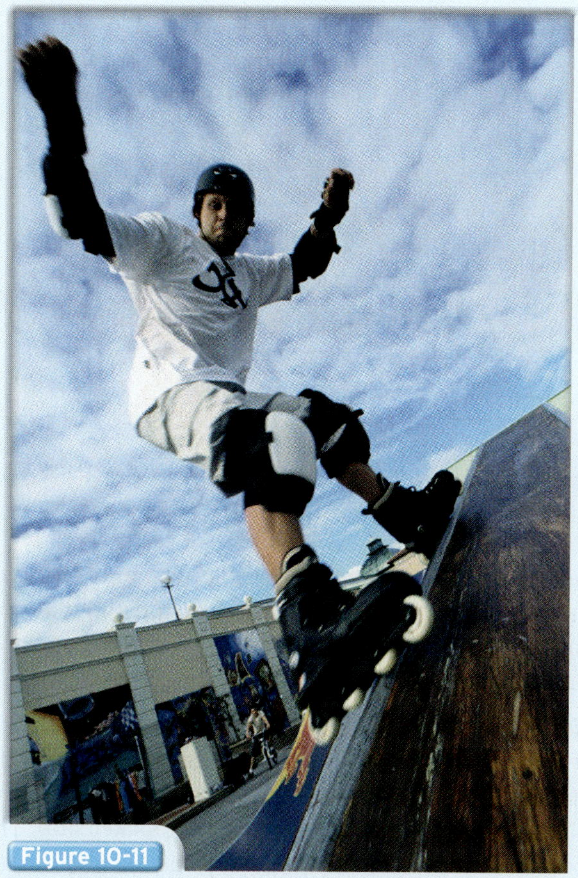

Figure 10-11

An in-line skater.

in-line skating is judged with a scoring system similar to that used in ice skating.

Environment

In-line skating races may be a few miles long or a full marathon. In-line speed skating takes place on tracks, or in-line skaters may compete on courses with ramps, steps, rails, and obstacles. Staircases are sometimes included for the skaters to jump over, or skaters may slide down the railings. Races may take place indoors but are more commonly held outdoors on closed-off streets and paths. Competitions are not usually held in the winter, as it is unsafe for in-line skaters to race through snow or ice. The paths or roads are usually in good condition and prepared for the event, but hazards

TIP

An extreme sporting event may include several subevents with different types of sports, such as in-line skating, BMX, and skateboarding. For these events, a course is prearranged so every athlete can be compared on the same terrain.

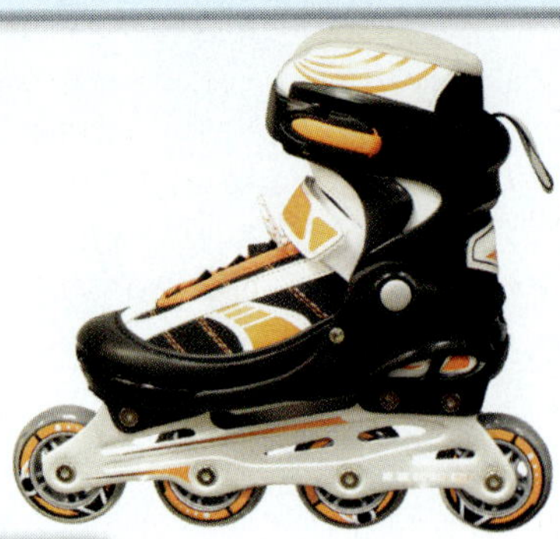

Figure 10-12

An in-line skating boot, or rollerblade.

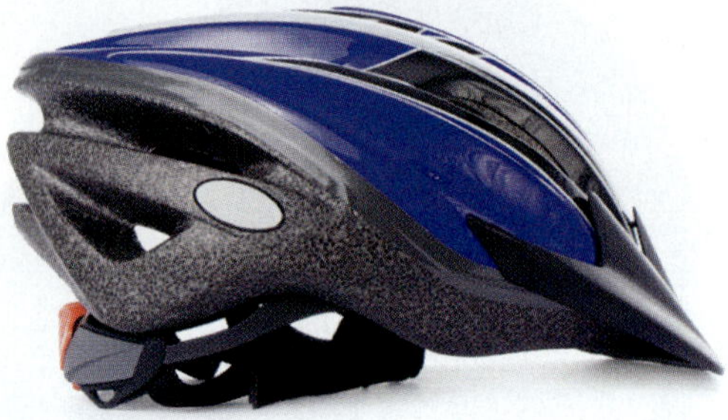

Figure 10-13

An in-line skating helmet.

such as fallen tree limbs, sewer grates, and potholes may present. Obstacle courses may include high ramps, stairs, and railings (called "rails"), which the skater jumps over or skates down.

Gear and Equipment

In-line skates vary in size and material but always have a straight line of wheels. They may include a small piece of plastic behind the last wheel to help the skater stop. The "boot" of the skate usually has clips across the tongue to tighten around the ankle; clips extend a few inches above the ankle Figure 10-12.

Skaters may wear knee pads, wrist guards, and elbow pads with a hard outer casing and a soft inside padding that fits against the skater's skin. These pads can reduce strains, sprains, and fractures but are not required gear. Helmets are often worn and include padding on the inside and rear. Some helmets are raised in the back of the head and include slits every few inches to allow air to reach the head, decreasing heat and sweating Figure 10-13. Other helmets have a high-impact plastic shell interlined with padding; this type is also used in BMX and skateboarding competitions. This type is not raised on the back of the head and is shaped more like the head's natural shape, with less plastic and padding.

Common Injuries and Conditions

The most common injuries for in-line skating occur from falls, including sprains and strains to the wrists and elbows, fractures, and head injuries. Falls to the rear may involve a bruised or chipped coccyx (tailbone). Extreme falls may cause internal hemorrhaging, extremity fractures, as well as spinal cord, back, head, groin, and shoulder injuries. If helmets are not worn (or not worn properly), the skater may experience head, facial, or neck trauma. When treating a patient with any of these injuries, follow local protocol governing immobilization for helmet removal and spinal immobilization. In addition to these considerations, SEMS providers should consider dehydration and heat exhaustion in outdoor races.

> **TIP**
>
> Keep in mind that participants in extreme sports events may have a cavalier attitude toward injury. While this should not affect the care given by SEMS providers, it is important for SEMS providers to expect this attitude and be prepared with strategies to deal with it. During preplanning, work with event organizers to specify who will decide if an injured participant can continue.

Bicycle Motocross

Bicycle motocross (BMX) is a sport in which athletes perform tricks on bicycles. BMX riders often compete at local skate parks, national extreme sports tours, and special events. Depending on the type of event, participants may be judged on time or style.

Environment

BMX tracks are usually on wooden ramps (often facing each other in a valley shape, called a **vert**), which may be as much as 27 feet off the ground Figure 10-14. Tricks can also be performed on trails, flat surfaces, streets, and parks. BMX events can be inside at arenas or stadiums or outside at parking lots. Ramps at these events vary in size and shape and are usually constructed for specific events.

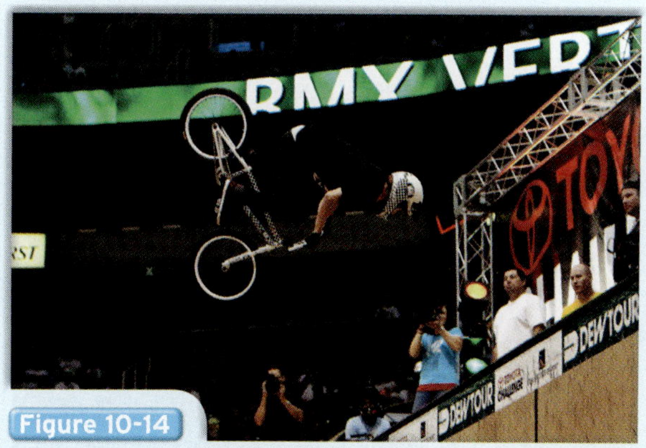

Figure 10-14

A vert, used in BMX courses.

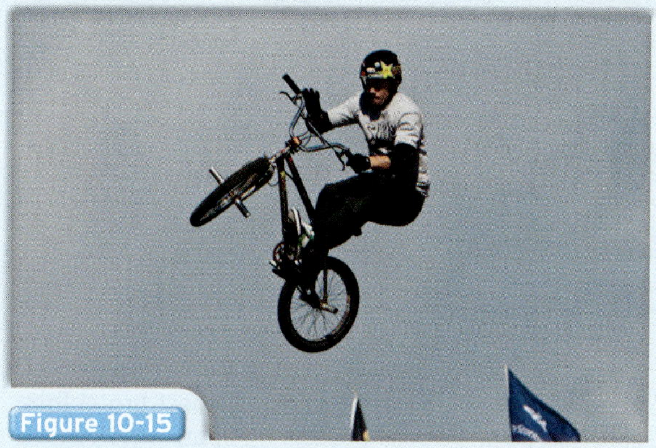

Figure 10-15

A BMX rider has a bike specially designed for the sport.

Gear and Equipment

Bikes are specially made for BMX from lightweight aluminum, alloys, and titanium. Handlebars rotate 360 degrees (for turns and flips), and a small bar (less than 8 inches) extends on each side from the back wheel (for the athlete's feet to be placed on during flips). Wheels range from 18 to 24 inches, depending on the size of the rider Figure 10-15.

Protective equipment varies. Most often, riders wear a helmet that covers the top, back, and sides of the head but not the neck, face, and jaw. Once a helmet has been dropped or a rider has fallen on it, it no longer can be used. Some riders (though very few) wear elbow and knee pads to prevent strains, breaks, and sprains as well as the tearing of clothes (which may cause road rash—a severe abrasion to the skin resulting from friction caused when sliding on the pavement).

TIP Because of frequent falls and recurrent injuries, extreme athletes may have a higher threshold for pain and may be unaware of the severity of their injuries.

Common Injuries and Conditions

The most common injuries for BMX riders occur after they lose control of the bike. Wrist sprains, strains, and breaks are common from falls. Handlebars may impact the abdomen, causing internal injuries such as a ruptured spleen and liver. If internal injuries are suspected, transport riders to a hospital as quickly as possible, as shock may quickly result from internal bleeding and multisystem organ failure may develop. Flips and falls may lead to bumps and bruises, open compound fractures, or brain and spinal injuries. As always, each rider should be evaluated after an incident occurs.

Motocross

Motocross is a sport that uses bikes with engines Figure 10-16. Events may be judged based on time or style; freestyle competitors do tricks instead of racing. Motocross riders may perform with professional tours. Some tours may feature motocross, skateboarding, and BMX competitions.

Environment

Motocross riders perform on dirt or mud tracks that often include hills of different sizes and heights

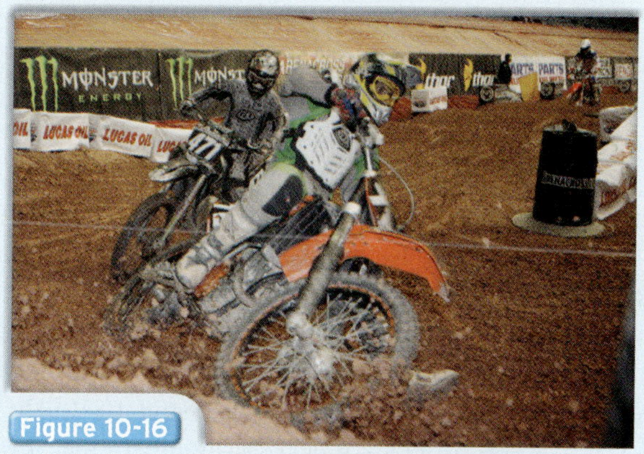

Figure 10-16

Motocross events involve bikes with engines.

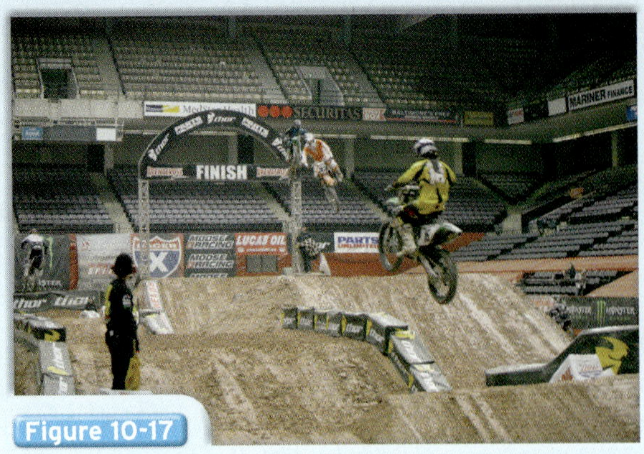

Figure 10-17

Motocross riders compete on dirt or mud tracks.

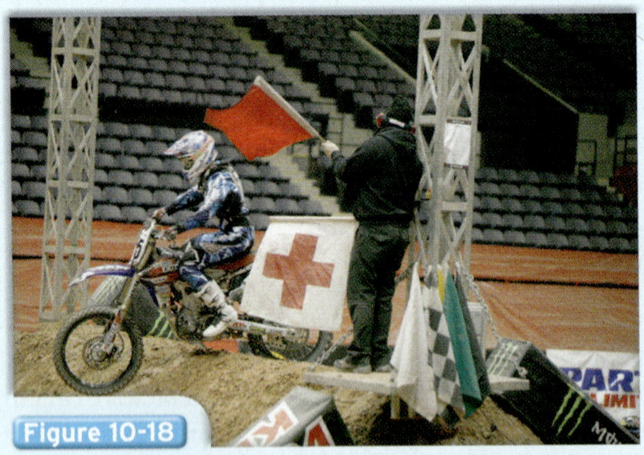

Figure 10-18

A red cross flag at a motocross event communicates that a rider is down in a blind spot and warns other riders not to go there. It does not necessarily mean that SEMS providers should respond.

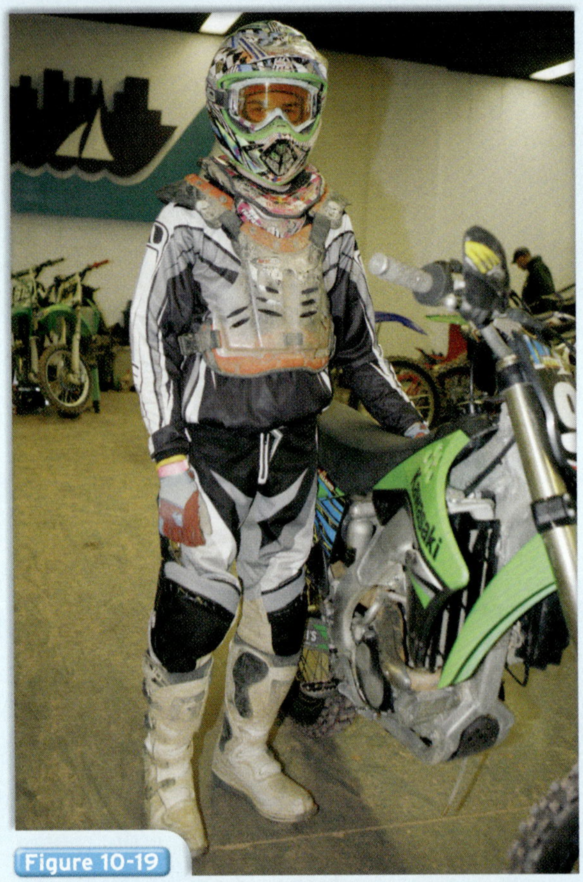

Figure 10-19

Motocross safety gear includes a motocross helmet, goggles, neck collars, neck braces, chest protectors, shin and wrist guards, gloves, and boots.

Figure 10-17. Only bikes of a similar size and riders of similar experience ride together. Professional motocross competitions may occur outdoors or in large indoor arenas where dirt is placed and packed for the races. Large foam blocks line the course to protect riders from leaving the track and hitting hard objects such as seats or gates. These may also protect the spectators from being hit by the riders.

A special flag system is used to communicate at motocross events. The SEMS provider should become familiar with the meanings of the various flags. For example, a red cross means that a rider is down in a blind spot and warns other riders not to go there Figure 10-18. It does not necessarily mean that SEMS providers should respond. SEMS providers should have a specific communication plan in place so that they know how and when their services will be requested.

Gear and Equipment

Motocross bikes are made out of lightweight, inexpensive metals such as aluminum. They are multispeed fuel-powered vehicles that include a clutch, brake, and accelerator.

Riders wear a wide variety of safety gear Figure 10-19 and Figure 10-20. Motocross helmets cover the entire head, including the back, most of the face, and the entire jaw. The outside of the helmet is usually made of a hard material such as polycarbonate;

TIP

There are many different types of helmets. Different types may be secured and removed in different ways. Prior to the event, familiarize yourself with any equipment being used at the event.

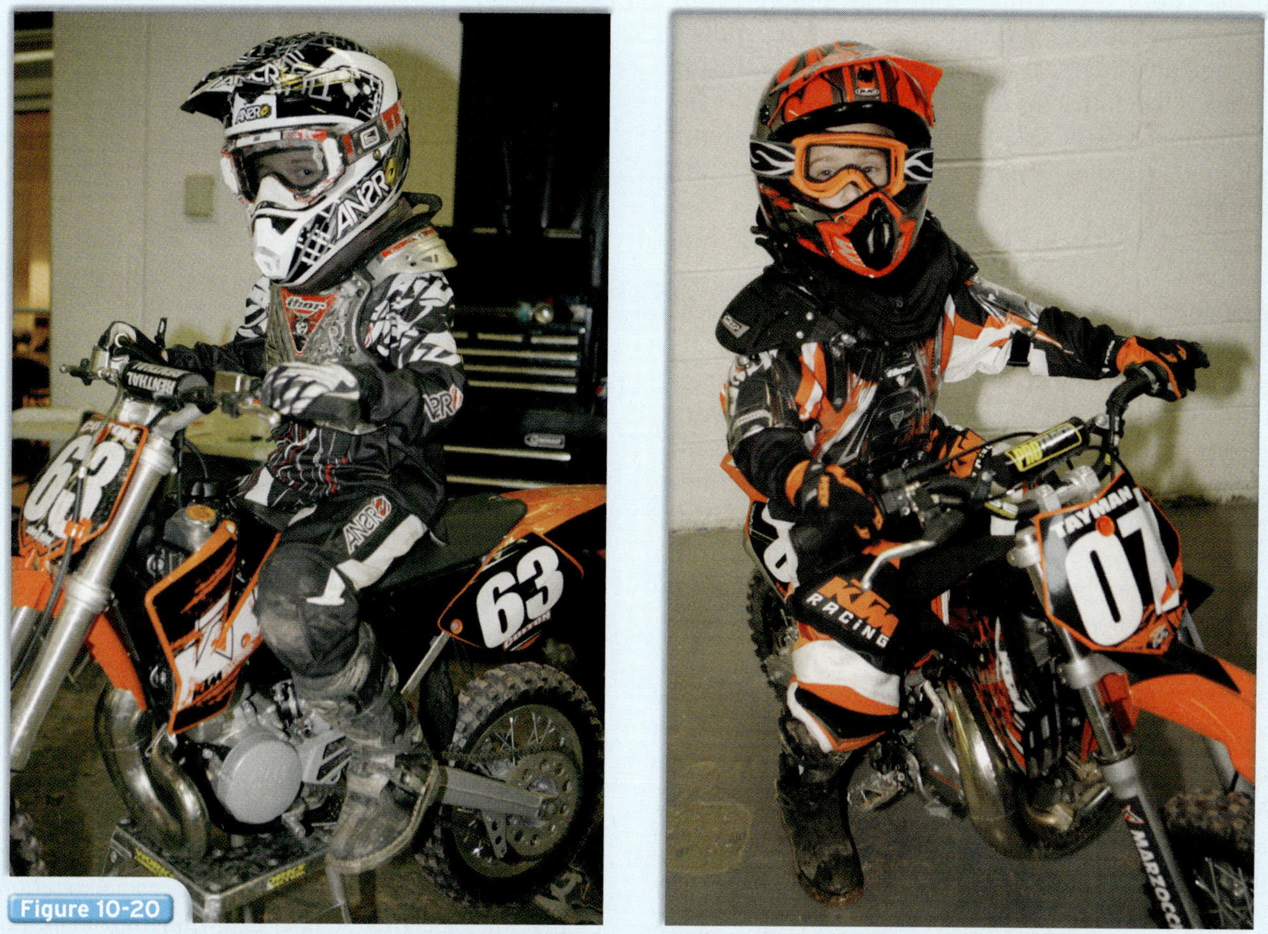

Figure 10-20

Children may also compete in motorcross and other extreme sporting events, and generally wear at least as much gear as adult competitors.

the inside is foamed and cushioned. Riders also wear goggles to protect their eyes from foreign bodies that may fly up during the competitions.

In some extreme sports including motocross, some participants wear a specialized device in their helmet called the Eject® Helmet Removal System Figure 10-21. This device is a small air bladder that is placed inside the top of the helmet. An air tube descends from the bladder down the right side of the helmet. Should it become necessary for an emergency provider to remove the helmet, he or she must first cut the helmet's chin strap and remove the patient's goggles and eyeglasses if he or she is wearing any. The provider attaches the inflator bulb to the Eject tube connector, inflating the bladder to gently lift the helmet off the patient's head.

Neck collars are worn, providing a soft cushion around the neckline. Neck braces are also worn and cover the neckline, extending over the top part of the back and chest to reduce sternal and spinal cord

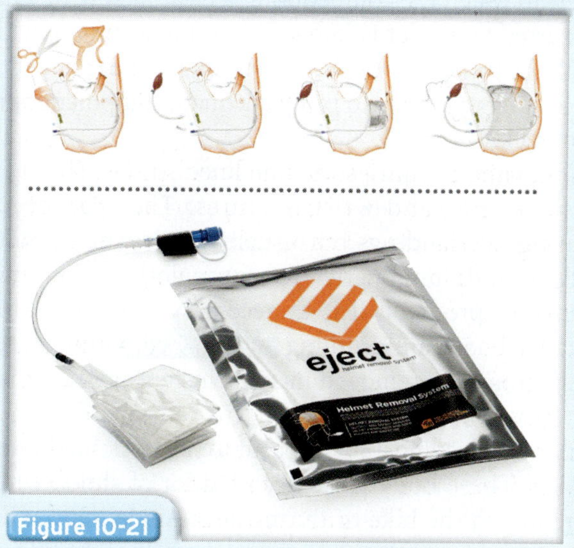

Figure 10-21

The Eject® Helmet Removal System.

injuries. Both neck collars and neck braces fill in the space created by the helmet between the rider's head and shoulders. If a rider were to fall on his or her head, the impact could push the helmet down, possibly injuring the shoulders and clavicles. With the neck protected, the helmet cannot be pushed into the shoulders.

Chest protectors are worn over jackets and clothes. They cover the deltoid muscles of the arms and the entire chest and stomach along with the entire back. This not only protects the body from impact but helps the rider sit properly on the bike with a good frame for stunts and jumps. Specialized pants and jackets are worn beneath protective devices.

Shin and wrist guards are worn to prevent fractures and sprains and ease impacts once riders safely finish jumps. Gloves are worn to prevent the hands from getting cold and help the rider to grip the handlebars. Boots for this sport are specialized to cover the entire foot, ankle, and lower shins. These boots are very hard on the outside yet comfortable enough to be worn for long periods of time.

Common Injuries and Conditions

Motocross competitions will have a **track crew** that monitors the competition and communicates with other personnel, including SEMS providers. During motocross competitions, SEMS providers should maintain contact with the track crew to find out the location of a fallen rider and when it is safe to enter the track.

Never race onto the course in an attempt to reach the rider. The track crew will point SEMS personnel in the best path of travel to reach the patient. By maintaining a crew to watch the competitions, a clear picture of what occurred to a rider is known. Communicating quickly with the track crew before responding to the emergency will allow providers to bring adequate equipment onto the track.

Common injuries include knee strains, shoulder dislocations, and wrist fractures. They can occur during safe landings but usually occur when a rider falls or lands improperly. Treat musculoskeletal injuries per local protocol. It is unnecessary to remove shin guards, boots, and clothing Figure 10-22, though the helmet may be removed in some instances depending on protocols.

Other leading injuries occur to the tibia, fibula, and ankle. These body parts absorb a lot of shock while landing on the bike or during falls. Ankle injuries are very common as the foot may hit the side of the bike or the ground. Unless there is a high risk of hypovolemia, it is suggested to leave the boots and shin guards just as they are when treating these injuries. The equipment stabilizes the injury, so removing the equipment can aggravate the injury and cause more pain.

When riders land on their head or back, paralysis and life-threatening injuries may occur. If an ALS crew is not on scene but is needed, it will be crucial to request them immediately. Remember to always preplan for how ALS care will be provided, should it be needed. The American College of Surgeons Committee on Trauma lists separation of a rider from a motorcycle or any crash at a speed of over 20 mph as a significant mechanism of injury, so suspect serious injuries at these events and preplan for them.

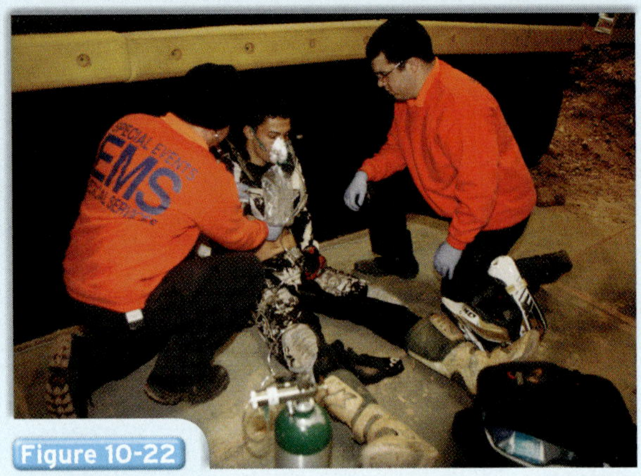

Figure 10-22

If spinal or head trauma is not suspected, remove the helmet and neck brace. It is unnecessary to remove other patient gear.

Rock Climbing

Rock climbing is a sport in which a person climbs rocks or a man-made rock climbing wall. The climber who reaches the top of the rock the fastest wins.

Environment

Rock climbing may be an outdoor or indoor event. The climbing surface may include ledges, tight crevices, and preset hand and foot holds. Climbers may have to determine the best route of travel, or the path may be set. Climbing times vary based on skill of the climber and height of the walls (which generally vary from 15 to 200 feet).

When held indoors, the rock climbing environment is controlled with safety systems in place and proper protective equipment. Outdoor rock climbing varies, based on the type of climb and weather conditions. Rain may cause slippery surfaces; cool weather may lead to

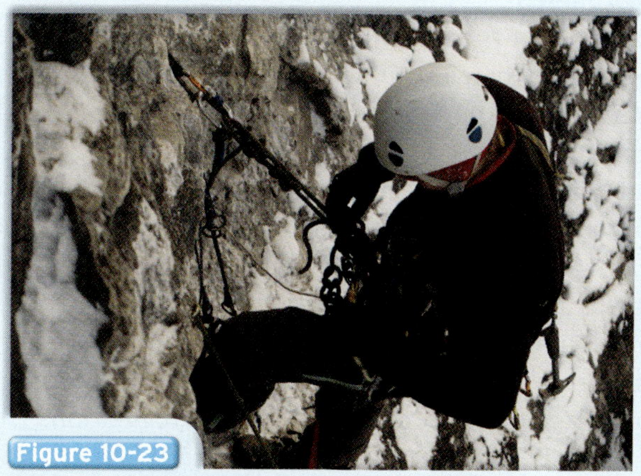

Figure 10-23

Anchors may be used to attach the rope to the rock climbing wall.

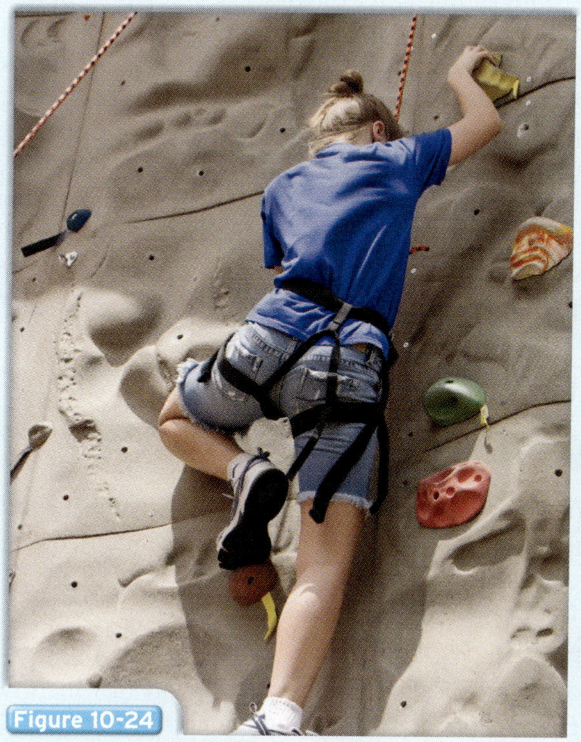

Figure 10-24

A rock climbing harness safety system.

hypothermia. Outdoor rock climbing competitions are commonly along hiking trails, which in many cases are a few miles away from any major roads.

Gear and Equipment

The type of equipment used varies depending on the type of rock climbing event. Some types of rock climbing use a harness and rope system (**belay system**) kept under control by an assistant (called a **belayer**) at the base or the top of the climb, while other rope systems are secured by anchors as the climber ascends Figure 10-23. Other types of climbing use installed handholds or no safety system at all. A belay system reduces the friction caused on climbing ropes if a climbing partner were to slip.

Harnesses are durable, lightweight, and flexible. Some harnesses wrap around the climber's legs and waist; others extend over the climber's torso and over the shoulders Figure 10-24. Harnesses loop around the waist, allowing the climber to secure himself or herself to safety ropes. Safety ropes are secured to the harness with carabineers (special clips) designed to quickly attach and hold ropes securely. Ropes may be held by a support person on the ground, a safety system along the climbing surface, or a belayer on the ground. When a support person is used, this person keeps the rope taut (so that the climber would not drop far if he or she falls off the wall).

All types of rock climbers generally wear helmets with a hard outer shell to protect themselves (and support persons) from falling debris and falls. Climbing gloves are universal to help the climber's hands firmly grip the climbing surface. Climbers who do not wear gloves may powder their hands with chalk to keep them dry; a chalk bag can be secured to the waist for this purpose. Special flexible shoes are worn to help climbers grip the rock and offer protection.

Common Injuries and Conditions

Extremity and trauma injuries are the most common rock climbing injuries. Injuries such as extremity sprains and fractures to the elbow, forearm, hand, and wrist are common, as are overuse injuries such as pulls, tears, and muscle strains. Muscles in the fingers may get pulled and strained when a climber uses only one or two fingers to hold onto the rock. Carpal tunnel syndrome is a very common occurrence in this sport—it results in wrist pain caused by a nerve in the wrist being compressed. The climber should rest for at least a few days and keep ice on the elevated injured arm. Trainers should be sought to teach preventive exercises and to prescribe special bandages to reduce carpal tunnel inflammations. Shoulder injuries sometimes occur when the muscles are torn. For this injury, the arm should be placed in a position of comfort and rested until the patient can be examined by a physician. Ankle injuries are rare, but sprains or fractures may occur. The ankle should be placed in a position of comfort and stabilized until the patient can get an x-ray.

Minor injuries may include scratches and bruises; severe falls may cause spinal cord and closed head injuries as well as concussions. Treating these athletes does not vary greatly from other sporting events, except for the challenge that transport may pose due to the rock climbing environment. Proper stabilization of musculoskeletal trauma is essential. Ensure that splints do not diminish circulation but also do not allow movement, which can cause further damage to the injury site.

Combat Sports

The following sections discuss common combat sports, their environment, gear and equipment, and frequently associated injuries or conditions.

Boxing

Boxing (also called pugilism) is a sport in which two fighters of similar weight punch each other with the goal of winning the fight by "knock out" (determined by a fighter's inability to rise from the floor within 10 seconds). A boxer may also win the match if an opponent is considered unable to continue due to injury. Boxing matches are divided into timed intervals (called **rounds**) that can last from 1 to 5 minutes.

Environment

Boxing occurs in a ring surrounded by a crowd of spectators. Therefore, it will be important to have a clear path for access and egress. During the event, you should have a designated location to allow yourself quick access to the ring. As always, when preplanning, also consider how you will access various sections of the crowd. As has been witnessed at several boxing events, crowd control issues can surface when a fighter is injured.

Note that when planning a first aid station for a boxing event, you may need to consult with the boxing commission, as there are sometimes regulations that determine where first aid stations should be situated. There may also be specific rules regarding where equipment can be stored; SEMS personnel may need to work with security personnel to access equipment.

Ambulance access/egress is also an important consideration at boxing events. Periodically, the SEMS provider will need to ensure that the ambulance unit's

> **TIP**
> Care must be taken to maintain a safe environment to avoid unnecessary injuries. For example, loose equipment or untied shoes may cause injuries. Spilled water or unsafe entrances and exits from the performance area can lead to falls.

You Are the SEMS Provider

CASE 2

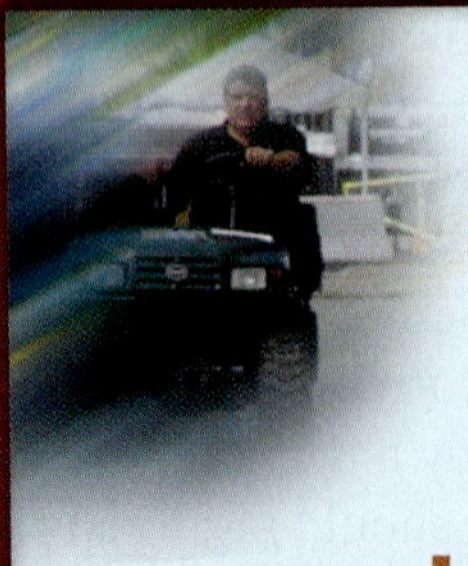

Two amateur boxers are in the ring, and one is getting tired. He is not blocking punches to his head. His posture deteriorates along with his hand-eye coordination. He receives powerful blows to his body and head. His feet stop pacing and his arms hang lower to his chest. His opponent lands an uppercut to his jaw, and he falls backward, straight onto his back, smacking his head on the mat and losing consciousness. The referee stops the match.

SEMS providers grab the necessary equipment and rush into the ring along with a doctor, trainer, and cut men. The doctor checks for responsiveness and finds that the boxer has the following vital signs:

- Glasgow coma scale score: 9
- Respiratory rate: 14 breaths/min
- Pulse: 120 beats/min
- Blood pressure: 140 by palpation
- Pupils are equal, round, and reactive to light

SEMS providers begin spinal immobilization and provide 100% high-flow oxygen via a nonrebreathing mask at a rate of 15 L/min. After 2 minutes, there is no change in the patient's vital signs, and he remains unconscious.

1. What should SEMS providers do to care for the patient?
2. What considerations should be given to transporting the patient?

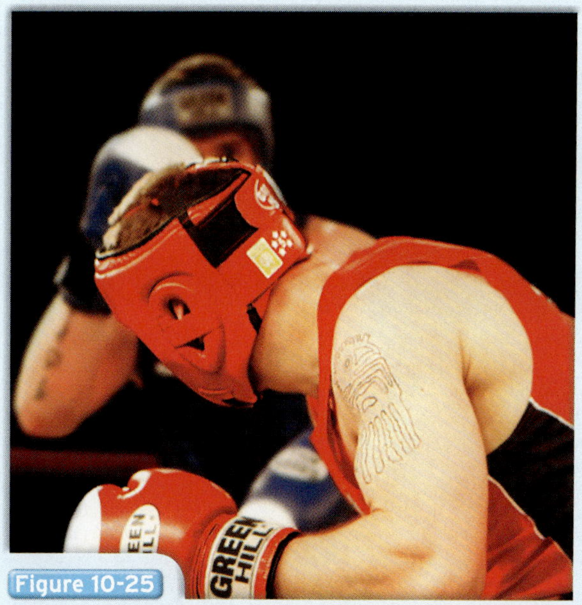

Figure 10-25

A boxer's headgear.

path of access and egress has not become blocked. Should it become blocked, SEMS providers will need to ensure that the path is cleared. This may involve requesting a public service announcement and working with security personnel.

Gear and Equipment

Amateur boxers are required to wear protective headgear, and professionals use protective headgear during training to reduce the number of injuries. The headgear is basically a pad covering the ears and encircling the head, held on by straps. It does not protect the boxer's chin. If necessary, boxing headgear can easily be cut away Figure 10-25.

Beginners who have not achieved amateur status wear kidney belts, headgear, mouth guards, shorts, and boxing shoes. Experienced boxers sometimes opt to not wear headgear or kidney belts. Most boxers wrap their hands with tape to prevent injuries by tightly securing the bones on the hand to each other.

Boxing gloves are padded to prevent injury to the boxer's hands but also allow the boxer to protect his or her head from trauma by blocking the opponent's punches. Gloves are laced around the wrists.

Common Injuries and Conditions

Common boxing injuries include the following:

- Fractures and dislocations
- Tearing injuries
- Lacerations
- Head injuries and concussions

Shoulder, wrist, hand, ankle, and head injuries are the most common boxing injuries. Dislocations may occur if a boxer becomes entangled in the rope surrounding the ring. Lacerations and contusions are common. More severe boxing injuries include closed head trauma and other forms of trauma to the body.

To treat strains, sprains, dislocations, and fractures, use proper splinting techniques to immobilize the injured extremity. Place an ice pack on the injury site and wrap it securely. In some jurisdictions, SEMS providers may provide analgesics to ease pain associated with these injuries.

One term specific to boxing is "cut men." This term refers to specialists trained to treat cuts and swelling that result in a boxing match. Usually SEMS providers will not be called in for minor injuries such as cuts and swelling. In fact, at boxing matches, cut men and other medical staff such as physicians generally take care of most injuries. While SEMS providers may be contracted to treat all emergencies in the crowd, SEMS providers may only be called upon to treat athletes when there is a significant injury or injuries. Again, this will depend on your contract with the event organizer.

Wrestling

Wrestling is a combat event in which two opponents battle one another using grappling, holds, and throws. There are many different styles of wrestling with slightly different rules and techniques, but the basic form of the sport and resulting injuries are all the same. Some forms of wrestling such as Japanese professional wrestling (or puroresu) involve strikes and incorporate elements of mixed martial arts styles (eg, karate, judo, and jujitsu), which increase the likelihood and severity of injuries. There are also "fake" wrestling events where contestants pretend to wrestle, and may perform extreme acts as a source of entertainment. These contestants can experience injuries as a result of their performance.

Environment

Usually wrestling matches take place on a well-padded mat that offers some shock absorption to cushion the wrestlers from throws. A unique form of wrestling called beach wrestling takes place on sand. At more professional events, an actual elevated platform is used, with the ring placed on top, allowing spectators to view from a distance.

Spectators at wrestling events can vary widely. Crowds at high school and college wrestling meets range from a few hundred people to thousands. Professional wrestling events can draw tens of thousands of very active and enthusiastic spectators. Alcohol can also

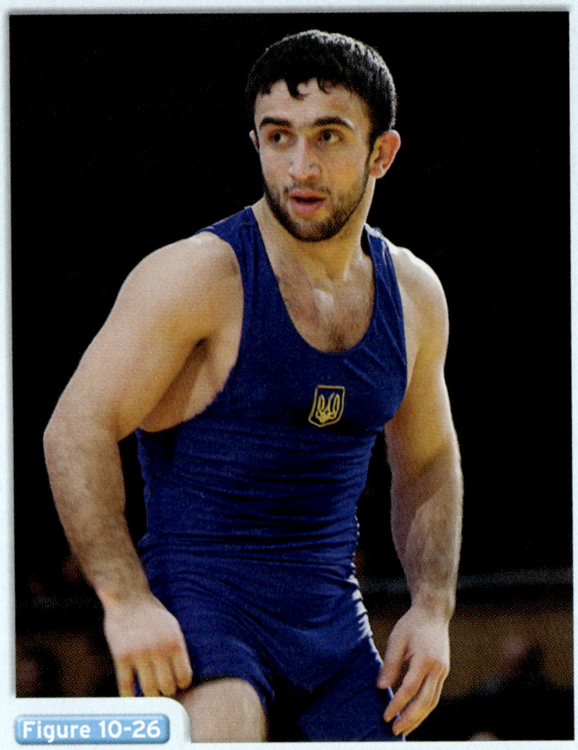

Figure 10-26

A wrestling outfit, or singlet.

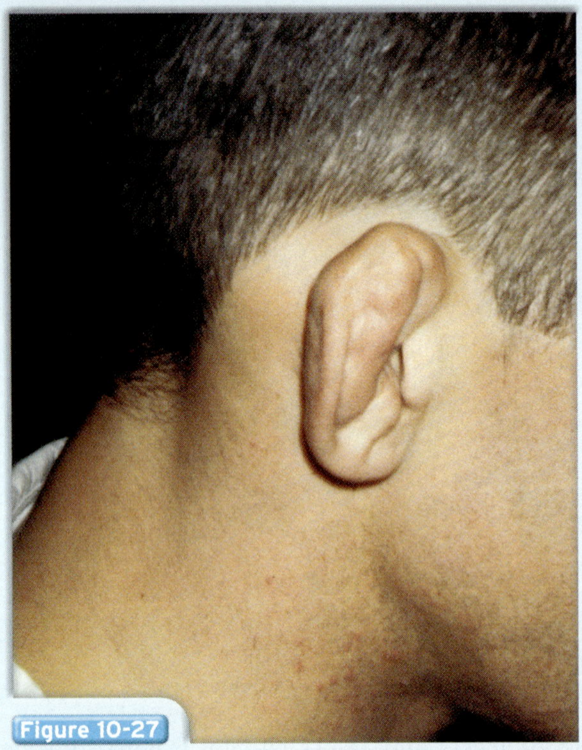

Figure 10-27

Cauliflower ear, the result of ear trauma.

play a factor at these larger events. Preplanning should determine staffing needs and whether you need first aid stations.

Gear and Equipment

Wrestlers generally wear a tight, elastic uniform called a **singlet** Figure 10-26. The uniform allows the referee to see each wrestler's body clearly to award points according to their moves; the uniform also prevents a wrestler from grabbing onto the opponent's clothing. However, in some forms of wrestling, athletes may wear swimsuits, spandex shorts, or athletic shorts. Wrestlers generally wear headgear and light, flexible sneakers that provide ankle support.

Common Injuries and Conditions

Wrestlers receive injuries similar to those experienced by boxers (dislocations, tearing injuries, lacerations, and head injuries), as well as the following:

- Spinal injuries
- Toe injuries
- Ear trauma

Shoulder, wrist, and knee injuries are the most common, as wrestlers are thrown onto extended shoulders, arms, or legs. Knee injuries include excessive swelling, ligament, and cartilage strains. As with boxing injuries, if qualified, consider providing analgesics to ease pain associated with these injuries.

Some wrestlers may experience a hematoma between the ear cartilage and the skin (known as cauliflower ear) marked by thickening of the entire ear. This may occur immediately upon injury, and the ear's appearance may remain this way if the injury is not properly treated Figure 10-27. To treat this condition, stop external bleeding (if any) and apply an ice pack to the ear.

Fencing

Fencing is a combat sport in which two opponents strike each other using sword-like weapons. Fencers do not aim to cause bodily harm, but rather demonstrate their technique, skill, and experience in the art. Fencing has many different forms including Kendo, Japanese sword fighting, and Filipino knife fighting.

Environment

Olympic-style fencing is normally performed on a mat of specific dimensions. The fencers are tethered in by a rope that only allows them to go to a certain specified distance. Other styles of fencing, such as Kendo, can take place anywhere. For example, it may be performed outdoors on a grass surface or indoors with boundaries marked on a floor with tape.

Gear and Equipment

Athletes are protected with several layers of material while they perform to reduce the risk of injuries Figure 10-28.

Fencers may use a variety of sword-like weapons (eg, foil, épée, and saber) to thrust and jab at their opponent. The points of the weapons have been blunted and capped to avoid injury. Fencing weapons may also have electronic components that allow judges to note where a fencer was struck and with how much force. To use this electronic equipment, fencers must wear special equipment on their clothing.

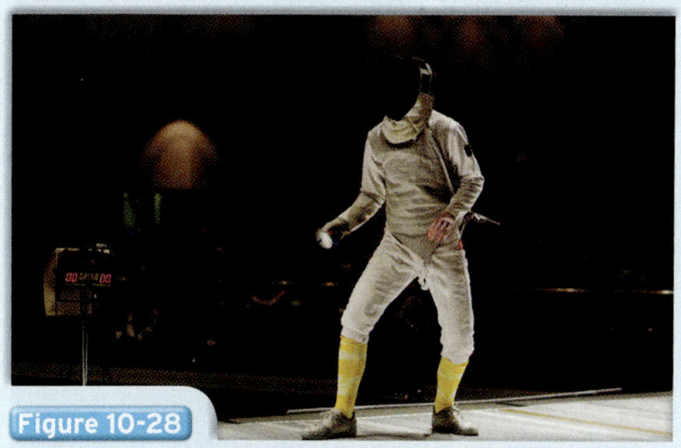

Figure 10-28

Fencing gear includes special clothing and a sword.

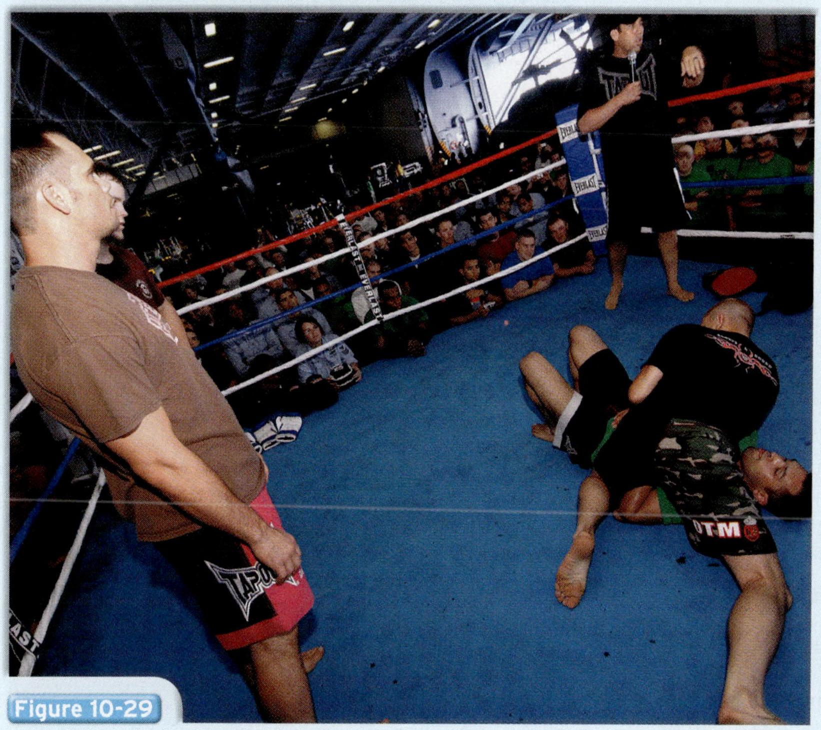

Figure 10-29

Martial arts are combat sports that involve striking and grappling but not weaponry.

TIP Some competitions include a mixture of martial arts. The types of moves used will dictate the types of injuries that SEMS providers should suspect.

Common Injuries and Conditions

Though the athletes wear plenty of padding, injuries still may occur from fencing. Common injuries include sprains, strains, and fractures, usually to the wrists or ankles. Bruising is very common. Head injuries also occur, including concussions.

Martial Arts

Martial arts are combat sports that involve striking and grappling but not weaponry Figure 10-29. Judo, jujitsu, karate, and muay thai are just some of the many variations of martial arts. Some forms of martial arts include kneeing, kicking, and punching. Others incorporate throwing opponents to the ground and holding them there.

As always, a basic knowledge of the language of the event will be helpful to the SEMS provider. In martial arts, **groundwork** refers to a martial arts fight that occurs on the ground. **Clinching** is holding an opponent while he or she is standing, preventing him or her from moving to the ground. A **takedown** is a move or combination of moves that forces the opponent to fall to the mat. **Defensive moves** slow an opponent's actions. Finally, a **submission hold** is a move or combination of moves that attacks an opponent's joint, muscle, or air and bloodflow to the brain, causing the opponent to surrender before any serious harm is done.

"Fake" wrestling, mentioned earlier, may allow certain vicious moves, but most martial arts prohibit the following:

- Head butting
- Eye gouging
- Hair pulling
- Biting
- Clawing or pinching skin
- Joint manipulation (twisting, extending, or compressing a joint)
- Spitting
- Attacking the groin, back of head, spine, kidneys, or trachea

Environment

Some competitions take place on a raised mat surrounded by a fence (resembling a cage) to prevent athletes from sliding off and becoming injured. During preplanning, SEMS providers should determine the best way to enter this cage, should they need to access an injured participant.

Gear and Equipment

Some martial artists wear open-fingered gloves to protect the hands. Some competitions require tight-fitting shirts or mid-thigh–length shorts. Socks and shoes are generally optional, and many martial artists prefer to participate barefooted.

Common Injuries and Conditions

Cuts to the head and scalp are common. The head and scalp are very vascular, so even superficial cuts to these areas will bleed significantly; however, this will not stop a fight. As always, SEMS providers should be careful to take appropriate body substance isolation precautions, including gloves, eye protection, and vigorous hand washing, as the martial artist may be covered with his or her own blood, and possibly the opponent's blood.

Sprains, strains, and tears, especially to the shoulder and elbow, may occur at martial arts competitions. Traumatic brain injury or closed head injury may result from sudden, violent hits to the head.

Remember to listen to your patient. It is important to acknowledge the injury that is the most painful or concerning to the athlete, even if it is different than what the SEMS provider believes is the most important concern. Conversely, be sure to properly assess for and treat all injuries. For example, an open head wound may look serious, but the athlete may be more concerned about a dislocated shoulder.

Other Sporting Events

Though they are not categorized as extreme sports, the next two sections cover cheerleading and paintball. Cheerleading is a leading cause of significant injuries and is therefore included. Paintball, while not an extremely common event, is becoming more popular and has specific injuries and hazards to be aware of.

> **TIP**
> At many sporting events, a physician will determine whether an athlete can continue participating. If SEMS providers will be providing medical care for athletes, establish during preplanning who will be making these decisions.

Cheerleading

As mentioned, cheerleading is a leading cause of catastrophic injuries. Cheerleading teams vary in size and skill level. Advanced cheerleaders may perform pyramids, aerial tosses, flips, and throws **Figure 10-30**. While cheerleaders may range widely in age, most

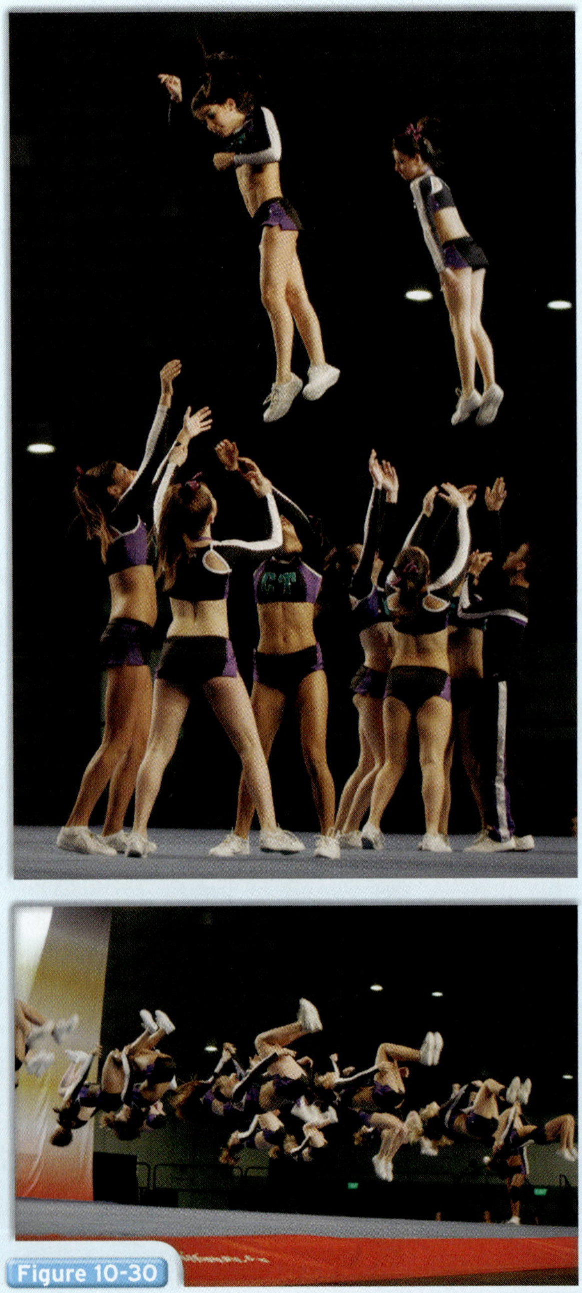

Figure 10-30 Cheerleaders can perform a wide variety of high-risk tricks.

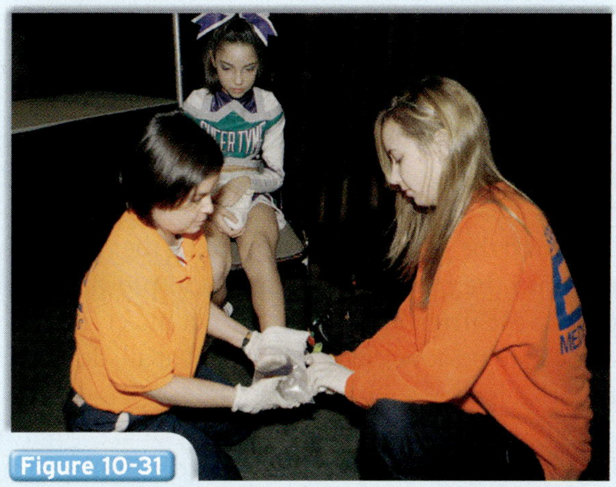

Figure 10-31

The most common cheerleading injuries are strains and sprains to the ankles and wrists.

cheerleaders are between 12 and 22 years old. A common misconception is that cheerleaders are only female; in fact more advanced cheerleading teams have many male cheerleaders.

Cheerleading often takes place on turf and usually on flat surfaces, so terrain is not a major consideration for these events. As with many other events, there are usually spectators surrounding the performance area. There may be a large number of participants if the competition involves multiple large teams. SEMS providers may also care for cheerleading injuries at sporting events if cheerleaders are part of the event.

Cheerleaders do not wear protective gear. Females tend to wear skirts; males often wear long pants or shorts.

The most common cheerleading injuries are strains and sprains to the ankles and wrists due to falls or missteps, or trauma injuries due to falls from a height Figure 10-31. Stabilize the injury in a position of comfort for the patient, and use rest, ice, compression, and elevation (RICE):

- Rest the injured area.
- Ice can be placed on the injury at 10- to 20-minute time intervals.
- Compression will alleviate swelling with tightly wrapped bandages used in stabilization.
- Elevate the injury above the heart.

Like other athletes, cheerleaders who sustain injuries should be referred to a certified athletic trainer and physician for a closer examination and prolonged treatment.

A cheerleader thrown into the air and not properly caught may fall onto his or her head and fracture cervical vertebrae. Take spinal cord precautions when treating falls from a height: maintain in-line stabilization, apply a properly fitted cervical collar, and use a backboard.

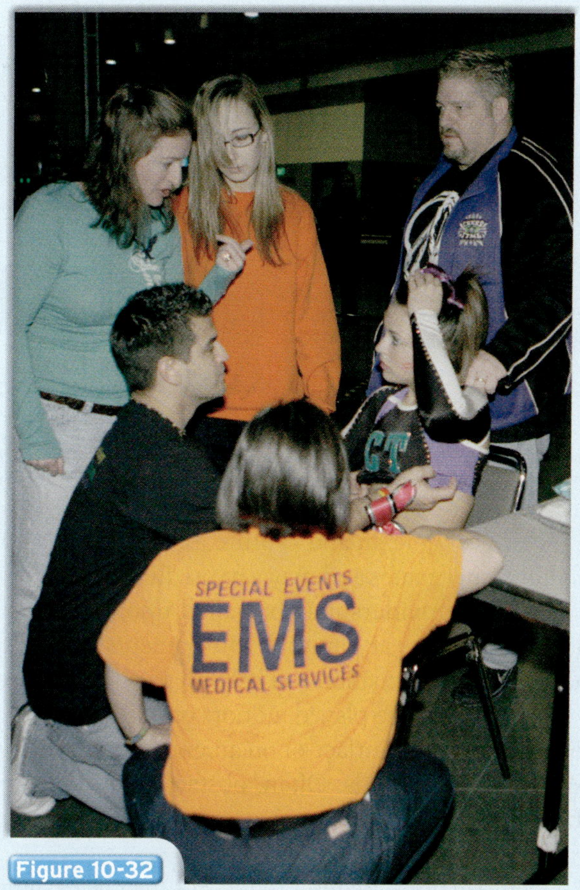

Figure 10-32

Remember to provide emotional support while providing care to patients.

When injured, adolescent cheerleaders may be very concerned about their appearance and their future in cheerleading. To ease their concerns, as always, tell them step by step what is going on and describe the course of treatment (eg, "We are moving you onto a hard board to keep your back safe while we take you to a doctor."). A coach, close friend, or parent may stay with the cheerleader to provide emotional support Figure 10-32. Other traumatic injuries may be noticed with falls at such heights but are secondary to the spinal cord injury unless they present as immediately life threatening. These injuries include extremity fractures with splinting, closed head injuries with spinal immobilization, and shoulder and hip injuries with stabilization.

Paintball

Paintball is a contest in which participants shoot each other with specialized guns that contain balls filled with paint Figure 10-33. Paintball is played by teams (of 1 to 1,000 players) who try to shoot all of the members

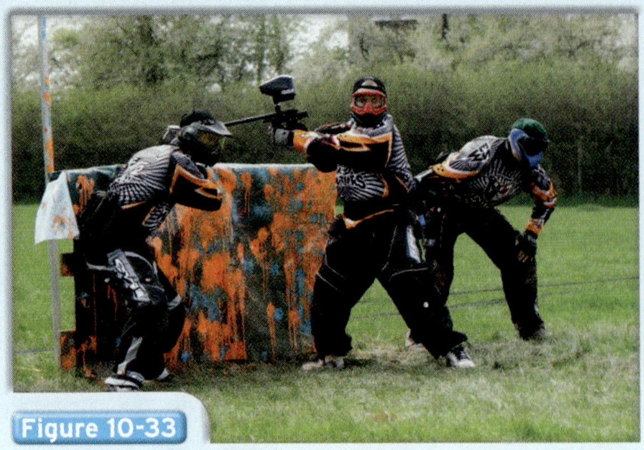

Figure 10-33

A paintball tournament.

of the opposing team and capture a flag. Tournaments include many games and may vary in duration. Though rare, SEMS providers may be called upon to provide medical coverage at paintball tournaments, and if so, the following information will help prepare the provider.

Paintball can be played indoors or outdoors. It may be played on a flat surface or on an uneven surface—for example in the woods. Often, obstacles and inflatable objects are added to the course for an additional challenge.

Paintball guns are required. Guns may be designed to fire long distances or to fire rapidly. Paintball guns cannot hold bullets; they are powered by refillable high-pressured air or carbon dioxide. The paintballs are held inside a hopper on top of the paintball gun. Paintballs are encapsulated balls containing nontoxic paint. Paintballs can cause injury, as they travel up to 300 feet per second and can be fired in rapid succession. Once a paintball has splattered, the paint resembles a piece of a balloon.

Face masks and goggles are strongly recommended for this sport to prevent damage to the eyes from paintballs. Clothing may include an outfit worn over the participant's regular clothes and is loose to allow greater mobility. Boots or sneakers may be worn depending on the course design and the player's preference.

Eye injuries, caused by paintballs hitting the eyes, are the major concern in this sport. Eye injuries may be as minor as a scratch to the cornea or as severe as losing an eye. Other injuries that may result from paintball include sprains, strains, bruises, welts, or bleeding from the site hit by the paintball, resulting from a paintball shot at close range. These injuries may lead to further and prolonged damage. Finally, paintballers may be trampled.

To manage eye injuries, it is critical for the player to cease playing so SEMS providers may assess the eye(s) for damage and treat appropriately. Injuries may include hemorrhage into the eye, fractures of the orbit, or even ocular injuries that require surgery. If any part of the paintball still remains in the eye, it is best to carefully rinse the area with sterile water by leaning the injured side toward the ground, thus preventing the runoff from going into the other eye. Follow local protocols with regard to eye irrigation; if an eye is not intact, irrigation may need to be done cautiously or not at all, depending on protocols.

If within your scope of practice, consider administering ALS anti-anxiety medications to any patient with an eye injury. Most patients with significant eye injury have other types of trauma as well and are usually anxious about losing the eye. However, use caution as some of these medications may increase intraocular pressure or may cause respiratory depression. Finally, remember to consider the need for spinal immobilization.

While treating the affected areas, document the eye's functioning. For example, the player may be able to see straight ahead but may not have peripheral vision, or the player's entire field of vision may be blurred. Cover both eyes to avoid involuntary movement of the affected eye when the uninjured eye moves. Explain to the patient what is going on, the treatment, and the course of action to help calm and reassure the patient. Never leave a patient alone with both eyes covered; patients are often scared, and even a momentary separation from the SEMS provider can cause severe anxiety. Remember the importance of communication when guiding a blindfolded patient; be sure to inform him or her of upcoming uneven surfaces, for example. Lead the patient by hand when walking, or transport the patient with a wheelchair or stretcher.

General Conditions Associated With Extreme and Combat Sports

Several common conditions such as heat injury, cold injuries, dehydration, hyponatremia, and closed head injuries occur at extreme and combat sporting events. SEMS providers should be aware of the signs, symptoms, and appropriate treatment for these conditions. As always, be sure to check local protocols and follow them when treating patients, as protocols may differ from region to region.

Heat Injury

Heat-related illness may progress quickly if it is not treated properly. **Heat cramps** can easily be treated with oral hydration and rest. **Heat exhaustion** will cause signs and symptoms of nausea, vomiting, and profuse sweating. IV fluids are the preferred method of rehydrating patients with heat exhaustion, since they may vomit if given anything by mouth.

Signs and symptoms of **heat stroke** include:

- Altered mental status
- Hot, dry skin
- Seizures
- Coma
- Tachycardia
- Low blood pressure
- Unusually fast or slow respiratory rate

To treat patients with heat exhaustion or heat stroke, rapidly remove all clothing, apply ice packs to the groin and armpits, aggressively hydrate with IV fluids, and rapidly transport to the nearest hospital. It is easy to miss these emergencies—for example, at sporting events such as baseball or soccer games—so stay alert for the signs of these emergencies and anticipate them during preplanning.

Cold Injuries

Cold injuries may occur during skiing events, snowboarding events, or any other event that occurs during cold weather. The human body can rapidly lose heat, causing hypothermia. Providers should consider the following questions:

- How long has the patient been exposed?
- What is the ambient outdoor temperature?
- What is the windchill?
- Has the patient become damp or wet?
- Was the patient using alcohol or drugs?

To treat hypothermia, remove the patient from the cold and remove any wet clothing. Treat cold emergencies according to initial training and local protocols.

Dehydration

Proper hydration of the body for a sporting event should begin 24 hours prior to the start of the event. When an athlete loses just 2% of his or her body weight in fluid, dehydration can occur. In general, athletes should be encouraged to replace the fluid at the same rate the body sweats—an average of 68 ounces an hour in hot weather or 34 ounces in cooler weather. While athletes may know this rule, bystanders may not be as careful to hydrate themselves or select adequate beverages for hydration.

Combat athletes are especially prone to dehydration because they are often matched for competition according to their weight and dehydrate themselves to **make weight** (also called cutting weight) to get into a specific weight category or class. An athlete may wear a rubber suit while exercising or may sit in a sauna for an extended period to sweat excessively and reduce the amount of water contributing to his or her body mass. Dehydration may lead to lethargy, hyperventilation, or cardiac dysrhythmia. Seek to rehydrate the athlete using room-temperature fluids. For severe dehydration, provide supportive care and consider IV fluids in accordance with your local protocol.

Closed Head Injuries

Extreme and combat athletes may experience closed head injuries such as a concussion, epidural hematoma, subdural hematoma, and chronic traumatic brain injury. A **concussion** is a mild traumatic brain injury; **epidural hematomas** and **subdural hematomas** are moderate to severe brain injuries caused by increased swelling in the brain.

A concussion is an injury to the brain caused by the brain striking the skull after a blow to the head. The brain floats inside the skull in a protective pool of spinal fluid and can be thrown violently against the skull's interior walls. All concussions are considered serious injuries, regardless of severity. Concussions are categorized into three grades, as follows:

- Grade 1 is a mild concussion. The patient does not lose consciousness.
- Grade 2 can be considered moderate. The patient does not lose consciousness but is confused and does not remember what happened.
- Grade 3 is a severe concussion. The patient loses consciousness for a brief time and does not remember the incident.

> **TIP** Despite popular belief, it is not necessary for a person to lose consciousness for an injury to be considered a concussion.

TIP A growing number of studies suggest that any new concussion can aggravate an older concussion and cause complications.

The signs and symptoms of a concussion may include some or all of the following:

- Dizziness
- Loss of consciousness
- Weakness on one side of the body
- Uneven dilation of pupils
- Nausea and vomiting
- Convulsions
- Retrograde or anterograde amnesia
- Confusion

Most healthy people recover from a mild concussion within hours, but it is not uncommon for patients to demonstrate residual effects related to vision, orientation, and memory for weeks.

Severe concussions present with an extended period of unconsciousness, headaches, mood swings, and depression. This level of concussion can usually be diagnosed through the use of MRI or CT scans soon after the incident. Not all bleeding or bruising of the brain is considered dangerous or life threatening, but a concussion can aggravate existing conditions not previously diagnosed. With **post-concussion syndrome**, a patient may experience lasting weakness on one side of the body, extreme mood swings, or problems with basic cognitive functions (eg, memory or orientation). Therefore, patients should be observed for 24 to 48 hours following a concussion. Repeated concussions can also have lasting long-term health consequences including mood swings, depression, and early onset of symptoms resembling Alzheimer's and Parkinson's diseases.

It is important for a concussion to be correctly diagnosed and treated accordingly. Always convey the patient's condition to the medical authority as well as any concussions suffered in the previous 2 years and especially those in recent months. As a general rule, until an athlete is symptom-free for 7 days, he or she should not participate in any sport or training.

Signs and symptoms of epidural and subdural hematomas are more life threatening (and often easier to recognize) as they progress. Headaches are the first sign of increased intracranial pressure. When an athlete experiences a headache after a hit or fall, take his or her vital signs and have the patient assessed by a physician as soon as possible, regardless of the patient's presenting mental status. **Unilateral pupils** (in which the pupil on the side of the injury is dilated and does not respond to light, while the pupil on the other side does not have this appearance) are often an indication of increased intracranial pressure. **Cushing's triad** (increased systolic blood pressure [with widening pulse pressure], bradycardia, and a change in respiratory pattern) is another common sign. The slowed respirations are classified as **Cheyne-Stokes respirations**; the patient will repeatedly stop breathing, then take quick deep breaths. Unconsciousness is a late symptom indicating an epidural or subdural hematoma.

Chronic traumatic brain injury may also result from sporting events. It is a traumatic brain injury that occurs as a result of a series of injuries to the brain that either (1) are not allowed to heal before the next injury occurs or (2) produce lasting effects to the brain (eg, repeated blows in boxing). This injury occurs in approximately 20% of boxers. The first stage of traumatic brain injury is the actual trauma to the brain at the moment of the hit, and is called primary brain injury. The second stage is the events occurring after the blow. Signs and symptoms may differ as time from the injury progresses; the second stage (secondary brain injury) refers to physiologic impairments that result from the primary injury. These include processes such as cerebral edema, increased ICP, cerebral ischemia and hypoxia, and infection. Secondary brain injury can occur anywhere from a few minutes to several days following the initial injury. Finally, residual symptoms of traumatic brain injury can include abnormal muscle tone, chronic pain, depression, anxiety, behavioral problems, seizures, or headaches.

TIP Sport equipment technology can change as frequently as every year, and when it changes, methods for equipment removal may change too. Before working at any sporting event, find out from the event promoter or coaching staff what equipment the athletes will be wearing, and learn how to take it on and off. For example, it is important to know how to remove specific types of helmets before working at the event.

You Are the SEMS Provider SUMMARY

CASE 1

1. **How do you manage the scene, keeping the crowd calm and controlled while ensuring that the patient receives necessary and adequate care?**
Preplanning for any event should always include considerations for how a crowd will be managed and how SEMS providers will communicate with other venue personnel such as security. Because this motocross event is taking place in a stadium, it is likely a large event and there should be a decent number of SEMS providers working. Ideally three SEMS providers should respond to this emergency so that two can care for the patient and a third can direct other incoming personnel, if applicable. SEMS providers should also ensure that they request assistance from security personnel to cordon off the crowd around the emergency scene. It is important that SEMS providers not be distracted by crowd control issues while caring for a patient.

2. **What should SEMS providers do to increase the patient's chance of survival?**
This patient must continue to receive CPR and must be transported as quickly as possible to the closest trauma center. If the responding providers are not certified in ALS care, they should immediately arrange for ALS providers to respond.

CASE 2

1. **What should SEMS providers do to care for the patient?**
Due to the lack of mental improvement, the patient must be transported. SEMS providers should move the patient onto the backboard and maintain c-spine stabilization. It is suspected that the patient has a concussion and possibly closed head trauma. SEMS providers move the boxer onto the stretcher and then out of the ring with assistance from the trainers and security personnel. Information is taken from the trainers and the boxer's medical folder. The patient's gloves and the wrapping on the boxer's hands may be cut off; one of the trainers can do this if needed.
A detailed head-to-toe exam is conducted. Findings include swelling and bruising at the site of the hit. There are no other apparent injuries except for a small cut to the right temporal area of the skull with little bleeding. Meanwhile, another SEMS provider establishes IV access per local protocol. When the ALS ambulance arrives, the patient and information about his care are transferred to the transporting crew.

2. **What considerations should be given to transporting the patient?**
At this event, transport is to occur via an outside emergency department; therefore, SEMS providers must contact the outside emergency department to ensure that the unit is en route as soon as possible. After the ambulance departs, SEMS providers continue to provide care to others at the boxing event during the next fight.

Ready for Review

- As with other events, preplanning measures are essential to effectively provide SEMS coverage at an extreme or combat sporting event.
- Each type of extreme and combat sporting event requires that the SEMS provider be familiar with the language of the event.
- When preplanning for an extreme or combat sporting event, SEMS providers should consider the types of events/competitions that will be taking place, the specific details of each event (such as distance and duration), and how to access different parts of the facility and course.
- SEMS providers should develop a detailed timeline of the extreme sporting event to ensure providers are where they need to be at the right time.
- As always, spectators should also be considered. Concerns include who will provide care for the spectators, whether there will be a separate first aid station for participants and spectators, whether alcohol is being served at the event and how this may affect SEMS providers (types of emergencies, security issues), and crowd management plans.
- When an emergency occurs, consider which equipment will be needed. The stretcher and bulky equipment should be stored next to an easily accessible area between the ambulance and performance area.
- SEMS providers must know how they will be alerted to respond to an emergency. This should be determined during the preplanning phase, as with any event.
- Staffing levels will vary depending on the size of the event and also on whether the SEMS team will be providing care for the spectators, participants, or both. During preplanning, determine whether BLS will suffice or whether ALS providers are required.
- Note that SEMS providers may need to work with physicians, nurses, and athletic trainers at sporting events. Predetermine roles and responsibilities.
- There must be a plan for who will transport the patient (SEMS providers or an outside transport unit?).
- Always factor the crowd into transportation decisions. Depending on the size of the arena, it may be necessary to consider using EMS carts to move around outside the arena.
- During combat events, athletes are usually backstage or in the performance area. SEMS providers must preplan how to access them. Performance areas may be surrounded by fences or steep slopes. Only powered vehicles can be used at these locations. Other events may be best accessed on foot.
- Consider how to best access a patient in a crowd. It may be easier and faster to use a battery-powered or small fuel-powered vehicles.
- On the day of the event, carefully examine the environment. Ensure that damaged equipment, loose objects, or unsafe areas are taken care of. Point out any problems you may find to the referees, officials, or the location manager.
- Extreme sports are those involving dangerous and high-risk activities.
- Extreme sports include many sports, and each has its own environment, gear and equipment, common injuries and conditions, and unique preplanning concerns. Discussed in this chapter are events involving skiing, snowboarding, skateboarding, in-line skating, BMX, motocross, cheerleading, rock climbing, and paintball.
- Skiing may be downhill or cross-country skiing. It is always an outdoor activity performed in the snow.
- At ski events, SEMS providers should determine the path for accessing and removing a patient as part of preplanning.
- The most common ski injuries and conditions are knee and thumb injuries, trauma, and hypothermia.
- Snowboarders use a snowboard to race downhill or perform tricks on an obstacle course outside in the snow.
- The most common snowboarding injuries and conditions are joint injuries, closed head injuries, and internal injuries. Hypothermia may also occur.
- Skateboarders compete by doing tricks, turns, and flips on a short wooden board with wheels.
- Skateboarding events may be inside arenas or stadiums or outside in parking lots. They usually include obstacle courses with ramps, railings, steps, and curbs.
- The most common skateboarding injuries are extremity, spinal cord, closed head, and internal injuries.
- In-line skating involves racing or performing tricks over ramps, steps, rails, and obstacles wearing hard-shelled boots with four or five wheels on the bottom of each one.
- In-line skating races may be on indoor tracks or obstacle courses or outside on closed-off streets.
- The most common in-line skating injuries are injuries to the extremities, head, internal organs, spinal cord, back, neck, groin, and shoulders.
- BMX athletes perform tricks over ramps and obstacle courses on specially built BMX bikes.
- BMX events can be inside arenas or stadiums or outside on parking lots.

- The most common BMX injuries are wrist sprains, strains, internal organ injuries, open compound fractures, or brain and spinal injuries.
- Motocross uses bikes with engines to race or perform tricks on dirt or mud tracks.
- Motocross requires a wide array of safety gear including helmets, goggles, neck collars, neck braces, chest protectors, shin and wrist guards, and boots.
- The most common motocross injuries are knee strains, shoulder dislocations, wrist fractures, and injuries to the tibia, fibula, ankle, head, and back.
- Rock climbers climb rocks or a man-made rock climbing wall indoors or outdoors.
- Many forms of rock climbing use safety systems and protective equipment with ropes, harnesses, and spotters.
- The most common rock climbing injuries are extremity and trauma injuries.
- Combat sports involve two fighters competing in a contact sport according to a set of specific rules, using striking, grappling, or weapons.
- Like extreme sports, combat sports include many sports, and each has its own environments, gear and equipment, common injuries and conditions, and unique preplanning concerns.
- Boxing occurs in a ring surrounded by a crowd of spectators. Therefore, it will be important to have a clear path for access and egress should SEMS providers need to reach the ring. As always, when preplanning, consider how you will access various sections of the crowd.
- Boxers may wear protective headgear. It is important for SEMS providers to be familiar with the headgear worn at various events and to know procedures and local protocols for headgear or helmet removal.
- Most boxers wrap their hands with tape to prevent injuries. Boxing gloves are padded to prevent injury to the boxer's hands and to allow the boxer to protect his or her head.
- Common boxing injuries include lacerations and contusions. More severe boxing injuries include closed head trauma and other forms of trauma to the body.
- Fencing is a combat sport in which two opponents strike each other using sword-like weapons. Fencers do not aim to cause bodily harm.
- Fencing gear and equipment include special clothing and sword-like weapons to thrust and jab the opponent. Fencing weapons may also have electronic components that allow judges to note where a fencer was struck and with how much force.
- Common fencing injuries include sprains, strains, and fractures, usually to the wrists or ankles. Bruising is very common, and head injuries also occur.
- Wrestling is a combat event in which two opponents battle one another using grappling, holds, and throws.
- Wrestling matches take place on a well-padded mat that offers some shock absorption to cushion the wrestlers from throws.
- Wrestlers generally wear a light elastic uniform; headgear; and light, flexible sneakers.
- Common wrestling injuries include fractures and dislocations, tearing injuries, lacerations, head injuries and concussions, spinal injuries, toe injuries, ear trauma, and shoulder injuries.
- Martial arts are combat sports that involve striking and grappling but not weaponry.
- Most martial arts prohibit vicious moves.
- Some martial arts competitions take place on a raised mat surrounded by a fence to prevent athletes from sliding off and becoming injured. SEMS providers should determine the best way to enter this cage, should they need to access an injured participant.
- Gear and equipment for martial arts may include open-fingered gloves, tight-fitting shirts, and mid-thigh–length shorts. Socks and shoes are generally optional; many martial artists participate barefooted.
- Common martial arts injuries include cuts to the head and scalp, sprains, strains, tears, or closed head injury.
- SEMS providers should be careful to take appropriate body substance isolation precautions, including gloves, eye protection, and vigorous hand washing; combat sports participants may be covered with their own blood and possibly the opponent's blood.
- Cheerleading involves athletes performing pyramids, aerial tosses, flips, and throws to compete or encourage spectators at a sporting event to cheer.
- The most common cheerleading injuries are strains and sprains to the ankles and wrists, and trauma injuries.
- Paintball is an event in which participants shoot each other with balls filled with paint using specialized guns. Paintball events may occur indoors or outdoors.
- The most common paintball injuries are eye injuries, though other injuries such as blunt trauma may occur.
- Remember to listen to your patient. Acknowledge the injury that is the most painful or concerning to the athlete, even if it is different than what you believe to be the most serious concern. Conversely, be sure to properly assess for and treat all injuries.

- Note that in some jurisdictions, SEMS providers may provide analgesics to ease pain associated with injuries.
- Several common conditions such as heat injury, cold injuries, dehydration, hyponatremia, and closed head injuries occur at extreme and combat sporting events. SEMS providers should be aware of the signs, symptoms, and appropriate treatment for these conditions.

Vital Vocabulary

belayer In rock climbing, a person who keeps the harness and rope system under control; may be located at the base or the top.

belay system A harness and rope system used in rock climbing, kept under control by an assistant at the base of the climb.

bicycle motocross (BMX) A sport in which athletes perform tricks on bikes.

Cheyne-Stokes respirations Respirations that are fast and then become slow, with intervening periods of apnea; commonly seen following brain stem injury.

chronic traumatic brain injury A traumatic brain injury that occurs as a result of a series of injuries to the brain that either (1) are not allowed to heal before the next injury occurs or (2) produce lasting effects to the brain.

clinching The term for holding an opponent while he or she is standing, preventing him or her from moving to the ground.

combat sport A competitive, combative contact sport in which two opponents battle using specific rules of engagement.

concussion A mild brain injury caused by the brain striking the skull after a blow to the head, which can be categorized ranging from mild to severe; symptoms may continue for several weeks after the incident.

Cushing's triad Hypertension (with widening pulse pressure), bradycardia, and irregular respirations; classic trio findings associated with increased intracranial pressure.

defensive move A move that slows an opponent's actions.

epidural hematoma An accumulation of blood between the skull and dura.

extreme sport Sporting events that involve dangerous and high-risk activities.

fencing A combat sport in which two opponents strike each other using sword-like weapons.

groundwork In martial arts, a term referring to a fight that occurs on the ground.

half-pipe Used in snowboarding, a U-shaped bowl that allows snowboarders to move from one wall to the other by making jumps and performing snowboarding tricks on each transition.

heat cramps Acute and involuntary muscle pains, usually in the lower extremities, the abdomen, or both, that occur because of profuse sweating and subsequent sodium loss.

heat exhaustion A clinical syndrome characterized by volume depletion and heat stress that is thought to be a milder form of heat illness on the continuum leading to heat stroke.

heat stroke The least common and most deadly heat illness, caused by a severe disturbance in thermoregulation, usually characterized by a core temperature of more than 104°F (40°C) and altered mental status.

make weight Meeting a body weight requirement to compete in a combat sport; sometimes achieved by the participant sweating excessively to reduce his or her weight; also called "cutting weight."

martial arts Combat sports involving striking and grappling such as judo, jujitsu, and karate.

motocross A sport in which athletes perform tricks on bikes with engines.

paintball A contest in which participants shoot each other with balls filled with paint using specialized guns.

post-concussion syndrome Due to jarring of the brain within the skull, the patient experiences weakness on one side of the body, extreme mood swings, and/or problems with basic cognitive functions, such as memory or orientation.

round A timed interval in a boxing match.

singlet A wrestling uniform.

subdural hematoma An accumulation of blood beneath the dura but outside the brain.

submission hold A move or combination of moves that attacks an opponent's joint, muscle, or air and bloodflow to the brain, causing the opponent to surrender before any serious harm is done.

takedown A move or combination of moves that forces the opponent to fall to the mat.

track crew Individuals who monitor the course during a competition and communicate with other personnel, including SEMS providers.

unilateral pupils A condition in which the pupil on the side of an injury is dilated and does not respond to light, while the pupil on the other side does not have this appearance.

vert A part of a BMX track that faces another ramp, creating a valley shape.

Case Studies

Case 1

Event Information

The local ski club, The Ski Nuts, is holding an amateur downhill skiing competition to raise money for a local youth program. It is hosted annually by the Ourtown Parks and Recreation Program. The contact for the event is the Program Director, Mrs. Ann Johnson. Her office phone number is (555) 555-1212. The event is to be held the third weekend of January, on the 19th and 20th, at the Snow Top Ski Lodge. The lodge is located at 2735 Blizzard Road. Total attendance for this annual event is around 2,000 people, including approximately 250 participants of varying experience levels. The event is held in the early afternoon and is followed by a large banquet and gala ball. While this is normally a local event, the governor is attending this year, using the event as a campaign stop.

The ski lodge has its own snow patrol teams that consist of three snowmobiles, each staffed with two BLS-level patrollers, to transport patients.

Approximately 3 months before the event, Mrs. Johnson contacts you and requests EMS coverage for the skiing portion of the event. She requests to meet with you for initial planning next week. She details that the event requires at least one ALS transport unit and one BLS unit by the sanctioning body. The local ski patrol has already been contracted to provide BLS coverage on the course itself, but your agency will transport any injuries to the hospital, since the ski patrol does not have that capability. Your agency will also be contracted to operate the standing first aid station located at the base of the mountain. Lastly, due to the governor's attendance, the security detail will need certain information from you about your staff that will be providing coverage for the event. With the data Mrs. Johnson has provided, you complete your preplanning forms as follows.

Preplanning Form

Figure A-1 shows a filled-out preplanning form for Case 1.

Part I: BASIC INFORMATION

1. Estimated attendance
   - ☑ Fewer than 5,000
   - ☐ 5,001–10,000
   - ☐ 10,001–25,000
   - ☐ 25,001 or more
2. Type of event (check all that apply)
   - ☑ Outdoor
   - ☐ Indoor
   - ☐ Concert
   - ☐ Festival
   - ☐ Stadium
   - ☑ Sport
   - ☐ Extreme sport
   - ☐ Combat sport
   - ☐ Equestrian
   - ☐ Rodeo
   - ☐ Event involving water
   - ☑ Political
   - ☐ Other: ____________
3. Nature of event
   - ☑ High profile
   - ☐ Potentially violent
   - ☐ High likelihood of drug/alcohol use
   - ☐ Event of national significance
   - ☑ Other: Local athletic fund-raiser
4. Location(s) of event

   Name of facility: Snow Top Ski Lodge

   Address: 2735 Blizzard Road

   City: Ourtown State: UT Zip: 99999
5. Organizational information

   Name of organization: Ourtown Parks and Recreation Department

   Address: 511 Sports Complex Way

   City: Ourtown State: UT Zip: 99999

   Contact person: Mrs. Ann Johnson

   Telephone:

   Work: (555) 555-1212

   Cell: ____________

   Other: ____________

   E-mail address: ajohnson@ourtownpr.co.any.us

Part II: RESOURCE NEEDS

6. Resources needed

	Type	Number
Personnel*	☐ Emergency medical responder	____
	☑ BLS	4 (this number represents SEMS providers only and does not include the ski patrol staff)
	☑ ALS	2
	☐ Registered nurse	____
	☐ Physician	____
	☐ Other: ____________	____
Vehicles†	☐ Carts	____
	☑ Other: Snowmobiles	3
	Transport units	2 (one BLS, one ALS)

Figure A-1

Preplanning form for Case 1.

Medical Equipment	☑ Gloves	Multiple boxes and sizes of gloves, plus standard first aid equipment
	☑ AED	3 (one for the first aid station and one per ambulance [there are two ambulances])
	☑ Stretcher	3 (one for the first aid station and one per ambulance [there are two ambulances])
	☑ Other: ______	Heat packs, thermal angel (to warm IV fluids)
	❑ Other: ______	____
First Aid Stations‡	☑ On-site	1 (will use the facility already on the event site)
	❑ Tent	____
	❑ Other: ______	____

***Personnel:**
Guidelines for staffing an event with fewer than 5,000 attendees are to have one to two providers. For this event, four BLS providers have been planned for. Two of these BLS providers will staff the BLS transport unit. Two BLS providers will staff the first aid station. The ALS providers will staff the ALS transport unit. Note that these staffing calculations do not include the ski patrol staff, which are not part of your staff and should not be part of your staffing calculations in this case.

†Vehicles:
For an event with fewer than 5,000 attendees, it may not be necessary to have a transport unit on site. For this event, two transport units are planned for due to the long transport time to the nearest hospital (1 hour and 15 minutes round-trip).

‡First aid stations:
For an event with fewer than 5,000 attendees, one first aid station should be sufficient. For this event, the plan is to use the first aid facility that is already on site.

7. Description of on-site first aid facilities

Small first aid building located on the premises. The building contains two cots in a treatment area, allowing for minor treatment procedures. It also has the ability to keep several blankets warm in multiple blanket warmers.

8. Copies of maps and schematics of facility and any other special areas (list areas here and check off once maps have been obtained and distributed to all personnel)
   - ☑ Facility
   - ❑ Parking areas
   - ☑ Access/egress routes
   - ❑ Surrounding streets
   - ☑ Other: Proposed ski run

Figure A-1

Preplanning form for Case 1.

(continues)

9. Description of patient transfer protocols and agreements that will be used

Usage of on-site ski patrol equipment and personnel to assist in the care and transport of any injured skiers from the mountain.

10. Communication needs and capabilities (indicate which type of communications matrix will be used and which channel each party will use)

The onsite EMS units will operate on the event radios on a single channel that will keep them in constant contact with event staff, security detail, and the ski patrol. Upon patient transport, they will switch to their transport radios.

Part III: RESEARCH AND ACTIONS TAKEN

11. Measures that have been or will be taken to coordinate SEMS for the event with local EMS and public safety agencies, such as ambulance, police, fire, rescue, and hospital agencies or organizations (if not yet taken, state actions to be taken and target dates for these to be accomplished)

Action: Meeting with security detail to discuss any security concerns with the governor's visit to event

Target date: Two weeks prior to the event

Action: Work with other parties to identify landing zone, should one be needed.

Target date: One month prior to the event

Action:

Target date:

12. Security concerns and plans for addressing them:

General security for ski area: to be addressed by lodge event staff.

Specific requirements for governor's visit to the event. Meeting with security detail to address any issues.

Due to the governor's visit, security may require an onsite command center. Discuss with security detail whether this is planned.

13. Weather history (consult 2–3 sources and list results here)

Source: Local weather data from the National Weather Service

Information: Average high, 28°F (−2°C); average low, 15°F (−9.4°C); average precipitation, 4.5 inches

Source: National Weather Service advance forecast

Information: Likely to be cold (19°F to 22°F [−7.2°C to −5.6°C], 60% chance of snow)

Source: Local newspaper archives

Information: The past 5 years' records show that the average temperature was 25°F (−3.9°C) and that snow fell during three of the five years.

Figure A-1

Preplanning form for Case 1.

14. Possible inclement weather
- ❑ Rain
- ☑ Snow
- ❑ Lightning
- ❑ Tornado
- ❑ Hurricane
- ☑ Other: Extreme cold

Preplanning measures taken:

Action: Monitor local weather forecast. Plan for possible cold exposure patients.

Target date: Begin approximately 2 weeks before the event.

15. Surface considerations

Type of surface:
- ❑ Grass
- ❑ Loose gravel
- ❑ Dirt
- ❑ Asphalt
- ❑ Concrete
- ❑ Temporary flooring
- ☑ Other: Snow-covered ski slopes

Condition of surface:
- ❑ Smooth
- ❑ Rough
- ☑ Slippery
- ☑ Other: Snow-covered and steep

Levelness:
- ❑ Even
- ☑ Uneven

Preplanning measures taken:

Action: Use existing snow patrol teams.

Target date: Day of event

16. Credentialing process

Describe the event's credentialing process:

Department ID badges will be sufficient.

Do SEMS providers need to bring a photo ID to be used for creating a badge?
- ☑ Yes
- ❑ No

17. Security clearance

Will security clearance be needed?
- ☑ Yes
- ❑ No

If so, how far in advance of the event is it needed?

A list of all personnel working the event will be sent to the security detail 2 weeks prior to the event. This is due to the governor's attendance of the event.

Preplanning measures taken:

Action: Provide list as required.

Target date: January 2

Figure A-1

Preplanning form for Case 1.

(continues)

Part IV: SPECIAL CONSIDERATIONS

18. Special concerns and considerations (describe what you know about the following factors)

Communication:

None

Attendees:

Various age groups will be in attendance. Participants vary in age from late teens to mid 60s.

Demographics:

(See above.) All ages expected: pediatrics, adults, and geriatrics.

Where are the spectators located?

Primarily at the bottom of the ski run, in an already-existing spectator area. Some are also located throughout the course.

How are the spectators contained?

Along the course by orange snow fence; at the end of the run by banners that double as advertising signs.

Access/egress:

All areas are accessible; however, climbing the mountain can be difficult. Use of snowmobiles provided by the lodge will address the issue.

Are there areas that cannot be easily viewed?

No

Where is the best vantage point?

The bottom of the run offers the best view of the crowd. On the ski run, no one place is better than another.

Treatment issues:

Typical concerns for trauma at a ski event, heightened by the fact that several participants are new skiers and the slope chosen by the promoter is of medium difficulty.

Transportation:

Two transport units. Even though one would suffice, distance from the nearest hospital will require two units to be present.

Other considerations:

Ensure that the lodge has a room that is large enough to handle overflow of the first aid station, if needed. Discuss with event promoter one month before event.

Figure A-1

Preplanning form for Case 1.

Rotation Schedule

None required.

Preplanning Timeline

Reference the preplanning timeline in Table A-1 for a breakdown of when the preplanning tasks for this case must be completed.

TABLE A-1 Preplanning Timeline for Case 1

Preplanning: Action or Activity	Days Prior to Event
Meet with event sponsor.	60
Determine staffing level. Review roles and responsibilities with all staff.	60
Select SEMS crew.	21
Submit to security detail a list of all personnel working at the event.	17
Meet with security detail.	14
Talk to event contact to obtain last-minute changes.	7
Meet with event official. Walk through the site.	7
Deliver all equipment.	1
Set up equipment and ensure that first aid facility is prepared.	1
Event Day: Action or Activity	**Hours Prior to Event**
Supervisor arrives. Prep supplies. Double check that first aid facility is arranged.	2
Crew arrives. Walk through, familiarize, and rehearse response.	1
Check radio.	1
Transport units arrive.	1
First aid station placed in service.	1
Event start time:	**1:00 pm**

During the Event

During the event, 11 skiers fall, with 2 requiring transport to the first aid station. One individual is treated for a minor wound and released. The other individual is transported to the local hospital for a possible dislocated shoulder. Also during the event, the wind speed increases, causing the temperature to decrease, and a heavy snow begins to fall.

Critical Thinking Questions

1. With the decreasing temperature, how will you address potential exposure problems?
   Discussion: Exposure to cold can become a serious problem quickly. During the planning process, you should have considered this possible issue. The first aid station only has two cots. While this can be used as a rewarming area, it is not large enough to service all of the potential patients. During the planning process, agreements should have been reached to use larger buildings on the premises in an emergency situation.
2. What measures could you have taken during the preplanning process regarding potential event cancellation?
   Discussion: During your meetings with the promoter, you should establish a good working relationship with all parties involved. In most cases, the event promoter will decide whether or not an event can continue, but depending on the promoter and the relationship, SEMS providers may be involved in the decision. If you feel that a situation is severe enough to consider cancelling the event, you may communicate this to the promoter if the opportunity arises.

Postevent Actions

After the event, as a standard procedure SEMS providers should meet with the event promoter and discuss how things went, including whether the promoter's expectations were met. A postevent analysis is helpful to ensure that you evaluate what went right, what went wrong, and most importantly, how to improve for future events.

Depending on your local regulations, you may need to fill out certain forms after the event has occurred. Be sure to find out if this is required and obtain the needed forms.

Case 2

Event Information

Over the last several years, the town of Bloomfield has become a mecca for the area's BMX enthusiasts. Three years ago a track was built at the municipal park. Since then, the Parks and Recreation Department has sponsored an annual all-day bike rodeo for youth of all ages. There are a total of six age groups ranging from ages 4 to 18. Among the older participants (ages 12 to 18), there are novices and experts.

This event has grown into a regional event and now draws an average crowd of over 8,000 attendees. Because this is an annual fund-raiser for the park, your volunteer fire department has agreed to provide a BLS ambulance for transport services for the event.

This event will take place on Saturday, May 29th, from 10:00 am to 3:00 pm.

Preplanning Form

Figure A-2 shows a filled-out preplanning form for Case 2.

Part I: BASIC INFORMATION

1. Estimated attendance
   - ❑ Fewer than 5,000
   - ☑ 5,001-10,000
   - ❑ 10,001-25,000
   - ❑ 25,001 or more
2. Type of event (check all that apply)
   - ☑ Outdoor
   - ❑ Indoor
   - ❑ Concert
   - ❑ Festival
   - ❑ Stadium
   - ❑ Sport
   - ☑ Extreme sport
   - ❑ Combat sport
   - ❑ Equestrian
   - ❑ Rodeo
   - ❑ Event involving water
   - ❑ Political
   - ❑ Other: ______
3. Nature of event
   - ❑ High profile
   - ❑ Potentially violent
   - ❑ High likelihood of drug/alcohol use
   - ❑ Event of national significance
   - ❑ Other: ______
4. Location(s) of event

   Name of facility: Bloomfield Municipal Bike Park

   Address: 3721 Williams Street

   City: Bloomfield State: MA Zip: 01234
5. Organizational information

   Name of organization: Bloomfield Parks and Recreation Department

   Address: 511 Sports Complex Way

   City: Bloomfield State: MA Zip: 01234

   Contact person: Ms. Beatrice Smith

   Telephone:

   Work: (781) 638-3838

   Cell: ______

   Other: ______

   E-mail address: bsmith@blmfldtown.ma

Figure A-2

Preplanning form for Case 2.

Part II: RESOURCE NEEDS

6. Resources needed

	Type	Number
Personnel*	❑ Emergency medical responder	____
	☑ BLS	2
	☑ ALS	2
	❑ Registered nurse	____
	❑ Physician	____
	❑ Other: ____	____
Vehicles†	☑ Carts	1
	☑ Other: Transport unit	2 (one BLS, one ALS)
Medical Equipment	☑ Gloves	Multiple boxes and sizes, plus standard first aid equipment
	☑ AED	2
	☑ Stretcher	2 (one in first aid tent, one in each ambulance)
Medical Equipment (cont.)	☑ Other: ____	MCI/triage kit
	❑ Other: ____	____
First Aid Stations‡	❑ On-site	____
	☑ Tent	1
	❑ Other: ____	____

***Personnel:**
Guidelines for staffing an event with 8,000 attendees are to have two to three providers. For this event, two BLS providers and two ALS providers have been planned for. While this may seem slightly high, an extra provider is warranted because this is an extreme sport and more injuries are expected. ALS providers may be needed for pain management. Also, extra providers are present so that there is still SEMS coverage if the single transport unit must leave.

†Vehicles:
An event with 5,000 to 25,000 attendees would normally require one transport unit. Though this event is expected to have 8,000 attendees, two transport units have been planned since this is an extreme sports event involving children; ALS capabilities will be available on scene.

‡First aid stations:
For an event with 8,000 attendees, one first aid station should be sufficient. For this outdoor event, a first aid tent is planned.

7. Description of on-site first aid facilities

A first aid tent will be set up on the event site.

Figure A-2

Preplanning form for Case 2.

(continues)

8. Copies of maps and schematics of facility and any other special areas (list areas here and check off once maps have been obtained and distributed to all personnel)
   - ☑ Facility
   - ❑ Parking areas
   - ☑ Access/egress routes
   - ❑ Surrounding streets
   - ❑ Other: ____________

9. Description of patient transfer protocols and agreements that will be used

   A first aid cart will respond to all reported incidents. If patient transport is indicated, the first aid cart will bring the patient to the transport unit. Because round-trip to local emergency department is only 30 minutes, no other transport unit will be requested to cover if the initial unit is off-site. This has been confirmed with the promoter.

10. Communication needs and capabilities (indicate which type of communications matrix will be used and which channel each party will use)

    All units will operate on the event radio system.

Part III: RESEARCH AND ACTIONS TAKEN

11. Measures that have been or will be taken to coordinate SEMS for the event with local EMS and public safety agencies, such as ambulance, police, fire, rescue, and hospital agencies or organizations (if not yet taken, state actions to be taken and target dates for these to be accomplished)

    Action: Work with other parties to identify landing zone, should one be needed.

    Target date: One month prior to the event

    Action: ____________

    Target date: ____________

    Action: ____________

    Target date: ____________

12. Security concerns and plans for addressing them:

    General security for event: to be provided by Parks and Recreation staff members.

13. Weather history (consult 2-3 sources and list results here)

    Source: Local weather data from the National Weather Service

    Information: Average high, 67°F (19.4°C); average low, 51°F (10.6°C); average precipitation, 1.9 inches

    Source: Local newspaper archives

    Information: The past 5 years' records show an average temperature of 65°F (18.3°C) and that it rained during one of the five years.

    Source: Local TV station extended forecast

    Information: Temperature expected to be a high of 58°F (14.4°C) and a low of 50°F (10°C), with a 60% chance of rain.

Figure A-2

Preplanning form for Case 2.

14. Possible inclement weather
- ☑ Rain
- ❑ Snow
- ❑ Lightning
- ❑ Tornado
- ❑ Hurricane
- ☑ Other: Possible cooler-than-normal temperatures

Preplanning measures taken:

Action: Monitor local weather forecast. Plan for possible weather exposure patients.

Target date: Begin approximately 2 weeks before the event.

15. Surface considerations

Type of surface:
- ☑ Grass
- ☑ Loose gravel
- ☑ Dirt
- ❑ Asphalt
- ❑ Concrete
- ❑ Temporary flooring
- ❑ Other: ______

Condition of surface:
- ❑ Smooth
- ☑ Rough (some areas of the park have gravel)
- ❑ Slippery
- ❑ Other: ______

Levelness:
- ☑ Even
- ☑ Uneven

Preplanning measures taken:

Action: Planned to place first aid tent on an even surface midway between the BMX course and the food vendor area.

Target date: (Done)

16. Credentialing process

Describe the event's credentialing process:

Normal work photo ID is sufficient.

Do SEMS providers need to bring a photo ID to be used for creating a badge?
- ❑ Yes
- ☑ No

17. Security clearance

Will security clearance be needed?
- ❑ Yes
- ☑ No

If so, how far in advance of the event is it needed?

N/A

Preplanning measures taken:

Action: N/A

Target date: N/A

Figure A-2

Preplanning form for Case 2.

(continues)

Part IV: SPECIAL CONSIDERATIONS

18. Special concerns and considerations (describe what you know about the following factors)

Communication:

None

Attendees:

Various age groups will be in attendance. Participants vary in age from 4 to 18 years. Attendees of all ages are expected (children, adults, geriatrics, though more pediatrics are expected than geriatrics due to the pediatric participant population).

Demographics:

(See above.)

Where are the spectators located?

Spectators will be located around the course, but will be concentrated in a small area of grandstands near the start/finish line.

How are the spectators contained?

All spectators will be separated from the course by plastic fencing.

Access/egress:

Four access points to the track will be created to allow the cart to enter. There will be one at each end of the front stretch area, and the other two will be strategically placed around the course. These will be reviewed at the site visit.

Are there areas that cannot be easily viewed?

No

Where is the best vantage point?

The front stretch grandstands.

Treatment issues:

Possible musculoskeletal injuries as well as head trauma. Nearest neurologic trauma center is 40 minutes by ground or 15 minutes by helicopter.

Transportation:

Two transport units on site: one BLS, one ALS.

Other considerations:

None

Figure A-2

Preplanning form for Case 2.

Rotation Schedule

None required.

Preplanning Timeline

Reference the preplanning timeline in Table A-2 for a breakdown of when the preplanning tasks for this case must be completed.

TABLE A-2 Preplanning Timeline for Case 2

Preplanning: Action or Activity	Days Prior to Event
Meet with event sponsor.	45
Determine staffing level. Review roles and responsibilities with all staff.	30
Select SEMS crew.	14
Talk to event contact to obtain last-minute changes.	7
Meet with event official. Walk through the site.	12 (perform walk-through early because you need to provide input on access points)
Deliver carts, tent, and all equipment.	3
Set up equipment, including first aid tent.	1
Fuel carts.	1
Event Day: Action or Activity	**Hours Prior to Event**
Supervisor arrives. Prep carts. Prep supplies. Arrange tent.	2
Crew arrives. Walk through, familiarize, and rehearse response.	1
Check radio.	1
Transport unit arrives.	1
First aid tent placed in service.	1
Event start time:	**10:00 am**

During the Event

During the event, early on several riders go down but receive only minor injuries. Then during the race with the 6- to 9-year-old participants, a large group of riders is involved in an incident. Three of the riders suffer possible extremity fractures, and one is unresponsive with possible head trauma.

Critical Thinking Questions

1. Did you plan for enough pediatric supplies on site?

   Discussion: For events that involve large numbers of youth, you must ensure that you have enough supplies designed to treat this group appropriately. Extra backboard and splinting materials of a proper size must be present, and should have been noted in the above preplanning form.

2. Do you have enough transport units on site?

   Discussion: Yes, there are enough transport units on site. Though an event of this size would normally have one transport unit, you planned for two transport units (one BLS, one ALS) because this is an extreme sporting event. Also, it is important to note that when working with other agencies, such as the fire department in this scenario, you must establish a good rapport and working relationship so that you can work professionally together.

Postevent Actions

After the event, as a standard procedure SEMS providers should meet with the event promoter and discuss how things went, including whether the promoter's expectations were met. A postevent analysis is helpful to ensure that you evaluate what went right, what went wrong, and most importantly, how to improve for future events.

Depending on your local regulations, you may need to fill out certain forms after the event has occurred. Be sure to find out if this is required and obtain the needed forms.

Case 3

Event Information

The town of Whiting has been selected as a stop on this year's July 4th America Runs for Health National Marathon. The event is a 2-week marathon that visits different cities. The athletes run 26 miles every third day, using the off days to rest. Whiting is the third stop on the tour. The event draws runners from around the world and averages 18,000 attendees each day the race is held. The event is so large that it will require both BLS and ALS services. The event promoter will be supplying water stations along the route, but your agency will need to cover any emergencies that occur along the route. Traffic control will be handled by the State Police. The event will begin at 9:00 am and finish at 1:00 pm.

Preplanning Form

Figure A-3 shows a filled-out preplanning form for Case 3.

Part I: BASIC INFORMATION

1. Estimated attendance
   - ☐ Fewer than 5,000
   - ☐ 5,001-10,000
   - ☑ 10,001-25,000
   - ☐ 25,001 or more
2. Type of event (check all that apply)
   - ☑ Outdoor
   - ☐ Indoor
   - ☐ Concert
   - ☐ Festival
   - ☐ Stadium
   - ☑ Sport
   - ☐ Extreme sport
   - ☐ Combat sport
   - ☐ Equestrian
   - ☐ Rodeo
   - ☐ Event involving water
   - ☐ Political
   - ☐ Other: ______
3. Nature of event
   - ☐ High profile
   - ☐ Potentially violent
   - ☐ High likelihood of drug/alcohol use
   - ☐ Event of national significance
   - ☐ Other: ______
4. Location(s) of event

   Name of facility: Roadways in the area, including Park St. Central Ave, San Miguel Rd, Water St, Main St, Springside St, and Lucille Ave (see map).

   Address: (see above)

   City: Whiting State: AL Zip: 55555
5. Organizational information

   Name of organization: America Runs for Health National Marathon

   Address: 2567 Runners Way, Suite 204

   City: Washington State: DC Zip: 20005

   Contact person: Mr. Bill Demond

   Telephone:

   Work: (202) 555-4444, ext 2513

   Cell: ______

   Other: ______

   E-mail address: bill.demond@americaruns.org

Figure A-3

Preplanning form for Case 3.

Part II: RESOURCE NEEDS

6. Resources needed

	Type	Number
Personnel*	☑ Emergency medical responder	4 (one at each water station)
	☑ BLS	7 (three among the first aid tents, two in each of the two BLS transport units)
	☑ ALS	3 (one in a first aid tent, two in the ALS transport unit)
	❑ Registered nurse	____
	❑ Physician	____
	❑ Other: ____	____
Vehicles†	☑ Carts	4 (one with each emergency medical responder)
	☑ Other: Transport units	3 (two BLS: one at halfway point and one at finish; one ALS: at finish)
Medical Equipment	☑ Gloves	Multiple boxes and sizes of gloves, plus standard first aid equipment
	☑ AED	3 (one in each ambulance)
	☑ Stretcher	3 (one in each ambulance)
	❑ Other: ____	____
	❑ Other: ____	____
First Aid Stations‡	❑ On-site	____
	☑ Tent (four small 10′ × 10′ at each water station; two 20′ × 20′, one at start and one at finish)	6
	❑ Other: ____	____

***Personnel:**
Guidelines for staffing an event with 18,000 attendees are to have two to four providers. For this event, four emergency medical responders have been planned for at each water station. This is in line with the general guidelines. Additionally, there are two BLS providers in the first aid tent at the starting line. In the first aid tent at the finish line, there is one BLS provider and one ALS provider. There are also providers in the transport units: four BLS providers (two in each of the two BLS transport units), and two ALS providers (in the ALS transport unit).

†Vehicles:
For an event with 5,000 to 25,000 attendees, normally you would plan for one transport unit. However, at this event, three transport units (two BLS, one ALS) have been planned for due to the high likelihood of heat emergencies as well as the potential injuries among participants and attendees.

‡First aid stations:
For an event with 18,000 attendees, the general guideline is to have one to two first aid stations. For this event, there are four small (10′ × 10′) tents that will serve as water stations, and there are two larger (20′ × 20′) tents that will serve as first aid stations at the start and finish lines.

Figure A-3

Preplanning form for Case 3.

(continues)

7. Description of on-site first aid facilities

There will be a small (10′ × 10′) tent at each of the four water stations, a 20′ × 20′ tent at the start line, and a 20′ × 20′ tent at the finish line.

8. Copies of maps and schematics of facility and any other special areas (list areas here and check off once maps have been obtained and distributed to all personnel)

- ❑ Facility
- ❑ Parking areas
- ❑ Access/egress routes
- ❑ Surrounding streets
- ☑ Other: Route of race with first aid stations and transport unit locations noted

9. Description of patient transfer protocols and agreements that will be used

A first aid cart will respond to all reported incidents. If patient transport is indicated, the first aid cart will bring the patient to the nearest appropriate transport unit.

10. Communication needs and capabilities (indicate which type of communications matrix will be used and which channel each party will use)

Due to the larger number of units and need to coordinate with the police, all units will use the county radio system and will operate off of the Mutual Aid Channel 1. The promoter's safety staff will be issued four radios with this frequency to allow them to contact EMS in the case of emergency.

Part III: RESEARCH AND ACTIONS TAKEN

11. Measures that have been or will be taken to coordinate SEMS for the event with local EMS and public safety agencies, such as ambulance, police, fire, rescue, and hospital agencies or organizations (if not yet taken, state actions to be taken and target dates for these to be accomplished)

Action: Work with other parties to identify landing zone, should one be needed.

Target date: One month prior to the event

Action: ____

Target date: ____

Action: ____

Target date: ____

Figure A-3

Preplanning form for Case 3.

12. Security concerns and plans for addressing them:

Roadways to be closed for safety reasons. Captain Howard from local State Police barracks will ensure this is completed.

13. Weather history (consult 2–3 sources and list results here)

Source: Local weather data from the National Weather Service

Information: Average high, 81°F (27.2°C); average low, 70°F (21.1°C); average precipitation, 3.5 inches

Source: Local newspaper archives

Information: The past 5 years' records show that the average temperature was 83°F (28.3°C) with an average of 70% humidity, but it did not rain during any of those years.

Source:

Information:

14. Possible inclement weather

- ☑ Rain
- ❑ Snow
- ☑ Lightning
- ❑ Tornado
- ❑ Hurricane
- ☑ Other: High heat and humidity

Preplanning measures taken:

Action: Monitor local weather forecast. Plan for possible heat-exposure patients.

Target date: Begin approximately 2 weeks before the event. If needed, contract additional personnel if concerns dictate an increased presence on site.

Action: Discuss the need for plenty of water with event promoter, to avoid heat emergencies. Suggest that water be available to attendees and participants free of charge (not just for sale from vendors). Also plan for a misting station to be included at each water station.

Target date: Two months before the event.

15. Surface considerations

Type of surface:

- ❑ Grass
- ❑ Loose gravel
- ❑ Dirt
- ☑ Asphalt
- ❑ Concrete
- ❑ Temporary flooring
- ❑ Other:

Figure A-3

Preplanning form for Case 3.

(continues)

Condition of surface:
- ☑ Smooth
- ❑ Rough
- ❑ Slippery
- ❑ Other: ______

Levelness:
- ☑ Even
- ❑ Uneven

Preplanning measures taken:

Action: None

Target date: N/A

16. Credentialing process

Describe the event's credentialing process:

Normal work photo ID is sufficient.

Do SEMS providers need to bring a photo ID to be used for creating a badge?
- ❑ Yes
- ☑ No

17. Security clearance

Will security clearance be needed?
- ❑ Yes
- ☑ No

If so, how far in advance of the event is it needed?

N/A

Preplanning measures taken:

Action: None

Target date: N/A

Part IV: SPECIAL CONSIDERATIONS

18. Special concerns and considerations (describe what you know about the following factors)

Communication:

None

Attendees:

Most attendees will be young adults.

Demographics:

(See above.)

Where are the spectators located?

Along the route.

How are the spectators contained?

There are no barriers along the route.

Figure A-3

Preplanning form for Case 3.

Access/egress:

No problems are anticipated.

Are there areas that cannot be easily viewed?

No

Where is the best vantage point?

There is no one area due to the length of the event.

Treatment issues:

Concerns for hyperthermia, dehydration, and hyponatremia/hypernatremia.

Transportation:

As noted earlier, there will be two BLS transport units placed as follows: one along the route and one at the finish. There will also be an ALS unit placed at the finish.

Other considerations:

None

Figure A-3

Preplanning form for Case 3.

Rotation Schedule

None due to length of event (4 hours maximum).

Preplanning Timeline

Reference the preplanning timeline in Table A-3 for a breakdown of when the preplanning tasks for this case must be completed.

TABLE A-3 Preplanning Timeline for Case 3

Preplanning: Action or Activity	Days Prior to Event
Meet with event sponsor.	45
Determine staffing level. Review roles and responsibilities with all staff.	30
Select SEMS crew.	14
Talk to event contact to obtain last-minute changes.	7
Meet with event official. Walk through the site.	5
Deliver carts, tent, and all equipment.	2
Set up equipment, including water stations and first aid tents.	1
Meet crew at facility. Walk through, familiarize, and rehearse response.	1
Fuel carts and generators.	1
Event Day: Action or Activity	**Hours Prior to Event**
Supervisor arrives. Crew arrives. Prep carts. Prep supplies. Arrange tent.	2
Radio check.	1
Transport units arrive.	1
First aid tents place in service.	1
Event start time:	**9:00 am**

During the Event

Race day dawns, and at 9:00 am the event begins. The temperature and humidity quickly rise during the morning. You observe that the runners are coping with the conditions, but your staff begins to report bystanders who are showing signs of minor hyperthermia. So far the SEMS staff is handling the patient load. Each water station also serves as a misting station and provides free water for attendees; additionally, the local vendors are selling food and drink. By midday, the vendors are selling out of water. Your staff continues to report seeing dehydrated patients on a constant basis. Thus far, the SEMS staff has been able to orally hydrate the patients with supplies on hand.

Critical Thinking Questions

1. What measures could you have taken to better plan for emergencies among the attendees?
   Discussion: Professional athletes are usually in better shape and at least somewhat able to handle extremes in weather conditions that their sports involve; however, bystanders are much more susceptible to extremes in weather conditions. In an event such as this, your focus must be split to cover both populations.

   Remember that bystanders may not be the focus of the event, but it is your responsibility to plan for them. They may need as many, if not more, resources than have been planned for the event participants. At an event with potential heat emergencies, it is important to have cooling stations with free water and to have misting tents. This case's preplanning form properly noted to discuss water availability and misting stations with the promoter before the event. It also would have been a good idea, with the weather expected, to preplan for a shelter along the route for spectators as well as the athletes. Finally, if possible, ensure that prior to the event the promoter communicates to participants and attendees to bring drinks with them; this can help prevent heat emergencies before they occur.
2. What options could you consider if the supply of water becomes low during the event?
   Discussion: For an event that is underway, your options may be limited, which is a reason why preplanning supplies and resources is so important. Consider whether there are buildings in the area that you can use as emergency cooling stations. Libraries, fire houses, police stations, and schools would all make great locations for temporary shelters from the weather. These would have areas where people could sit, and they also have restrooms.

Postevent Actions

After the event, as a standard procedure SEMS providers should meet with the event promoter and discuss how things went, including whether the promoter's expectations were met. A postevent analysis is helpful to ensure that you evaluate what went right, what went wrong, and most importantly, how to improve for future events.

Depending on your local regulations, you may need to fill out certain forms after the event has occurred. Be sure to find out if this is required and obtain the needed forms.

Finally, if a temporary overwhelming patient load occurs, you may be required to write an after action report.

Case 4

Event Information

The town of Derry will play host to this year's 33rd annual National Science Fiction Convention and Trade Show. This week-long event is attended by science fiction fans of all ages from around this world. The event averages over 30,000 people each day, with a peak of 45,000 people on Friday and Saturday, when international celebrities from the science fiction genre attend the show. In anticipation of this event, local hotels and businesses expect large numbers of clients to frequent their establishments. All hotels in the area are booked solid for the event.

You have been contacted by Mr. James L. Pike, organizer for this event, about providing standby EMS coverage for the event. All events are being held inside at Memorial Hall in the downtown business district. There are also several smaller events not directly associated with your coverage, which will be occurring at local venues throughout the town.

Preplanning Form

Figure A-4 shows a filled-out preplanning form for Case 4.

Part I: BASIC INFORMATION

1. Estimated attendance
   - ❑ Fewer than 5,000
   - ❑ 5,001-10,000
   - ❑ 10,001-25,000
   - ☑ 25,001 or more
2. Type of event (check all that apply)
   - ❑ Outdoor
   - ☑ Indoor
   - ❑ Concert
   - ❑ Festival
   - ❑ Stadium
   - ❑ Sport
   - ❑ Extreme sport
   - ❑ Combat sport
   - ❑ Equestrian
   - ❑ Rodeo
   - ❑ Event involving water
   - ❑ Political
   - ❑ Other: ____________
3. Nature of event
   - ❑ High profile
   - ❑ Potentially violent
   - ❑ High likelihood of drug/alcohol use
   - ❑ Event of national significance
   - ❑ Other: ____________
4. Location(s) of event

   Name of facility: Memorial Convention Hall

   Address: 127 Convention Way

   City: Derry State: ID Zip: 65432
5. Organizational information

   Name of organization: International Science Fiction Convention Supporters

   Address: 1701 Starship Drive

   City: Ressick State: NV Zip: 98765

   Contact person: James L. Pike

   Telephone:

   Work: (666) 555-1701

   Cell: ____________

   Other: ____________

   E-mail address: james.pike@scificlub.org

Figure A-4

Preplanning form for Case 4. *(continues)*

Part II: RESOURCE NEEDS

6. Resources needed

	Type	Number
Personnel*	❑ Emergency medical responder	____
	☑ BLS	4
	❑ ALS	____
	❑ Registered nurse	____
	❑ Physician	____
	❑ Other: ____	____
Vehicles†	☑ Carts	2
	☑ Other: Transport unit	1 (BLS)
Medical Equipment	☑ Gloves	Multiple boxes and sizes of gloves, plus standard first aid equipment
	☑ AED	2 (one on the transport unit, one that belongs to the convention hall)
	☑ Stretcher	1 (in the transport unit)
	☑ Other: Cots	4 (to be placed in first aid station)
	❑ Other: ____	____
First Aid Stations‡	❑ On-site	____
	❑ Tent	____
	☑ Other: Table and cot area	1 (on convention room floor)

***Personnel:**
An event with more than 25,000 attendees will require a minimum of four BLS providers. At this event, exactly four BLS providers are planned for, because it is a convention and there is not a high likelihood of injury or illness. The four BLS providers will all work in the first aid station. If a patient needs to be transported, two of the BLS providers will transport the patient while the other two BLS providers remain on site at the first aid station.

†Vehicles:
Generally, an event with between 25,001 and 55,000 attendees would require two BLS ambulances and an ALS ambulance if available. Because this event has a low likelihood of illness or injury, one BLS ambulance has been planned for, and there are plans in place for how to request additional assistance should it be needed.

‡First aid stations:
Generally, an event with more than 25,000 attendees would require a minimum of two first aid stations; however, since this event has a low likelihood of illness or injury, only one has been planned.

7. Description of on-site first aid facilities

The first aid station will be located on the convention floor and will be denoted on the map of the event by a red cross symbol. Transport from the area will be made by one of the two on-site teams. No ALS will be on site due to nature of event. The first aid cots will be separated by curtains from the main convention floor. This area will be set up by the convention center staff.

Figure A-4

Preplanning form for Case 4.

8. Copies of maps and schematics of facility and any other special areas (list areas here and check off once maps have been obtained and distributed to all personnel)
   - ☑ Facility
   - ☑ Parking areas
   - ❑ Access/egress routes
   - ☑ Surrounding streets
   - ☑ Other: Map of convention show floor with booths numbered for reference. Also showing the location of the first aid station.

9. Description of patient transfer protocols and agreements that will be used

   As noted, one transport unit will be on site, and two of the crew members will transport a patient from the event. If needed, additional transport units may be requested through agency radio channel.

10. Communication needs and capabilities (indicate which type of communications matrix will be used and which channel each party will use)

    Department radios will be used; Derry 1 will be the operational channel. If needed, can request ALS through county Channel 1.

Part III: RESEARCH AND ACTIONS TAKEN

11. Measures that have been or will be taken to coordinate SEMS for the event with local EMS and public safety agencies, such as ambulance, police, fire, rescue, and hospital agencies or organizations (if not yet taken, state actions to be taken and target dates for these to be accomplished)

    Action: Meeting with promoter and convention center staff on site to coordinate response plan, including access and egress issues and the setup of the first aid station.

    Target date: Two weeks prior to the event

    Action: ______

    Target date: ______

    Action: ______

    Target date: ______

12. Security concerns and plans for addressing them:

    All security issues are being handled by the promoter and on-site convention security staff.

13. Weather history (consult 2-3 sources and list results here)

    Source: N/A (indoor event)

    Information: ______

    Source: ______

    Information: ______

    Source: ______

    Information: ______

Figure A-4

Preplanning form for Case 4.

(*continues*)

14. Possible inclement weather
    - ❑ Rain
    - ❑ Snow
    - ❑ Lightning
    - ❑ Tornado
    - ❑ Hurricane
    - ❑ Other: ______

    Preplanning measures taken:

    Action: N/A (indoor event)

    Target date: ______

15. Surface considerations

    Type of surface:
    - ❑ Grass
    - ❑ Loose gravel
    - ❑ Dirt
    - ❑ Asphalt
    - ☑ Concrete
    - ❑ Temporary flooring
    - ❑ Other: ______

    Condition of surface:
    - ☑ Smooth
    - ❑ Rough
    - ❑ Slippery
    - ❑ Other: ______

    Levelness:
    - ☑ Even
    - ❑ Uneven

    Preplanning measures taken:

    Action: N/A

    Target date: ______

16. Credentialing process

    Describe the event's credentialing process:

    Department-issued credentials are adequate for this event. On-site security staff will be given a list of personnel 2 weeks prior to the event.

    Do SEMS providers need to bring a photo ID to be used for creating a badge?
    - ❑ Yes
    - ☑ No

17. Security clearance

    Will security clearance be needed?
    - ❑ Yes
    - ☑ No

    If so, how far in advance of the event is it needed?

    ______

    Preplanning measures taken:

    Action: ______

    Target date: ______

Figure A-4

Preplanning form for Case 4.

Part IV: SPECIAL CONSIDERATIONS

18. Special concerns and considerations (describe what you know about the following factors)

Communication:

None

Attendees:

All ages will be in attendance.

Demographics:

Where are the spectators located?

Throughout the convention center.

How are the spectators contained?

N/A

Access/egress:

Attendees will use main entrance. Vendors and show personnel may also use rear entrance. Transport ambulance will be parked at door adjacent to the first aid station. EMS personnel will use the main entrance for initial entry to the event. All other access and egress may be made through entrance near first aid station.

Are there areas that cannot be easily viewed?

Yes, the convention center is a large, flat area with booths, but this is unavoidable and not as large a concern because of the low likelihood of injury.

Where is the best vantage point?

N/A

Treatment issues:

None

Transportation:

One BLS transport unit is all that will be used due to nature of the event.

Other considerations:

None

Figure A-4

Preplanning form for Case 4.

Rotation Schedule

No rotation required. Shifts will be from 9:00 am to 8:00 pm. Show times are from 10:00 am to 7:00 pm each day. Meals, drinks, and snacks will be provided by the promoter for all staff.

Preplanning Timeline

Reference the preplanning timeline in Table A-4 for a breakdown of when the preplanning tasks for this case must be completed.

TABLE A-4 Preplanning Timeline for Case 4

Preplanning: Action or Activity	Days Prior to Event
Meet with event sponsor.	45
Determine staffing level. Review roles and responsibilities with all staff.	30
Contact medical center to coordinate care.	From 20 to 2
Select SEMS crew.	14
Talk to event contact to obtain last-minute changes.	7
Meet with event official. Walk through the site.	5
Deliver carts and all equipment.	3
Set up equipment, including first aid stations or tents.	1
Meet crew at facility. Walk through, familiarize, and rehearse response.	1
Fuel carts.	1
Event Day: Action or Activity	**Hours Prior to Event**
Supervisor arrives. Prep carts. Prep supplies. Arrange first aid station.	2
Crew arrives.	1/2
Check radio.	1/2
Transport units arrive.	1/2
First aid station place in service.	1/2
Event start time:	**10:00 am**

During the Event

Your week begins with little in the way of emergencies. Band-Aids, medications for headaches, and information on where certain booths are located are your main issues the first 2 days. On day 3, however, you see four people with nausea and vomiting. This begins at 11:00 am. Each is allowed to rest but feels no better. You transport one and have to call for additional resources through your dispatch to transport the other three. By 1:00 pm, 15 people have come to you within 20 minutes complaining of the same signs and symptoms, stretching your resources. You manage to acquire additional chairs for these patients and request more transport units from your agency, as well as the county dispatch center. You request two ALS units to assist two dehydrated patients. As you speak to the county dispatcher, he informs you that they have also received several other calls from the Ivory Tower Hotel for patients with the same symptoms. They are all from a group called the Sci-Fi Lovers. You begin to inquire from your patients where they are staying and each informs you they are staying at the same hotel. You relay this information to County General Hospital, which has received each of your patients. As the day ends, you have transported 28 total patients in a 12-hour period with these signs and symptoms, all who were staying at that hotel. You requested four total ALS units and used your own on-site unit 12 times. During the rest of the week, the patient load returns to normal and no other transports are needed.

Critical Thinking Questions

1. Was this an MCI?
   Discussion: No, this was not an MCI because the event was able to continue. These events caused a TOPL. Although you and your staff were overwhelmed at the time, you were able to handle the issue and the event was not affected.
2. What are the potential causes of this event?
   Discussion: When EMS providers treat a group of patients who exhibit the same signs and symptoms, they must consider that this could be caused by a terrorist event. Relaying this information to the hospital is a proper step in addressing your concerns. Also notifying your local police agency would be appropriate, stating what you have experienced and the

information you were able to obtain from the patients. However, there are certainly other, more common causes of an event like this. Did they all eat a common meal? In this case, the patients were all part of a particular group staying at a particular hotel, so they were likely all exposed to something that caused their illness. This group all spent a day together in a bus coming to the event. Later you learn that one of the group's members was sick the first 2 days in town. The hospital contacts Public Health about this issue. It is learned that the original patient had a virus and infected the group during the bus ride. Each patient made a complete recovery. From this example you can see how one incident can quickly impact your event coverage. You may be wondering if you should have staffed more SEMS providers on site just in case this happens. The answer is no. While an event like this can cause a TOPL, it is not a common incident.

Postevent Actions

After the event, as a standard procedure, SEMS providers should meet with the event promoter and discuss how things went, including whether the promoter's expectations were met. A postevent analysis is helpful to ensure that you evaluate what went right, what went wrong, and most importantly, how to improve for future events.

Depending on your local regulations, you may need to fill out certain forms after the event has occurred. Be sure to find out if this is required and obtain the needed forms.

Case 5

Event Information

The town of Jessup is all abuzz with the announcement that the latest hit group The Teen Idols will be performing at Jessup Convention Hall this year. The group is scheduled to perform two shows on Friday and Saturday night, starting at 8:00 pm. The group is currently on a world tour and is playing to sellout venues all around the world. Their biggest and most energetic fans are young teenage girls who attend each show, numbering usually in the tens of thousands, screaming for their favorite musicians.

Your agency has been contacted to provide EMS coverage for this event. The convention center manager, Ms. Jane McAllen, feels this event will be a sellout early on and informs you to expect 55,000 attendees. The promoter for The Teen Idols, Mr. Dorsey, has also contacted you to provide coverage for the band itself during the event. The crew and ambulance for the musicians is to be separate from the crew and ambulances that will be covering the event.

Preplanning Form

Figure A-5 shows a filled-out preplanning form for Case 5.

Part I: BASIC INFORMATION

1. Estimated attendance
   - ☐ Fewer than 5,000
   - ☐ 5,001-10,000
   - ☐ 10,001-25,000
   - ☑ 25,001 or more
2. Type of event (check all that apply)
   - ☐ Outdoor
   - ☑ Indoor
   - ☑ Concert
   - ☐ Festival
   - ☐ Stadium
   - ☐ Sport
   - ☐ Extreme sport
   - ☐ Combat sport
   - ☐ Equestrian
   - ☐ Rodeo
   - ☐ Event involving water
   - ☐ Political
   - ☐ Other: ____________
3. Nature of event
   - ☑ High profile
   - ☐ Potentially violent
   - ☐ High likelihood of drug/alcohol use
   - ☐ Event of national significance
   - ☐ Other: ____________
4. Location(s) of event

   Name of facility: Jessup Convention Hall

   Address: 127 Convention Way

   City: Jessup State: CO Zip: 99999
5. Organizational information

   Name of organization: Jessup Convention Hall

   Address: 127 Convention Way

   City: Jessup State: CO Zip: 99999

   Contact person: Ms. Jane McAllen

   Telephone:

   Work: (111) 555-8888

   Cell: (111) 555-6565

   Other: ____________

   E-mail address: janemcallen@jessuphall.net

   Name of organization: Big Teen Productions

   Address: 24 Gammy Drive

   City: Los Angeles State: CA Zip: 99999

   Contact person: Mr. John Dorsey

   Telephone:

   Work: (777) 555-7171

   Cell: (777) 555-0202

   Other: ____________

   E-mail address: starmaker@bigteen.com

Figure A-5

Preplanning form for Case 5.

Part II: RESOURCE NEEDS

6. Resources needed

	Type	Number
Personnel*	❑ Emergency medical responder	
	☑ BLS	6
	☑ ALS	2
	❑ Registered nurse	
	❑ Physician	
	❑ Other:	
Vehicles†	☑ Carts	2
	☑ Other: Transport units	1 BLS 1 ALS
Medical Equipment	☑ Gloves	Multiple boxes and sizes of gloves, plus standard first aid equipment
	☑ AED	3 (one in each of the two transport units, one at a first aid station)
	☑ Stretcher	3 (one in each of the two transport units, one at a first aid station)
	☑ Other: Cots for first aid stations	10 (four for each, plus two for stage first aid)
	❑ Other:	
First Aid Stations‡	☑ On-site	3 (Utilize two rooms off of main concert hall for crowd's first aid stations, plus an extra dressing room for porformer and stage personnel first aid station.)
	❑ Tent	
	❑ Other:	

***Personnel:**
Generally for an event with more than 25,000 attendees, you will need a minimum of four SEMS providers. To help ensure a quick response time to various parts of the stadium, and because SEMS providers will care for performers as well as the crowd, more providers have been planned.

Each of the three first aid stations will have two BLS providers. The two ALS providers will be allocated as follows: There will be one ALS provider in each first aid station devoted to the crowd (there are two of these). There will be no ALS provider stationed at the backstage first aid station, but an ALS provider will be summoned there if needed.

†Vehicles:
Generally, an event with between 25,001 and 55,000 attendees requires two BLS ambulances and an ALS ambulance if the expected emergencies warrant it. For this event, one BLS ambulance and one ALS ambulance have been planned because few injuries are expected.

The two carts will be stationed at the two main first aid stations and will be sent to handle emergencies in the crowd as needed.

‡First aid stations:
An event with more than 25,000 attendees generally requires at least two first aid stations. At this event, there will be three first aid stations: two for the crowd and one for the performers and stage personnel.

Figure A-5

Preplanning form for Case 5. *(continues)*

7. Description of on-site first aid facilities

There will be a total of three first aid stations. Two meeting rooms just off of the concert hall will be used for two first aid stations for the crowd. One is located near the rear of the hall; the other is located just to the left of the front stage area. The third first aid station will be located in an extra dressing room backstage; it will be for performers and backstage personnel.

8. Copies of maps and schematics of facility and any other special areas (list areas here and check off once maps have been obtained and distributed to all personnel)
   - ☑ Facility
   - ☑ Parking areas
   - ☑ Access/egress routes
   - ☑ Surrounding streets
   - ☑ Other: Seating chart, map of backstage area

9. Description of patient transfer protocols and agreements that will be used

Standard protocols will be followed.

10. Communication needs and capabilities (indicate which type of communications matrix will be used and which channel each party will use)

County mutual aid Channel 1 will be used.

Part III: RESEARCH AND ACTIONS TAKEN

11. Measures that have been or will be taken to coordinate SEMS for the event with local EMS and public safety agencies, such as ambulance, police, fire, rescue, and hospital agencies or organizations (if not yet taken, state actions to be taken and target dates for these to be accomplished)

Action: Meeting with promoter and convention center staff on site to coordinate response plan, including access and egress issues, and to coordinate first aid station locations and setup.

Target date: One month prior to the event.

Action: ______

Target date: ______

Action: ______

Target date: ______

12. Security concerns and plans for addressing them:

All security issues are being handled by the promoter and on-site convention security staff.

Figure A-5

Preplanning form for Case 5.

13. Weather history (consult 2-3 sources and list results here)

Source: N/A (indoor event)

Information:

Source:

Information:

Source:

Information:

14. Possible inclement weather

- ❑ Rain
- ❑ Snow
- ❑ Lightning
- ❑ Tornado
- ❑ Hurricane
- ❑ Other:

Preplanning measures taken:

Action: N/A (indoor event)

Target date:

15. Surface considerations

Type of surface:

- ❑ Grass
- ❑ Loose gravel
- ❑ Dirt
- ❑ Asphalt
- ☑ Concrete
- ❑ Temporary flooring
- ❑ Other:

Condition of surface:

- ☑ Smooth
- ❑ Rough
- ❑ Slippery
- ❑ Other:

Levelness:

- ☑ Even
- ❑ Uneven

Preplanning measures taken:

Action: N/A

Target date:

16. Credentialing process

Describe the event's credentialing process:

When EMS providers arrive, the promoter will issue a supplemental photo ID that allows for all access to the venue, including backstage areas and dressing rooms.

Do SEMS providers need to bring a photo ID to be used for creating a badge?

- ☑ Yes
- ❑ No

Figure A-5

Preplanning form for Case 5. *(continues)*

17. Security clearance

    Will security clearance be needed?

    ☐ Yes

    ☑ No

    If so, how far in advance of the event is it needed?

    Preplanning measures taken:

    Action: N/A

    Target date:

Part IV: SPECIAL CONSIDERATIONS

18. Special concerns and considerations (describe what you know about the following factors)

    Communication:

    None

    Attendees:

    Mostly teenagers and young adults

    Demographics:

    Where are the spectators located?

    Concert hall.

    How are the spectators contained?

    Metal barricades and security personnel will keep fans back from the stage.

    Access/egress:

    Access to concert floor is by walking. All SEMS personnel will work at the first aid stations, and teams of two providers will be sent in carts to handle crowd emergencies as needed.

    Are there areas that cannot be easily viewed?

    Difficult to see into crowd as they stand during the event.

    Where is the best vantage point?

    No vantage point is ideal, but the best is at the far end of the concert hall, from the middle level. From this point, most of the seating area can be seen, as well as the stage area.

Figure A-5

Preplanning form for Case 5.

Treatment issues:

None

Transportation:

Transport units will be stationed outside the exit doors by the first aid stations. The two BLS providers from each transport unit will work in the two first aid stations unless a transport is required. ALS providers will only accompany the patient if medically required; otherwise they will remain at the first aid stations.

Other considerations:

None

Figure A-5

Preplanning form for Case 5.

Rotation Schedule

None required; event is 4 hours long.

Preplanning Timeline

Reference the preplanning timeline in Table A-5 for a breakdown of when the preplanning tasks for this case must be completed.

During the Event

Friday night's event goes off without an incident. Only 10 patients are taken to the first aid stations, all with heat problems due to crowd and activity level. None are transported. Saturday's concert begins the same. Suddenly you hear screams over the loud music as a crowd rushes the barricades. A section of the barricade has collapsed and many people have fallen. People are being crushed by others. The SEMS supervisor sends two carts each with two providers to the incident site. The SEMS supervisor communicates the incident to the event promoter, but the band continues to play. You estimate that there are 30 to 40 injured people. You request that the transport units assigned to the backstage first aid station assist you.

Critical Thinking Questions

1. Should the event continue?

   Discussion: In most states, some type of legal authority is granted to police, fire, and/or EMS allowing them, should an MCI occur, to take command of a scene. Such would be the case here. It would be appropriate to halt the event, but the event would continue unless the incident prevented patients from receiving EMS care. Note that in this scenario, the event promoter

TABLE A-5 Preplanning Timeline for Case 5

Preplanning: Action or Activity	Days Prior to Event
Meet with event sponsor.	45
Determine staffing level. Review roles and responsibilities with all staff.	30
Contact medical center to coordinate care.	From 20 to 2
Select SEMS crew.	14
Talk to event contact to obtain last-minute changes.	7
Meet with event official. Walk through the site.	5
Deliver carts and all equipment.	3
Set up equipment, including first aid stations or tents.	2
Meet crew at facility. Walk through, familiarize, and rehearse response.	2
Fuel carts.	1
Event Day: Action or Activity	**Hours Prior to Event**
Supervisor arrives. Prep carts. Prep supplies. Arrange first aid station.	2
Crew arrives.	2
Check radio.	3
Transport units arrive.	1
First aid station place in service.	1
Event start time:	**8:00 pm**

could deny your request that the personnel and transport units dedicated for performers/stage personnel assist with this incident, as one of their responsibilities is to ensure that care is available for the performers and stage personnel. Therefore, it may be more appropriate to request assistance from outside resources. This is also common when assisting with political events to ensure that politicians and event personnel have medical care available. Be sure that details regarding additional assistance are preplanned and noted in an incident action plan prior to large events such as this one.

2. How will you access the patients in this scenario? How will you obtain extra units and supplies?
   Discussion: Access in these cases can be nearly impossible. Security staff will need to clear the area where the injured patients are located before you can begin caring for them. It is generally a good idea to set up a treatment area in a location that is accessible to where the incident occurred. Most venues like this have large parking areas, including limited-access areas such as loading docks, which could be used for staging if needed. As always, preplan what areas could be used for staging should an MCI occur. It is also important to predeploy MCI equipment. Departmental guidelines on when you will predeploy may vary. As a general rule, any event with the potential to produce a large-scale MCI should have MCI supplies predeployed.

Postevent Actions

After the event, as a standard procedure, SEMS providers should meet with the event promoter and discuss how things went, including whether the promoter's expectations were met. A postevent analysis is helpful to ensure that you evaluate what went right, what went wrong, and most importantly, how to improve for future events.

Depending on your local regulations, you may need to fill out certain forms after the event has occurred. Be sure to find out if this is required and obtain the needed forms.

Finally, when a TOPL or MCI occurs, you will likely be required to write an after action report.

References

Chapter 5: Safety Concerns

Fruin J. *The Causes and Prevention of Crowd Disasters*. Courtesy of the crowdsafe.com Crowd Library. © 1993 Elsevier Science Publishers, BB. Accessed 1/21/2010 at: http://www.crowdsafe.com/FruinCauses.pdf.

Hyponatremia "Water Intoxication." TheDEA.org. Accessed 1/21/2010 at: http://thedea.org/hyponatremia.html.

National Institute of Health. *Young Adults: Alcohol Use and Violence*. © 2009 eNotAlone.com. Accessed 11/30/09 at: http://www.enotalone.com/article/11145.html.

Still K. *The Science of Crowd Dynamics—Education/Resources Website*. Crowd Dynamics Ltd. Accessed 1/12/2010 at:http://www.crowddynamics.co.uk/.

Chapter 7: Weather and Outdoor Events

Ikeda T, Ashida H. *Is Recreational Diving Safe?* Rubicon Foundation. UHMS meeting abstracts. Issue date: 2000. Accessed 2/23/10 at: http://archive.rubicon-foundation.org/6770.

Chapter 8: Stadium Events and Mega-events

FEMA. *Special Events Contingency Planning: Job Aids Manual*. March 2005. U.S. Department of Homeland Security. Accessed 2/9/2010. Available at: http://training.fema.gov/EMIWeb/downloads/is15aSpecialEventsPlanning-JAmanual.pdf.

Chapter 9: Equestrian Events and Rodeos

American Medical Equestrian Association News. April 1993, Volume III, Number 2. The University of Vermont. Accessed 12/8/09 at: http://asci.uvm.edu/equine/law/amea/apr93nws.htm.

Exadaktylos AK, Eggli S, Inden P, Zimmermann H. Hoof kick injuries in unmounted equestrians. Improving accident analysis and prevention by introducing an accident and emergency based relational database. *Emerg Med J*. 2002;19:573-575. doi:10.1136/emj.19.6.573. Accepted January 31, 2002. Accessed 12/8/09 at: http://emj.bmj.com/cgi/content/abstract/19/6/573.

Moss PS, Wan A, Whitlock MR. A changing pattern of injuries to horse riders. *Emerg Med J* 2002;19:412–414. doi:10.1136/emj.19.5.412. Accepted February 8, 2002. Accessed 12/8/09 at: http://emj.bmj.com/cgi/content/abstract/19/5/412.

Silver JR. Spinal injuries resulting from horse riding accidents. *Spinal Cord*. June 2002;40(6):264–271. Accessed 12/8/09 at: http://www.nature.com/sc/journal/v40/n6/full/3101280a.html.

Glossary

after action report (AAR) A report consisting of a summary of lessons learned from an incident; it should include recommendations for improvements for decision makers and agency personnel to consider.

anterograde amnesia Loss of memory relating to events that occurred after an injury or episode of drug use.

attendability The likelihood that sick people will attend an event, usually related to the importance of the event to a person's life.

bareback riding An event in which no saddle is used to ride a bucking horse until the rider is thrown or falls off.

barefoot water skiing A type of water skiing that is done without water skis and at higher speeds.

barotrauma Injury resulting from pressure disequilibrium across body surfaces.

barrel man A rodeo performer who entertains the crowd, works to keep riders safe, and uses a padded barrel for protection if needed.

barrel racing A race in which a horse and rider maneuver in a cloverleaf pattern around three barrels placed in a triangle.

barricade operations Generally taught to security personnel, a skill set on how to safely protect and remove distressed individuals who may be pinned against a barricade, such as near a stage.

base station Assembly of radio equipment consisting of at least a transmitter, receiver, and antenna connection at a fixed location.

belay system A harness and rope system used in rock climbing, kept under control by an assistant at the base of the climb.

belayer In rock climbing, a person who keeps the harness and rope system under control; may be located at the base or the top.

bicycle motocross (BMX) A sport in which athletes perform tricks on bikes.

bound event A special event that is contained within set perimeters, such as walls, fences, or natural barriers such as lakes or ponds.

bull in the ring A modified form of moshing that occurs when one person is surrounded by a crowd and must break through the crowd by smashing into people.

bull poker An event in which four to six participants attempt to be the last one sitting around a card table while a bull is in the ring.

bull riding A sport in which a rider attempts to sit on a bull for 8 seconds while the bull attempts to buck the rider off.

bull rope In bull riding, a rope that wraps under the bull behind its front legs.

bullfighters People who round up the bull to move it to the exit chute in bull riding.

calf roping An event in which a cowboy attempts to lasso a calf, roll it over, and tie at least three of its feet together.

calf scramble A rodeo event in which something is tied to a calf and children compete to pull it off.

camp on The term in bull riding for a bull throwing a rider off and running him or her over.

catapult injury A type of injury unique to harness racing in which the cart, or sulky, launches over the horse and rider, causing injury when it lands.

cells on wheels (COWs) Temporary cell phone towers that can be brought in to increase cellular site availability.

Cheyne-Stokes respirations Respirations that are fast and then become slow, with intervening periods of apnea; commonly seen following brain stem injury.

choke point Any area that prohibits the crowd from moving freely and can cause a pedestrian backup, such as doorways, riot gates, or places where people naturally stop to talk, blocking the pathway of others.

chronic traumatic brain injury A traumatic brain injury that occurs as a result of a series of injuries to the brain that either (1) are not allowed to heal before the next injury occurs or (2) produce lasting effects to the brain.

chute box The area where the rider mounts the bull.

classical style A rider position in which the rider's head is held high and the rider's body is perpendicular to the horse's back; in this position, the rider is more likely to fall onto his or her buttocks.

clinching The term for holding an opponent while he or she is standing, preventing him or her from moving to the ground.

combat sport A competitive, combative contact sport in which two opponents battle using specific rules of engagement.

comfort station A station that is designated for rehabilitation, cooling, or warming of staff and patients, as needed; for example, this station may be air conditioned or heated, if needed, and is ideally indoors.

communications matrix The configuration of a radio system, which can be simple, tiered, or complex; which includes multiple channels for different groups to communicate with other members of their group, or other groups; and may be configured to accommodate one frequency or several frequencies depending on the communication needs for the event.

concussion A mild brain injury caused by the brain striking the skull after a blow to the head, which can be categorized ranging from mild to severe; symptoms may continue for several weeks after the incident.

cross-country equestrian jumping A riding event that tests endurance and includes obstacles such as water, logs, and fences that the horse must jump; horses are started at different times and do not compete with one another to clear an obstacle; a component of eventing.

crowd demographics Statistical characteristics of a crowd, such as age, race, and sex distribution.

crowd panic The occurrence of widespread alarm in a group of people; responses of people in the group may vary or be amplified because of the fact that they are in a group.

crowd surfing Laying on top of a crowd of people and being passed around; this often begins with stage diving (diving off a stage into a crowd).

crowd surging Crowd movement as a group, for example to overtake security personnel to jump onto the stage at a performance.

crowd syndrome A collection of physical symptoms that may occur when a person feels anxious in a crowd; symptoms include sweating, shortness of breath, and feeling hot, faint, or paranoid.

Cushing's triad Hypertension (with widening pulse pressure), bradycardia, and irregular respirations; classic trio findings associated with increased intracranial pressure.

cutting A rodeo event in which a horse and rider attempt to separate an animal, usually a cow, from a herd for a set amount of time.

cyclical attendance The number of attendees as it rises and falls during an event's operational period.

decompression sickness A broad range of signs and symptoms caused by nitrogen bubbles in blood and tissues coming out of solution on ascent; also called the bends.

deep water blackout A loss of consciousness that occurs while ascending to the surface after a dive of at least 32 feet, and which is the result of a rapid drop in the partial pressure of oxygen on ascent.

defensive move A move that slows an opponent's actions.

dispersed Injuries or illnesses that occur in more than one place.

dressage A riding discipline in which horse and rider perform a sequence of movements and are scored on specific criteria such as style and obedience; a component of eventing.

duplex Radio system using more than one frequency to permit simultaneous transmission and reception.

ecstasy (MDMA) A drug officially named methylenedioxymethamphetamine and generally sold as a capsule or tablet; it alters and intensifies a person's sensory perception, producing stimulant and hallucinogenic effects and lowering individuals' inhibitions; may lead to hyperthermia or hyponatremia.

epidural hematoma An accumulation of blood between the skull and dura.

evacuation plan Plan created during the preplanning stage that outlines the method of evacuating the entire crowd from an event in an emergency situation.

eventing A type of equestrian event that includes three phases: cross-country, dressage, and jumping.

Event of National Significance An event classification assigned by the US government, which means that FBI, ATF, and Homeland Security will be stakeholders in the event and in the planning stages.

extreme sport Sporting events that involve dangerous and high-risk activities.

Federal Communications Commission (FCC) The federal agency that has jurisdiction over interstate and international telephone and telegraph services and satellite communications, all of which may involve EMS activity.

Federal Emergency Management Agency (FEMA) An independent agency of the US government that provides a single point of accountability for all federal emergency preparedness and mitigation and response activities.

fencing A combat sport in which two opponents strike each other using sword-like weapons.

festival seating A style of seating that is usually assigned on a first-come, first-served basis, rather than being preassigned.

first aid station A specific enclosure that is dedicated to the medical aid of attendees and comes in many different forms, ranging from tents to 32-foot mobile homes.

flank strap A strap that wraps around the bull's underside to provoke the bull to buck more.

free diving An extreme water sport in which divers hold their breath for as long as possible while diving, without using any device to assist breathing.

frequency In radio communications, the number of cycles per second of a signal, inversely related to the wavelength.

gamma-hydroxybutyric acid (GHB) A central nervous system depressant that is colorless and has a salty taste; it has sedating and intoxicating effects and is used to perpetrate date rape.

groundwork In martial arts, a term referring to a fight that occurs on the ground.

half-pipe Used in snowboarding, a U-shaped bowl that allows snowboarders to move from one wall to the other by making jumps and performing snowboarding tricks on each transition.

hanging up A situation that occurs when a bull or horse continues to buck after the rider begins to fall off, but has not gotten loose from the rope or saddle.

harness racing A type of horse racing in which the horses pull a type of cart called a sulky, and the horses race in a specified gait.

heat advisory A notice issued within 12 hours of the onset of extreme heat conditions, including a heat index of at least 105°F (40.6°C) but less than 115°F (46.1°C) for less than 3 hours per day, and nighttime lows remaining above 80°F (26.7°C) for 2 consecutive days.

heat cramps Acute and involuntary muscle pains, usually in the lower extremities, the abdomen, or both, that occur because of profuse sweating and subsequent sodium loss.

heat exhaustion A clinical syndrome characterized by volume depletion and heat stress that is thought to be a milder form of heat illness on the continuum leading to heat stroke.

heat index The apparent temperature of skin exposed to air with high moisture content.

heat stroke The least common and most deadly heat illness, caused by a severe disturbance in thermoregulation, usually characterized by a core temperature of more than 104°F (40°C) and altered mental status.

herd mentality A situation in which people in a crowd react as a herd does when startled or enraged, initiating violence or generally becoming dangerous and unpredictable.

hertz (Hz) Unit of frequency equal to one cycle per second.

hurdling A type of steeplechase racing often used to train horses for more challenging courses; it involves jumping hurdles.

hydroplane racing A type of boat racing in which a specially designed watercraft with a jet-powered turbine engine is raced around a course.

incident commander The overall leader of the incident command system to whom commanders or leaders of incident command system divisions report.

jockey style A rider position in which the rider's body is relatively parallel to the horse's neck and the rider's head is forward; in this position, the rider is more likely to sustain cervical injury accompanied by head injury.

joint operations center (JOC) The central location from which all operations of a large-scale event are managed.

ketamine hydrochloride A veterinary anesthetic and a phencyclidine hydrochloride (PCP) derivative; street names include special K, vitamin K, cat Valium, and Fort Dodge; can be absorbed through another person's skin.

kiss the rider In bull riding, when the bull uses its head and horns to throw the rider and draw him or her into the area beneath the bull.

local Injuries or illnesses that occur in one location only.

lysergic acid diethylamide (LSD) Also called acid, a hallucinogen that alters a person's perception and can cause intense hallucinations; it can transfer through another person's skin.

make weight Meeting a body weight requirement to compete in a combat sport; sometimes achieved by the participant sweating excessively to reduce his or her weight; also called "cutting weight."

martial arts Combat sports involving striking and grappling such as judo, jujitsu, and karate.

mass-casualty incident (MCI) An event in which a large number of casualties are produced in a relatively short period, exceeding local logistic support capabilities. MCIs are usually the result of a single incident such as a military aircraft accident, hurricane, flood, earthquake, or armed attack.

mass gathering A situation (event) during which crowds gather and where there is the potential for a delayed response to emergencies because of limited access to patients or other features of the environment and location.

maximum cycle rate The turnover of the crowd, meaning how many people leave versus how many arrive.

mega-event An event that has an on-site attendance of over 55,000 people at any given time.

methamphetamine A highly addictive stimulant drug that affects mood, energy, and appetite; it comes as a white, crystalline powder and is made out of common over-the-counter medications and common household products.

misting station A place that includes sprinkler-like equipment that provides a gentle water vapor with the intention of cooling event participants.

mobile aid station A specific enclosure that is dedicated to the medical aid of attendees and has the ability to move around the event.

mobile team A group of medical providers that leaves a posted position to assist, assess, and if needed, transport patients to either a first aid station or to a transport vehicle for further care and transport to a hospital.

money the hard way A rodeo event in which participants attempt to grab a pouch of money that is tied around the horn of a bull.

mosh pit An area, usually in front of a stage, where members of the audience flail and smash into each other.

moshing A modern version of the punk tradition of slam dancing wherein dancers start flailing around wildly and smashing into each other.

motocross A sport in which athletes perform tricks on bikes with engines.

multilevel emergent care (MLEC) facility A more permanent type of medical care station generally used at a mega-event, whose staffing may include physicians, nurses, paramedics, and professional sports technicians.

multiplex Method by which simultaneous transmission of voice and electrocardiogram (ECG) signals can be achieved over a single radio frequency.

multi-tiered response system A type of staffing structure that can be expanded to meet the needs of even the largest event.

mutton busting An event in which a child, usually between ages 6 and 10 years, climbs atop a sheep and holds on for as long as possible.

National Incident Management System (NIMS) A Department of Homeland Security system designed to enable federal, state, and local governments and private-sector and nongovernmental organizations to effectively and efficiently prepare for, prevent, respond to, and recover from domestic incidents, regardless of cause, size, or complexity, including acts of catastrophic terrorism.

nitrogen narcosis A state resembling alcohol intoxication produced by nitrogen gas dissolved in the blood at high ambient pressure; also called rapture of the deep.

noise In radio communications, interference in a radio signal.

objective factors Proven, unbiased facts about the event, such as the type of event, duration, and crowd size.

open swim Any swimming event that occurs on the open water.

open water sports Water sports held on the seas.

outgate In bull riding, the gate through which the bulls are supposed to exit the arena.

oxygen toxicity A condition that occurs when oxygen in the body exceeds a safe partial pressure (PPO_2); in extreme cases, the central nervous system becomes affected, causing a seizure.

pack mentality A situation that occurs when individuals in a crowd base their decisions on what they believe to be the collective standpoint, rather than basing decisions on their own beliefs and thought processes; can lead to members of a group performing unthinkable actions.

paintball A contest in which participants shoot each other with balls filled with paint using specialized guns.

passive interaction interviewing A technique used to interview a potential patient using everyday questions that reveal key patient data, such as mental status.

patient load The number of patients who require care at a given time.

peak attendance rate The maximum number of people attending in a span of a single hour of an event.

pens The areas where bulls are held to separate them from each other before a bull riding event.

pick-up man In rodeo, a professional cowboy on a horse who assists the rider if he or she is thrown or needs to be removed from a bucking horse, or after dismounting the horse; may also rope a bull to assist it in exiting an arena.

point-to-point racing A type of amateur horse racing that involves hunter horses jumping fences.

polar bear plunge An event in which participants jump into frigid water.

pole bending A race in which a horse and rider move around five poles in a slalom or serpentine pattern; also called equine slalom.

portable radio A handheld radio that can be carried on a person and is used for communications away from a vehicle.

post-concussion syndrome Due to jarring of the brain within the skull, the patient experiences weakness on one side of the body, extreme mood swings, and/or problems with basic cognitive functions, such as memory or orientation.

postevent stage Analysis stage that allows all involved parties to assess the performance of resources and plans that were developed to cover the event.

pre-event stage A period before a gathering when meetings and planning cycles occur.

preplanning A process that involves all interested parties and develops event response plans and needs.

public safety answering point (PSAP) An official term for a dispatch center; a designated location where incoming calls to public safety are routed during an event; helps ensure that all incidents are communicated to SEMS providers.

push-to-talk A method of communication that uses a half-duplex communications system. By pushing a button on the communication device, a person can send; by releasing the button, a person can receive.

rank bull A bull known for trying to injure riders.

relative humidity The ratio of the amount of water vapor actually in the air compared to the amount of water vapor the air can hold at a particular temperature and pressure.

repeater Miniature transmitter that picks up a radio signal and rebroadcasts it, extending the range of a radio communications system.

rigging The rope used in rodeos that allows the performer or rider to hold on.

riptide A current that runs perpendicular to the beach and that can pull a person out to sea very quickly.

riverboarding An extreme water sport in which an athlete lies prone on a board and travels down river rapids.

rodeo A type of event that showcases cowboy skills such as riding, racing, roping, and working with livestock; includes a number of subevents.

rodeo clown A rodeo performer who entertains the crowd and works to keep riders safe.

Rohypnol A benzodiazepine sometimes used to perpetrate date rape because it can cause memory loss; commonly called rophie or roofies; produces incapacitatory effects that last up to 12 hours.

round A timed interval in a boxing match.

rule of three A policy that three SEMS providers should respond to and handle each emergency at an event.

saddle bronc An event in which a rider rides a saddled, bucking horse until he or she is thrown or falls off; also called bronco.

SALT triage A triage method that first identifies which patients can understand verbal instructions, then involves performing several lifesaving interventions.

shallow water blackout A loss of consciousness that occurs while underwater in depths of about 15 feet or less, and which is caused by hypoxia from holding one's breath.

show jumping A type of equestrian event in which horses jump obstacles and are judged on different criteria depending on whether the event is a hunter event or a jumper event; a component of eventing.

simplex Method of radio communication using a single frequency that enables transmission or reception of voice or an electrocardiogram (ECG) signal but is incapable of simultaneous transmission and reception.

singlet A wrestling uniform.

somersaulting A dangerous situation in which a horse's chest collides with a fence or object, causing the horse to flip over, either taking the rider with it or causing the rider to fall off.

special event A gathering of people for a specific reason, such as music, sports, or politics.

special event log A record of patient interactions that occur at a particular event.

stadium A facility that consists of a center where an event takes place, which is surrounded by rows of seats or bleachers on all sides; may be home to a variety of special events.

START triage A triage method that uses a limited assessment of the patient's ability to walk, respiratory status, hemodynamic status, and neurologic status.

static attendance The term used to describe a predetermined number of attendees that cannot change, such as attendees at a preticket sales–only event.

steeplechase horse racing A form of horse racing that involves obstacles such as fences, water features, and jumps.

steer wrestling An event in which a cowboy attempts to jump from a horse onto a steer and wrestle the steer onto its back.

stunt riding An event in which a rider performs acrobatic moves while riding a horse.

subdural hematoma An accumulation of blood beneath the dura but outside the brain.

subjective factors Information that is not made up of provable facts; examples include crowd mentality and memories from previous experience.

submission hold A move or combination of moves that attacks an opponent's joint, muscle, or air and bloodflow to the brain, causing the opponent to surrender before any serious harm is done.

sulky A two-wheeled cart that is pulled behind a horse in harness racing.

takedown A move or combination of moves that forces the opponent to fall to the mat.

temporary overwhelming patient load (TOPL) A brief period during which there is a larger number of victims than the available resources can handle (though additional resources may need to be brought in), but this does not prevent the event from continuing and subsides without external resources being required.

thoroughbred racing A type of horse racing that occurs over a flat, even track; this race is a set distance.

track crew Individuals who monitor the course during a competition and communicate with other personnel, including SEMS providers.

transceiver A radio transmitter and receiver housed in the same radio; a two-way radio.

transport unit-wise number The estimated number of transports expected per day, determined using the total number of people, the expected number of days, and additional factors that could affect the number of emergencies, such as temperature, comfort provisions, age of attendees, and health of attendees.

triathlon An event that consists of a road race, a bike race, and an open water swim.

trunking Sharing of radio frequencies by multiple agencies or systems.

ultrahigh frequency (UHF) band The portion of the radio frequency spectrum between 300 and 3,000 MHz.

unbound event A special event that has no or very few structured perimeters, such as road races, marathons, charity walks, and outdoor festivals.

unified command system A command system used in larger incidents in which there is a multiagency response or multiple jurisdictions are involved.

unilateral pupils A condition in which the pupil on the side of an injury is dilated and does not respond to light, while the pupil on the other side does not have this appearance.

vert A part of a BMX track that faces another ramp, creating a valley shape.

very high frequency (VHF) band The portion of the radio frequency spectrum between 30 and 150 MHz.

walk-through The opportunity for the SEMS team to evaluate the physical space where an event will take place; it can be theoretical or actual (physical).

well In bull riding, the area beneath the bull.

wild horse racing An event in which a team of cowboys attempts to catch and ride an untamed horse.

windchill The apparent temperature of the air on exposed skin.

Index

D

E

F

Photo Credits

Title Page © Jim Bourg/Reuters

You are the SEMS Provider Courtesy of Doug Poore, NREMT-P and David Mick, NREMT-P

Chapter 1

Opener Courtesy of Doug Poore, NREMT-P and David Mick, NREMT-P; **1-5** © MIEMSS; **1-9** © Reuters/Robin Utrecht/Pool Netherlands

Chapter 2

2-1A © Pixel4 Images/ShutterStock, Inc.; **2-3** Courtesy of Doug Poore, NREMT-P and David Mick, NREMT-P; **2-9A** Courtesy of Doug Poore, NREMT-P and David Mick, NREMT-P; **2-9B** Courtesy of Doug Poore, NREMT-P and David Mick, NREMT-P; **2-13** Courtesy of Dover International Speedway

Chapter 3

Opener Courtesy of Doug Poore, NREMT-P and David Mick, NREMT-P; **3-1** Courtesy of Doug Poore, NREMT-P and David Mick, NREMT-P; **3-3** Courtesy of Doug Poore, NREMT-P and David Mick, NREMT-P; **3-4** © MIEMSS; **3-5A** Courtesy of Captain David Jackson, Saginaw Township Fire Department; **3-5B** Courtesy of FEMA/Mark Wolfe; **3-6** Courtesy of Doug Poore, NREMT-P and David Mick, NREMT-P; **3-7** Courtesy of Doug Poore, NREMT-P and David Mick, NREMT-P; **3-8** Courtesy of Doug Poore, NREMT-P and David Mick, NREMT-P; **3-9** © AP Photo/Ross D. Franklin; **3-10** © sonya etchison/ShutterStock, Inc.; **3-11** Courtesy of Doug Poore, NREMT-P and David Mick, NREMT-P; **3-12** Courtesy of Doug Poore, NREMT-P and David Mick, NREMT-P; **3-13** Courtesy of Doug Poore, NREMT-P and David Mick, NREMT-P

Chapter 4

4-1 Courtesy of Doug Poore, NREMT-P and David Mick, NREMT-P

Chapter 5

Opener © MIEMSS; **5-1** © MIEMSS; **5-2** © Robin Tomaszewski/Dreamstime.com; **5-3** © MIEMSS; **5-4** Courtesy of Doug Poore, NREMT-P and David Mick, NREMT-P; **5-6A** © Pavel Losevsky/Dreamstime.com; **5-6B** © MIEMSS; **5-7** © MIEMSS; **5-8** © MIEMSS; **5-9** © MIEMSS; **5-10** Courtesy of Steve Zeidler; **5-12** © MIEMSS; **5-13** © Nzgmw2788/Dreamstime.com; **5-15** Courtesy of Doug Poore, NREMT-P and David Mick, NREMT-P; **5-16** Courtesy of Doug Poore, NREMT-P and David Mick, NREMT-P

Chapter 6

Opener © Reuters/Mike Blake/Landov; **6-1** © AP Photo/Ken Cedeno; **6-3** © AP Photo/M. Spencer Green; **6-4** Courtesy of FEMA/George Armstrong; **6-5** Courtesy of FEMA/Greg Henshall; **6-6** Courtesy of Doug Poore, NREMT-P and David Mick, NREMT-P

Chapter 7

Opener © AP Photo/The Daily Record, Tyson Trish; **7-1** © AP Photo/Ross D. Franklin; **7-2** © David Park/Dreamstime.com; **7-3** © AP Photo/The Denver Post, Helen H. Richardson; **7-5A** Courtesy of Billy Heatter/U.S. Air Force; **7-5B** © Ron Hilton/ShutterStock, Inc.; **7-6** Courtesy of Josh Galt, Face Level Industries LLC; **7-7** Courtesy of Connie Groah, Barefoot Photography; **7-8** © BartlomiejMagierowski/ShutterStock, Inc.; **7-9** Courtesy of Carol B. Guerrero; **7-10A** © MIEMSS; **7-10B** Courtesy of Karen Turner; **7-11** Courtesy of Vision Racing LLC; **7-12** Courtesy of James Perryman

Chapter 8

Opener © MIEMSS; **8-1A** © MIEMSS; **8-1B** © Marcelo Saavedra/ShutterStock, Inc.; **8-3** Courtesy of Wally Gobetz; **8-4C** Courtesy of Doug Poore, NREMT-P and David Mick, NREMT-P; **8-7** © Alexandru Chiriac/ShutterStock, Inc.; **8-8** © MIEMSS

Chapter 9

Opener © AP Photo/The Daily Times, Lindsay Pierce; **9-1** © Cheryl Ann Quigley/ShutterStock, Inc.; **9-2** © Jeff Schultes/ShutterStock, Inc.; **9-3** © Dennis Donohue/ShutterStock, Inc.; **9-4** © Perry Correll/ShutterStock, Inc.; **9-5** © PA Photos/Landov; **9-6** © Margo Harrison/ShutterStock, Inc.; **9-7** © muzsy/

ShutterStock, Inc.; **9-9** © Alpha/Landov; **9-10** © Cheryl Ann Quigley/ShutterStock, Inc.; **9-11** © Kondrashov Mikhail Evgenevich/ShutterStock, Inc.; **9-12** © PA Photos/Landov; **9-13** © Cosmin-Constantin Sava/Dreamstime.com; **9-14** © Joy Brown/ShutterStock, Inc.; **9-15** Courtesy of Phoenix Performance Products; **9-16** © topal/ShutterStock, Inc.; **9-18** © Algecireño/ShutterStock, Inc.; **9-20** © MIEMSS; **9-21** © steve estvanik/ShutterStock, Inc.; **9-22** © Sergei Bachlakov/ShutterStock, Inc.; **9-23** © Shawn Hine/ShutterStock, Inc.; **9-24** © Christopher Halloran/ShutterStock, Inc.; **9-25** © J.T. Lewis/ShutterStock, Inc.; **9-26** © joyfuldesigns/ShutterStock, Inc.; **9-27** © Ron Hilton/ShutterStock, Inc.; **9-28** © Ron Hilton/ShutterStock, Inc.; **9-29** © Lincoln Rogers/ShutterStock, Inc.; **9-30** © Michael Klenetsky/ShutterStock, Inc.

Chapter 10

10-2 Courtesy of Lance Cpl. Lydia L. Collison/U.S. Navy; **10-6A** © Sportsphotographer.eu/ShutterStock, Inc.; **10-6B** © Vojta Herout/ShutterStock, Inc.; **10-7** © Maxim Petrichuk/ShutterStock, Inc.; **10-8A** © Troscha/ShutterStock, Inc.; **10-8B** © dean bertoncelj/ShutterStock, Inc.; **10-9** © Ryan McVay/Photodisc/Getty Images; **10-10** © BMCL/ShutterStock, Inc.; **10-11** © Photos.com; **10-12** © Vereshchagin Dmitry/ShutterStock, Inc.; **10-13** © ZTS/ShutterStock, Inc.; **10-14** © Ben Haslam/Haslam Photography/ShutterStock, Inc.; **10-15** © Ben Haslam/Haslam Photography/ShutterStock, Inc.; **10-21** Courtesy of Shock Doctor, Inc.; **10-23** © Auddmin/Dreamstime.com; **10-24** © LindyCro/ShutterStock, Inc.; **10-25** © Karina Maybely Orellana Rojas/ShutterStock, Inc.; **10-26** © Alexander Ishchenko/ShutterStock, Inc.; **10-27** © Wellcome Images/Custom Medical Stock Photo; **10-28** © Howard Grill/ShutterStock, Inc.; **10-29** Courtesy of Seaman Kevin T. Murray Jr./U.S. Navy; **10-33** © JanJar/ShutterStock, Inc.

Unless otherwise indicated, all photographs and illustrations are under copyright of Jones & Bartlett Learning, courtesy of Maryland Institute for Emergency Medical Services Systems, or have been provided by the author.